Special Tests for Neurologic Examination

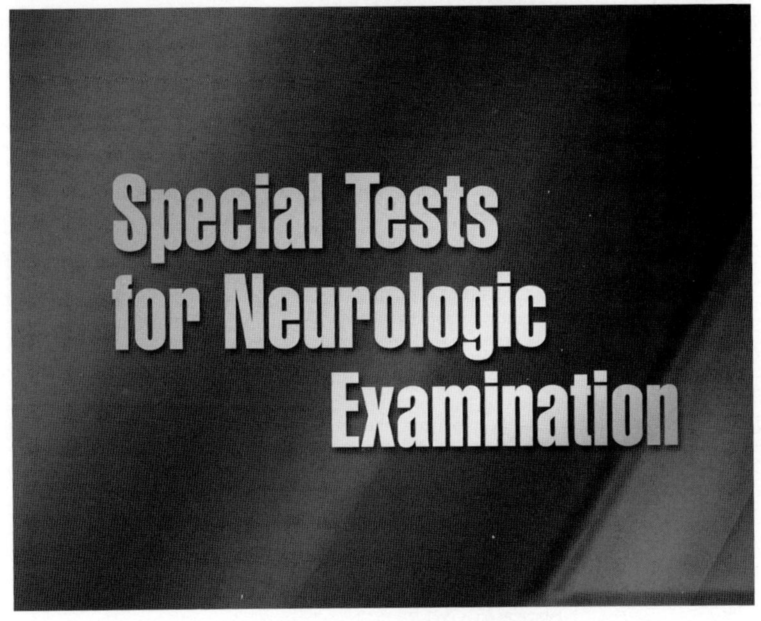

James R. Scifers, DScPT, PT, SCS, LAT, ATC
Associate Professor, School of Health Sciences
Associate Professor, Department of Physical Therapy
Program Director, Athletic Training Education Program
Western Carolina University
Cullowhee, NC

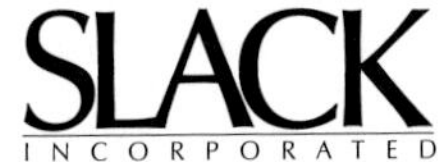

Delivering the best in health care information and education worldwide

www.slackbooks.com

ISBN: 978-1-55642-797-8

The procedures and practices described in this book should be implemented in a manner consistent with the professional standards set for the circumstances that apply in each specific situation. Every effort has been made to confirm the accuracy of the information presented and to correctly relate generally accepted practices. The authors, editor, and publisher cannot accept responsibility for errors or exclusions or for the outcome of the material presented herein. There is no expressed or implied warranty of this book or information imparted by it. Care has been taken to ensure that drug selection and dosages are in accordance with currently accepted/recommended practice. Due to continuing research, changes in government policy and regulations, and various effects of drug reactions and interactions, it is recommended that the reader carefully review all materials and literature provided for each drug, especially those that are new or not frequently used. Any review or mention of specific companies or products is not intended as an endorsement by the author or publisher.

Published by: SLACK Incorporated
6900 Grove Road
Thorofare, NJ 08086 USA
Telephone: 856-848-1000
Fax: 856-853-5991
www.slackbooks.com

Contact SLACK Incorporated for more information about other books in this field or about the availability of our books from distributors outside the United States.

Library of Congress Cataloging-in-Publication Data

Scifers, James R.

Special tests for neurologic examination/James R. Scifers
p. ; cm.
Includes bibliographical references and index.
ISBN 978-1-55642-797-8 (alk. paper)

1. Neurologic examination. 2. Nervous system--Diseases--Diagnosis.
3. Physical therapists. I. Title.

[DNLM: 1. Neurologic Examination--methods--Handbooks. WL 39 S416s 2008]

RC348.S396 2008
616.8'0475--dc22

2007038940

Printed in the United States of America.

Last digit is print number: 10 9 8 7 6 5 4 3 2 1

Dedication

This book is dedicated to my wife Michelle and my children, Jacob, Jonathan, and Katherine, whose love, support, and patience consistently provided me with the inspiration and dedication necessary to complete this project.

Contents

Acknowledgments

The concept for this text was provided by Dr. Jeff Konin, PhD, ATC, PT, who was gracious enough to share his vision and guidance during the completion of this project. Jeff's continual professional support and advice were critical components to the completion of this textbook.

Furthermore, the completion of this text would not have been possible without the assistance of a number of individuals. First, I would like to thank my colleague, Jill Manners, MS, LAT, ATC, for her contribution as a coauthor and content reviewer for the project. Additionally, Jill dedicated a significant amount of time to assisting in the completion of the photographs contained in the book. I would also like to express my sincerest thanks to Krispen Burns, Mark Green, Katlyn Joyner, and Stephenie Stark for taking time out of their busy schedules to pose as subjects for the photographs contained in this text. Also, a special thanks to Katie Martin for her assistance with the formatting of several of the photographs.

Most importantly, I would like to thank Jennifer Briggs, Carrie Kotlar, Kimberly Shigo, Michelle Clerici, Stephanie Doherty, and Debra Toulson at SLACK Incorporated, who assisted me throughout the completion of this project. Without their assistance and guidance, this project would never have come to fruition.

About the Author

James R. Scifers, DScPT, PT, SCS, LAT, ATC is the founding Program Director for the Western Carolina University Athletic Training Education Program. He also serves as an Associate Professor in the School of Health Sciences and the Department of Physical Therapy at Western Carolina University.

Dr. Scifers received his bachelor of science degree in athletic training from East Stroudsburg University, his master of physical therapy degree from Emory University, and his doctor of science in physical therapy degree from the University of Maryland School of Medicine. He is a North Carolina licensed athletic trainer and physical therapist and holds certification as a Board Certified Specialist in Sports Physical Therapy.

Dr. Scifers has more than 18 years of clinical practice in the professional, collegiate, secondary school, and clinical settings. He has served as Program Director for the Athletic Training Education Programs at Salisbury University and Lock Haven University and also as a professor in the University of Kentucky Department of Physical Therapy.

About the Contributor

Jill A. Manners, MS, LAT, ATC is an Associate Professor in the School of Health Sciences and the Coordinator of Clinical Education for the Western Carolina University Athletic Training Education Program.

Ms. Manners received her bachelor of science degree in athletic training/exercise science from Ithaca College and her master of science degree in athletic training from West Virginia University. She is a North Carolina licensed athletic trainer, with more than 15 years of clinical practice in the professional, collegiate, secondary school, and clinical settings. In addition to her roles at Western Carolina University, Jill also serves as a Primary Health Care Provider for the United States Tennis Association.

Jill has previously served as both Program Director and Coordinator of Clinical Education at Salisbury University and as an Instructor in the Athletic Training Education Program at West Virginia University.

Preface

Special Tests for Neurologic Examination was originally the brainchild of Dr. Jeff Konin, who envisioned this text as a companion to his already popular *Special Tests for Orthopedic Examination*. Jeff was kind enough to share his project vision with me and to give me ownership of the project during a visit to the SLACK booth at the annual meeting and clinical symposia of the National Athletic Trainers' Association.

Jeff's idea, coupled with my inability to say no, launched the project later that year. Over the next 2 years, the project took on a life of its own, growing beyond its original vision of a compilation of neurologically-based special tests into a text that included discussion of cranial nerve assessment; dermatome, myotome, and reflex testing; concussion grading scales; sideline and computerized concussion testing; and neuropsychological testing, along with a large number of neurologic special test procedures.

Although no single text can be comprehensive in nature, the primary goal of this text is to provide the reader with clear images and simple, yet detailed, descriptions of the most commonly used examination techniques for patients with neurologic dysfunction. In compiling the material contained in this text, the authors considered the prevalence of the tests in other published materials; the availability of published research regarding the reliability, validity, sensitivity, and specificity of the various tests; and the usage of the tests in clinical practice. In some cases, there is little to no evidence to support or refute the clinical use of procedures contained in this text. In these instances, the examination procedures were included due to their prevalence in other published textbooks, their prevalence of use in clinical practice, and the continuous inclusion of these examination procedures in entry-level education programs. The lack of evidence to support such tests continues to stand as a challenge to researchers, educators, and clinicians alike to conduct clinical studies to support or refute their efficacy.

References are provided along with each special test in order to allow the reader to easily locate both historical materials and evidence-based research relating to the test being described. These references are not comprehensive, but provide the reader with a focused view of much of the data available for each test procedure.

Additionally, historical notes are provided, when applicable, to give the reader a basic background regarding the test's development, history, and origin. All information regarding historical materials for test procedures was retrieved from the website Who Named It at www.whonamedit.com.

In many cases, special tests are known regionally by various titles. In order to decrease confusion when referring to specific examination procedures, alternate names have been provided for many of the test included in this textbook. The Special Considerations section provides valuable clinical pearls and application-specific information aimed at allowing the practitioner to maximize the test procedure findings, while minimizing testing error and false-positive or false-negative findings.

Finally, in the spirit of the ever-growing move toward evidence-based practice, data is included for exam reliability, specificity, and sensitivity, as well as positive and negative likelihood ratios where specific outcome data is available. Instances where no published data was available at the time of publication are also noted. These gaps in our collective knowledge provide the reader with the opportunity to initiate research studies to validate these test procedures for future generations of practitioners.

In conclusion, this textbook attempts to pay homage to history with an eye to the future of clinical practice. This project has been a fun, challenging, and enlightening experience for all those involved in its creation. In completing this text, I hoped to consolidate an assortment of neurological assessment materials into one useful resource for students, educators, and practitioners alike. I hope that I was successful in this endeavor and that each of you find this text of value in your present and future clinical practice.

James Scifers, DScPT, PT, SCS, LAT, ATC

Foreword

It is a great honor and pleasure to write the foreword for *Special Tests for Neurologic Examination* by Dr. James Scifers. By providing students with a clear, concise, and well-illustrated text on neurologic examination techniques, Dr. Scifers has filled an obvious void in the athletic training, physical therapy, and allied health literature. This book will be an excellent companion text to *Special Tests for Orthopedic Examination, Third Edition,* also published by SLACK Incorporated.

The publication of this text is both timely and appropriate. *Special Tests for Neurologic Examination* will be particularly helpful to athletic trainers as they look to further enhance their ability to evaluate and treat physically active patients with a variety of musculoskeletal and neurological conditions. The text offers students and sports health care practitioners an overview of the neurologic examination tests that are necessary to formulate an informed and evidenced-based clinical diagnosis. Most importantly, the tests and techniques included in this manual have been selected and are presented based on their diagnostic accuracy, sensitivity, and specificity. Dr. Scifers sets the stage for the presentation of the specific tests with an excellent discussion of evidence-based practice in his Introduction.

Special Tests for Neurologic Examination is much more than a collection of special tests and examination techniques. The descriptions and figures have been carefully selected and the inclusion of alternate (regional) names for selected techniques minimizes the confusion experienced by students who are often required to master a large number of tests. Educators who couple this manual with a comprehensive physical examination textbook and their own expertise will find students can master these psychomotor competencies more easily. Most importantly, students who are challenged to critically analyze these techniques will not only be able to execute the necessary skills, but they will also be equipped to defend their selection by providing an appropriate rationale.

Jay Scifers has done an outstanding job of extending the work of Konin, Wiksten, Isear, and Brader by providing us with a text that is long overdue. True to form, Jay has utilized his keen insight as a clinician and educator to complete this latest project in superior fashion. His detailed approach has culminated in an outstanding resource for all of us to use and enjoy.

In summary, *Special Tests for Neurologic Examination* will quickly take its place among the other primary textbooks and manuals in our professional libraries. It will also be found in a large number of student backpacks and athletic training kits!

John M. Hauth, EdD, ATC
Professor of Athletic Training
East Stroudsburg University of Pennsylvania

Introduction

The world of medicine has undergone a shift toward evidence-based practice over the last decade. Evidence-based medicine relies on the integration of the best available research, coupled with clinical expertise to guide clinicians to the best practice patterns. Evidence is used in all areas of clinical practice, including examination, diagnosis, and intervention. In the areas of examination and diagnosis, evidence-based practice assists the clinician in selecting the most appropriate examination procedures to distinguish between patients who present with or do not present with various dysfunctions. Although only one piece of the evaluation process, special test procedures provide the clinician with valuable information in the formation of a differential diagnosis. Therefore, evidence identifying the most reliable and valid special test procedures to perform can help direct the clinician's evaluation procedure. Every portion of the evaluation process should be helpful to the clinician in determining the probability of the patient suffering from various conditions.

Textbooks have traditionally provided the learner with a multitude of clinical exam techniques and testing procedures with little or no emphasis placed on diagnostic accuracy or test utility. When examination procedures are presented in this light, the clinician is left to believe that a positive test is always indicative of the patient suffering from the specific disorder for which the test was designed. In reality, however, many widely-accepted and heavily-utilized examination procedures exhibit diagnostic accuracy of less than 50%. This means that a positive test finding when performing the exam technique is no more likely to indicate a positive diagnosis than would flipping a coin with heads assigned as one diagnosis and tails assigned as another diagnosis. Knowledge of the diagnostic accuracy of the various techniques employed in the clinical setting is crucial to the clinician formulating an accurate diagnosis and, consequently, an appropriate treatment plan.

In keeping with the trend toward evidence-based practice, *Special Tests for Neurologic Examination* strives to provide data regarding the clinical utility of the various procedures described herein. In meeting this goal, the authors provide data regarding specificity and sensitivity for testing procedures, where data exists. Unfortunately, medicine is in its infancy in terms of evidence-based practice and, therefore, many examination procedures that are practiced daily in the clinical setting lack any evidence to support their application. This glaring gap in our collective clinical knowledge is narrowing; however, we have a long road ahead of us in terms of validating many of our clinical assessment and treatment procedures. Perhaps the lack of evidence available to today's practitioners will inspire future researchers to investigate the effectiveness of various techniques and procedures.

Diagnostic tests can be assessed in a number of ways. Reliability determines the test's ability to produce precise, accurate, and reproducible information. Diagnostic accuracy assesses the test's ability to discriminate between patients with or without a specific disorder. Clinical utility of various examination techniques requires that test results be compared to referenced standards such as diagnostic imaging or surgical diagnosis.

Pre-test probability, the likelihood that a patient has a specific disorder, is determined based on the patient's medical history, examination findings, and the clinician's experience. The performance of various examination procedures hinges on the patient's pre-test probability. For example, with a patient reporting a medical history consistent with carpal tunnel syndrome, demonstrating visual inspection and palpation findings consistent with carpal tunnel syndrome, and given a clinician with previous experience assessing patient's suffering from carpal tunnel syndrome, the clinician should assume a high pre-test probability that the patient is indeed suffering from carpal tunnel syndrome. From this pre-test probability, the clinician can select special test procedures aimed at confirming or refuting this potential diagnosis. When armed with evidence supporting testing procedures with the highest clinical utility, the clinician can now select the most appropriate special test procedures to facilitate the most accurate diagnosis. The patient's post-test probability is the likelihood that a patient has a specific disorder after all evaluation procedures have been performed.

Special tests must demonstrate a high degree of reliability to be considered clinically useful. Reliability determines the extent to which an examination procedure demonstrates a true representation and the proportion that is the result of measurement error. Stated another way, reliability is a measure of the consistency with which an instrument or examiner measures a particular attribute.

For reliability to remain high, testing procedures must be performed in an identical manner from one clinician to another and one test session to the next. Additionally, the definitions of positive and negative findings must also remain constant between clinicians and between test sessions. Reliability between examiners is termed inter-tester reliability, while reliability within a single examiner is termed intra-tester reliability. Numerous errors exist that can threaten reliability of special tests procedures. These errors commonly include inappropriate application of testing procedures (varying test application from accepted norms), inappropriate interpretation of test results (misinterpreting test findings) and equipment error (uncalibrated or faulty test equipment).

Reliability data is most often expressed as either a kappa coefficient (k), a Pearson correlation coefficient (r), or an intraclass correlation coefficient (ICC). When kappa or intraclass correlation coefficient values are used, the following scale can be applied to determine the strength of the coefficients: below .50 represents poor reliability, .50 to .75 represents moderate reliability, and greater than .75 indicates good reliability. When using a Pearson correlation coefficient, values range from -1 to +1. Negative values indicate an inverse relationship while positive values indicate direct relationships. A value of zero indicates that no relationship exists.

The diagnostic accuracy of a clinical exam technique is determined by comparing the test findings to a referenced standard, such as diagnostic imaging. Diagnostic accuracy compares the number of patients correctly diagnosed by the test procedure in comparison to those diagnosed using the referenced or "gold" standard. The percentage of patients correctly diagnosed becomes the test's diagnostic accuracy. Diagnostic accuracy is often described using positive and negative predictive values, sensitivity, specificity, and likelihood ratios.

In determining a test's diagnostic accuracy, a 2 x 2 contingency table is commonly utilized. The figure below illustrates a typical 2 x 2 contingency table.

	Positive Referenced Standard	Negative Referenced Standard
Positive Clinical Exam	True-Positive Findings (a)	False-Positive Findings (b)
Negative Clinical Exam	False-Negative Findings (c)	True-Negative Findings (d)

After gathering the data necessary to complete a 2 x 2 contingency table, the clinical utility, or usefulness, of the examination technique can be determined in terms of overall accuracy, positive or negative predicative value, sensitivity, specificity, and likelihood ratio.

Overall accuracy of the test is calculated by adding all true findings (true positive and true negative findings) and dividing by the total number of patients examined using the technique. Using the 2 x 2 contingency table, this equation can be expressed as:

Overall Accuracy = 100% x ([a+d] / [a+b+c+d])

Ideal test accuracy would be 100%, meaning that every patient assessed using the examination technique is appropriately identified as either having or not having the specific condition. Overall accuracy values of 100% are not attainable when utilizing clinical examination procedures.

Positive and negative predictive values estimate the likelihood that a patient with a positive test actually has the disorder for which the exam tests (positive predictive value [PPV]) or the likelihood that a patient with a negative test result is free of the disorder for which the exam technique assesses (negative predictive value [NPV]). Using the 2 x 2 contingency table, the following equations can be used to determine predictive values:

$$PPV = 100\% \times (a / [a+b])$$

$$NPV = 100\% \times (d / [c+d])$$

When positive predictive values approach 1, the examiner can be relatively sure that a positive test result indeed indicates the presence of the disorder. Conversely, as negative predictive values approach 1, the examiner can reasonably rule out the condition being assessed.

Sensitivity describes the test's ability to detect those patients who actually have the disorder as indicated by the referenced standard. Sensitivity is also referred to as the true-positive rate. Tests with high sensitivity are good at ruling out a specific condition. The acronym SnNOut reminds the clinician that high sensitivity, coupled with a negative result, indicates that the test is good for ruling out a disorder. When using the contingency table, sensitivity is calculated as:

$$\text{Sensitivity} = 100\% \times (a / [a+c])$$

Specificity, on the other hand, describes the test's ability to detect patients who are not suffering from a specific disorder, compared to the referenced standard. Specificity is also known as the true negative rate. Test procedures with high specificity are good for ruling in a specific disorder. The acronym SpPin is useful in assisting the clinician in remembering that a high specificity, coupled with a positive result is beneficial in ruling in a disorder. Specificity can be calculated using the equation:

$$\text{Specificity} = 100\% \times (d / [b+d])$$

While sensitivity and specificity can be easily utilized by the clinician in determining a special test's diagnostic utility, it should be noted that test procedures rarely demonstrate high scores for both sensitivity and specificity. Therefore, most special test procedures prove more useful for either ruling in a condition or ruling out a condition. This phenomenon often requires that the clinician perform multiple test procedures and correctly interpret the results in order to successfully complete the differential diagnosis.

Likelihood ratios combine a test sensitivity and specificity to determine the shift of probability that a patient has or does not have a specific disorder. Likelihood ratios are valuable to the clinician in altering clinical decision making. A positive likelihood ratio indicates an increased likelihood that a patient has a disorder given a positive test, while a negative likelihood ratio indicates a decreased likelihood that the patient has a disorder in the presence of a negative test. The formulas for calculating likelihood ratios are:

Positive Likelihood Ratio = sensitivity / (1 – specificity)

Negative Likelihood Ratio = (1 – sensitivity) / specificity

Positive likelihood ratios greater than 10 and negative likelihood ratios less than 0.1 indicate large and conclusive shifts in probability. Positive likelihood ratios between 5 and 10 and negative likelihood ratios between 0.1 and 0.2 generate moderate shifts in probability. Positive likelihood ratios of 2 to 5 and negative likelihood ratios ranging from 0.2 to 0.5 generate small, sometimes important shifts in probability. Finally, positive likelihood ratios between 1 and 2 and negative likelihood ratios between 0.5 and 1 alter probability to a small degree and are rarely important.

References

Cleland J. *Orthopedic Clinical Examination: An Evidence-Based Approach for Physical Therapists*. Carlstadt, NJ: Icon Learning Systems; 2005.

Domholdt E. *Physical Therapy Research*. 2nd ed. Philadelphia, PA: W.B. Saunders; 2000.

Fritz JM, Wainner RS. Examining diagnostic tests: an evidence based perspective. *Journal of Physical Therapy*. 2001;81:1546-1564.

Greenhalgh T. Papers that report diagnostic or screening tests. *British Medical Journal*. 1997;315:540-543.

Hagen MD. Test characteristics: How good is that test? *Primary Care*. 1995;22:213-233.

Jaeschke R, Guyatt GH, Sackett DL. How to use an article about a diagnostic test: what are the results and will they help me in caring for my patients? *JAMA*. 1991;271:703-707.

Jaeschke R, Guyatt GH, Sackett DL. How to use an article about a diagnostic test: are the results of the study valid? *JAMA*. 1994;271:389-391.

Maher CG, Sherrington C, Elkins M, Herbert RD, Moseley AM. Challenges for evidence-based physical therapy: Accessing and interpreting high-quality evidence on therapy. *Journal of Physical Therapy*. 2004;84:644-654.

Portney LG, Watkins MP. *Foundations of Clinical Research: Applications to Practice*. 2nd ed. Upper Saddle River, NJ: Prentice Hall Health; 2000.

Rothstein JM, Echternach JL. *Primer on Measurement: An Introductory Guide to Measurement Issues*. Alexandria, VA: American Physical Therapy Association; 1999.

Sackett DL. A primer on the precision and accuracy of the clinical examination. *JAMA*. 1992;267:2638-2644.

Sackett DL, Straws SE, Richardson WS, Rosenberg W, Haynes RB. *Evidence-Based Medicine: How to Practice and Teach EBM*. 2nd ed. London: Harcourt Publishers; 2000.

Schwartz JS. Evaluating diagnostic tests: what is done and what needs to be done. *J Gen Intern Med*. 1986;1:266-267.

Section ONE

Head

Chapter

1

Cranial Nerve Assessment

Table 1-1 summarizes the names, types, and functions of each of the cranial nerves. The remainder of this chapter is dedicated to various evaluation techniques used for cranial nerve assessment.

Table 1-1

CRANIAL NERVES

Cranial Nerve	*Type*	*Function*
I Olfactory	Sensory	Smell
II Optic	Sensory	Vision, Contralateral pupil reaction to light
III Oculomotor	Motor	Motor control of eye muscles, Ipsilateral pupil reaction to light
IV Trochlea	Motor	Motor control of superior oblique muscle
V Trigeminal	Sensory & Motor	Sensation to face, Motor control of muscles of mastication
VI Abducens	Motor	Motor control of lateral rectus muscle
VII Facial	Sensory & Motor	Taste to anterior one-third of tongue, Motor control of facial muscles
VIII Auditory	Sensory	Hearing and Balance (inner ear)
IX Glossopharangeal	Sensory & Motor	Taste on posterior portion of tongue, Motor control of pharynx

continued

Table 1-1, continued

CRANIAL NERVES		
Cranial Nerve	*Type*	*Function*
X Vagus	Sensory & Motor	Sensation and motor of the pharynx and larynx, Autonomic muscle control of thoracic and abdominal viscera
XI Spinal accessory	Motor	Motor control of the trapezius muscles and the sternocleidomastoid muscles
XII Hypoglossal	Motor	Motor control of the muscles of the tongue

REFERENCES

Magee DJ. *Orthopedic Physical Assessment.* 4th ed. Philadelphia, PA: W.B. Saunders; 2002.

Reese NB. *Muscle and Sensory Testing.* 2nd ed. Philadelphia, PA: W.B. Saunders; 2005.

Starkey C, Ryan JL. *Evaluation of Orthopedic and Athletic Injuries.* 2nd ed. Philadelphia, PA: FA Davis; 2002.

Cranial Nerve I: Olfactory Nerve

Materials Required

A food item or other item with a strong, distinct odor. Commonly used items for completing this test include a piece of hard candy, a stick of gum, lip balm, or an alcohol swab.

Cranial Nerve Function

Smell

Test Position

The patient is position in sitting, standing, or supine.

Action

The clinician instructs the patient to close his eyes. The clinician then holds the object under the patient's nose and asks the patient to identify the smell (Figure 1-1).

Positive Finding

A positive finding is the inability of the patient to perceive or distinguish the odor.

Special Considerations

The clinician should avoid using materials with unpleasant or pungent odors, especially in the case of a suspected cervical spine injury. This is due to the risk of the patient moving his head away from the object when presented.

References

Magee DJ. *Orthopedic Physical Assessment.* 4th ed. Philadelphia, PA: W.B. Saunders; 2002.

Meadows JTS. *Orthopedic Differential Diagnosis in Physical Therapy.* New York: McGraw-Hill; 1999.

Reese NB. *Muscle and Sensory Testing.* 2nd ed. Philadelphia, PA: W.B. Saunders; 2005.

Starkey C, Ryan JL. *Evaluation of Orthopedic and Athletic Injuries.* 2nd ed. Philadelphia, PA: F.A. Davis; 2002.

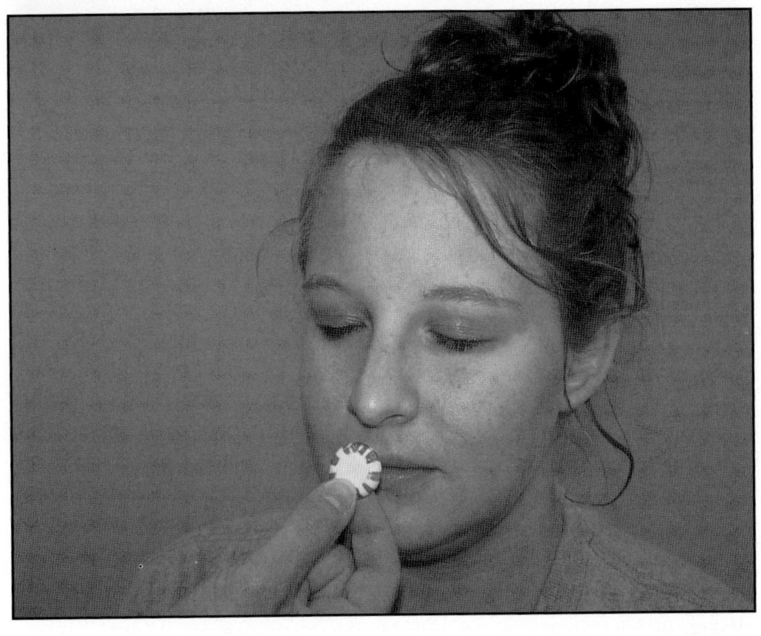

FIGURE 1-1

Cranial Nerve II: Optic Nerve

Materials Required

A Snellen eye chart or other object of reasonable size to use for assessing visual acuity and a penlight.

Cranial Nerve Function

Vision and contralateral pupil reflex.

Test Position

The patient is positioned in sitting.

Action

The clinician instructs the patient to read an object to assess for visual field deficits (Figure 1-2). The clinician also uses a penlight to assess contralateral pupillary reflex. For this test, the clinician shines a light in the patient's right eye while assessing for constriction of the left eye (Figure 1-3). The test is repeated bilaterally to assess for normal function.

Positive Finding

The patient is unable to read the object selected. The patient does not demonstrate normal contralateral pupil reaction (constriction) when the penlight is shown in his or her contralateral eye.

Special Considerations

The clinician must screen the patient for past medical history of visual impairment that might result in a false-positive test. Additional tests for assessing cranial nerve II include the confrontation test and visual field assessment looking for deficits in one or more fields.

References

Magee DJ. *Orthopedic Physical Assessment.* 4th ed. Philadelphia, PA: W.B. Saunders; 2002.

Meadows JTS. *Orthopedic Differential Diagnosis in Physical Therapy.* New York: McGraw-Hill; 1999.

Reese NB. *Muscle and Sensory Testing.* 2nd ed. Philadelphia, PA: W.B. Saunders; 2005.

Starkey C, Ryan JL. *Evaluation of Orthopedic and Athletic Injuries.* 2nd ed. Philadelphia, PA: F.A. Davis; 2002.

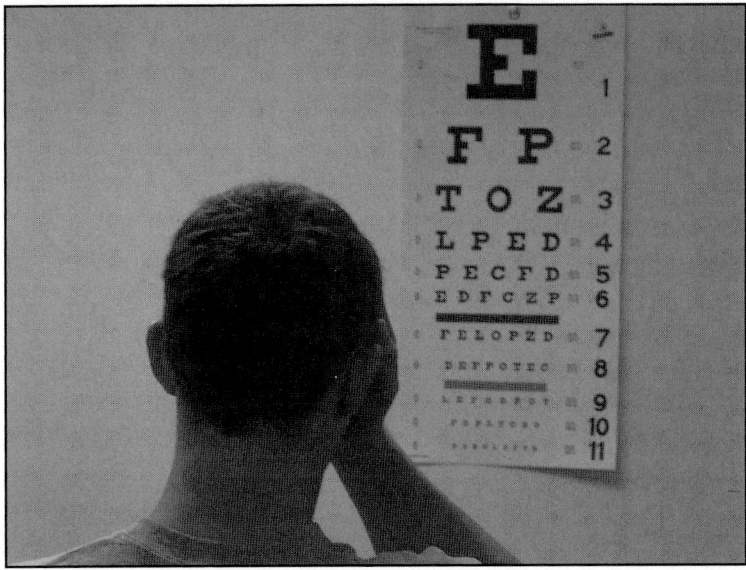

FIGURE 1-2

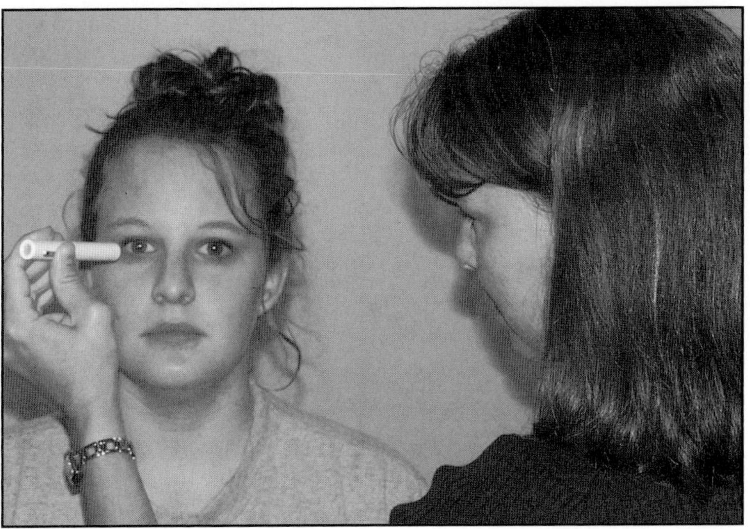

FIGURE 1-3

Cranial Nerve III: Oculomotor Nerve

Materials Required

Penlight

Cranial Nerve Function

Ipsilateral pupil reflex; motor control of the levator palpebrae; the superior, inferior, and medial recti; and the inferior oblique eye muscles.

Test Position

The patient is positioned in sitting.

Action

The clinician instructs the patient to elevate his or her eyelid (Figure 1-4) and also assesses for deficits in elevation, depression, and adduction motion of the eye (Figures 1-5a, 1-5b and 1-6). The clinician also uses a penlight to assess ipsilateral pupillary reflex. For this test, the clinician shines a light in the patient's right eye while assessing for constriction of the right eye (Figure 1-7). The test is repeated bilaterally to assess for normal function.

Positive Finding

The patient is unable to elevate the eyelid or is unable to follow the clinician's finger through eye elevation, depression, and adduction. The patient does not demonstrate ipsilateral pupil reaction (constriction) when the penlight is shown in his or her eye.

Special Considerations

End-point nystagmus is a normal finding when assessing this cranial nerve.

References

Magee DJ. *Orthopedic Physical Assessment.* 4th ed. Philadelphia, PA: W.B. Saunders; 2002.

Meadows JTS. *Orthopedic Differential Diagnosis in Physical Therapy.* New York: McGraw-Hill; 1999.

Reese NB. *Muscle and Sensory Testing.* 2nd ed. Philadelphia, PA: W.B. Saunders; 2005.

Starkey C, Ryan JL. *Evaluation of Orthopedic and Athletic Injuries.* 2nd ed. Philadelphia, PA: F.A. Davis; 2002.

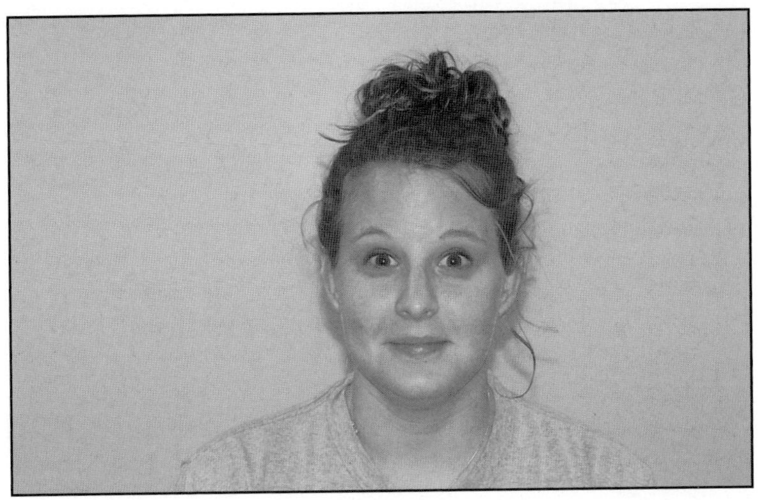

FIGURE 1-4

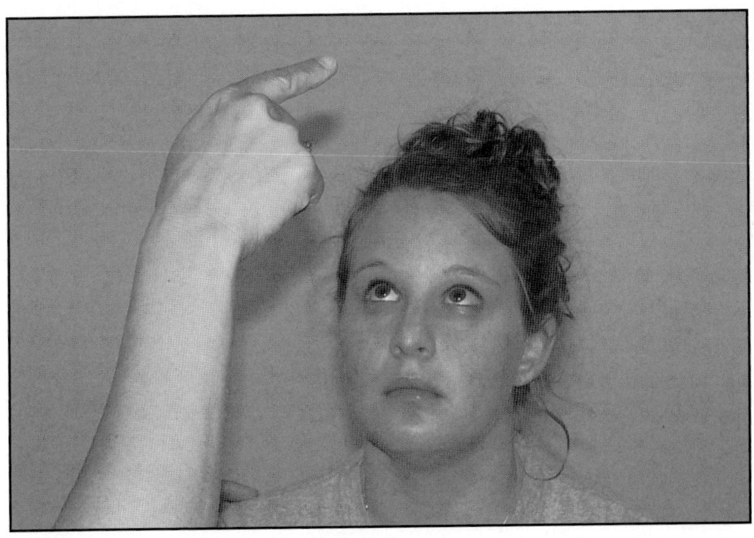

FIGURE 1-5A

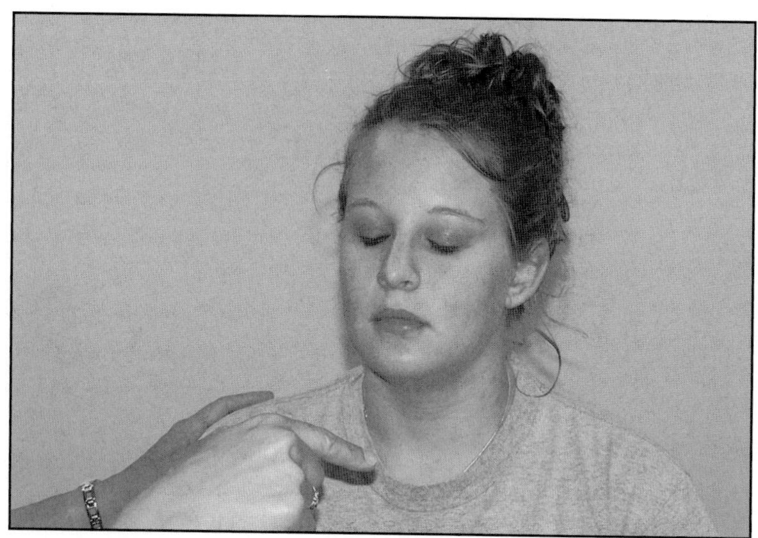

FIGURE 1-5B

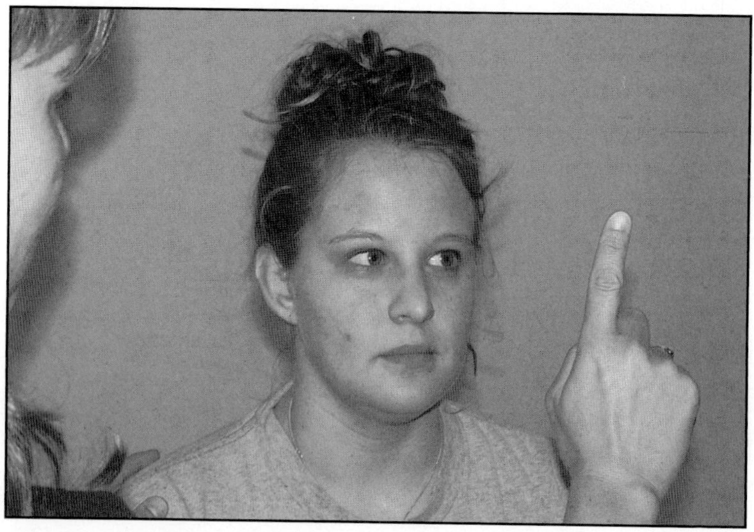

FIGURE 1-6

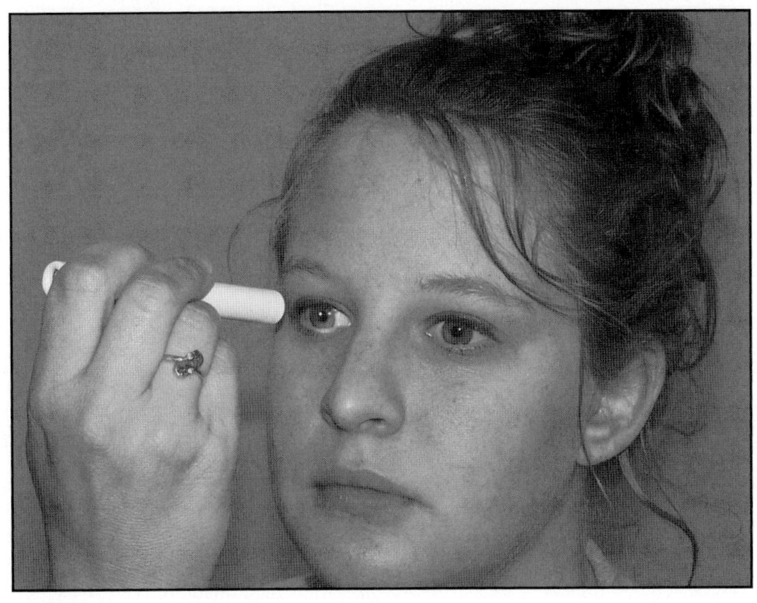

FIGURE 1-7

Cranial Nerve IV: Trochlear Nerve

Materials Required

None

Cranial Nerve Function

Motor control for the superior oblique muscle.

Test Position

The patient is positioned in sitting.

Action

The clinician instructs the patient to elevate his or her eyes (Figure 1-8).

Positive Finding

The patient is unable to elevate his or her eyes.

References

Magee DJ. *Orthopedic Physical Assessment.* 4th ed. Philadelphia, PA: W.B. Saunders; 2002.

Meadows JTS. *Orthopedic Differential Diagnosis in Physical Therapy.* New York: McGraw-Hill; 1999.

Reese NB. *Muscle and Sensory Testing.* 2nd ed. Philadelphia, PA: W.B. Saunders; 2005.

Starkey C, Ryan JL. *Evaluation of Orthopedic and Athletic Injuries.* 2nd ed. Philadelphia, PA: F.A. Davis; 2002.

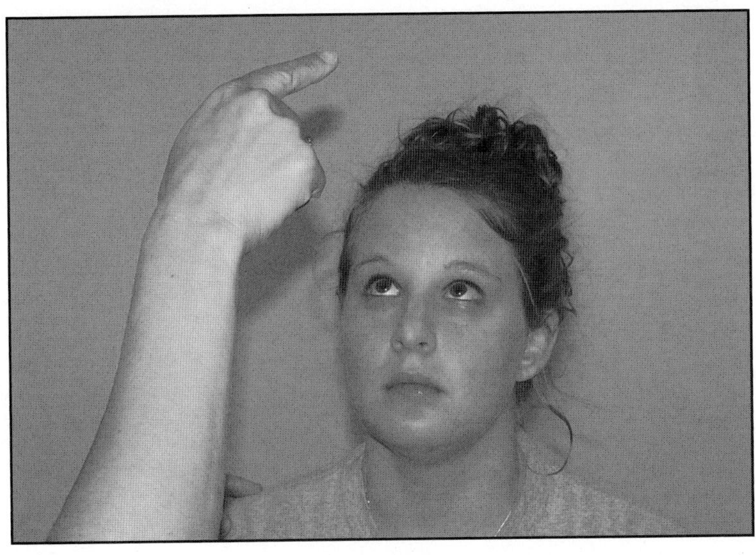

FIGURE 1-8

Cranial Nerve V: Trigeminal Nerve

Materials Required

None

Cranial Nerve Function

Sensation to the face and motor control to the muscles of mastication.

Test Position

The patient is positioned in sitting.

Action

The clinician assesses light touch of the skin of the face, comparing bilaterally for deficits (Figures 1-9 through 1-11). The clinician also instructs the patient to perform depression, elevation, and lateral excursion of his or her temporomandibular joint in order to assess the function of the muscles of mastication (Figures 1-12 through 1-14).

Positive Finding

A positive finding would be decreased sensation to light touch on one side of the face or inability to actively contract the muscles of mastication.

References

Magee DJ. *Orthopedic Physical Assessment*. 4th ed. Philadelphia, PA: W.B. Saunders; 2002.

Meadows JTS. *Orthopedic Differential Diagnosis in Physical Therapy*. New York: McGraw-Hill; 1999.

Reese NB. *Muscle and Sensory Testing*. 2nd ed. Philadelphia, PA: W.B. Saunders; 2005.

Starkey C, Ryan JL. *Evaluation of Orthopedic and Athletic Injuries*. 2nd ed. Philadelphia, PA: F.A. Davis; 2002.

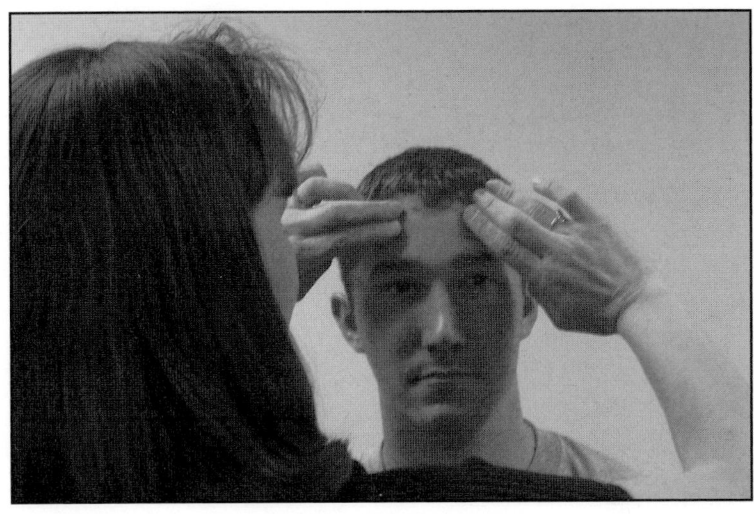

FIGURE 1-9

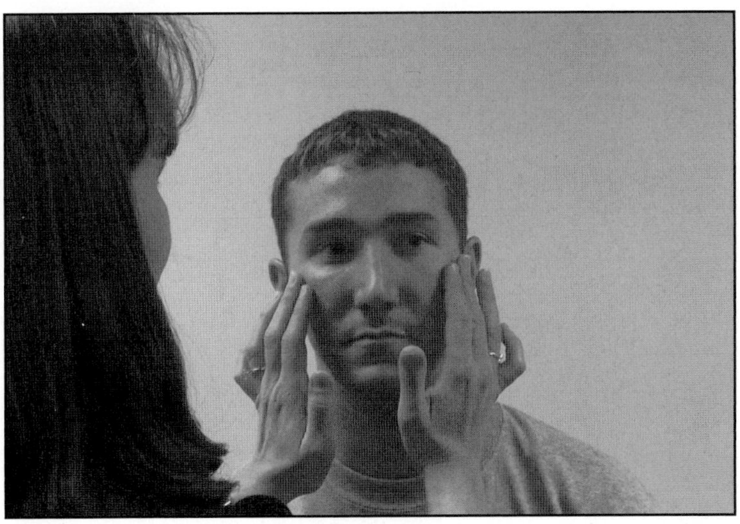

FIGURE 1-10

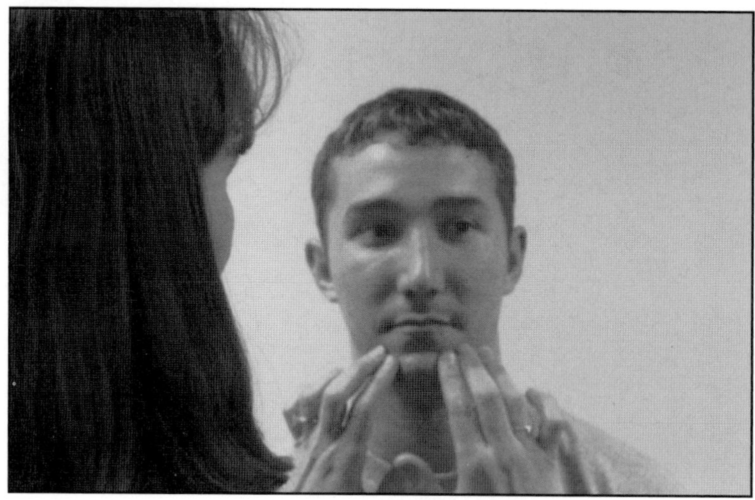

FIGURE 1-11

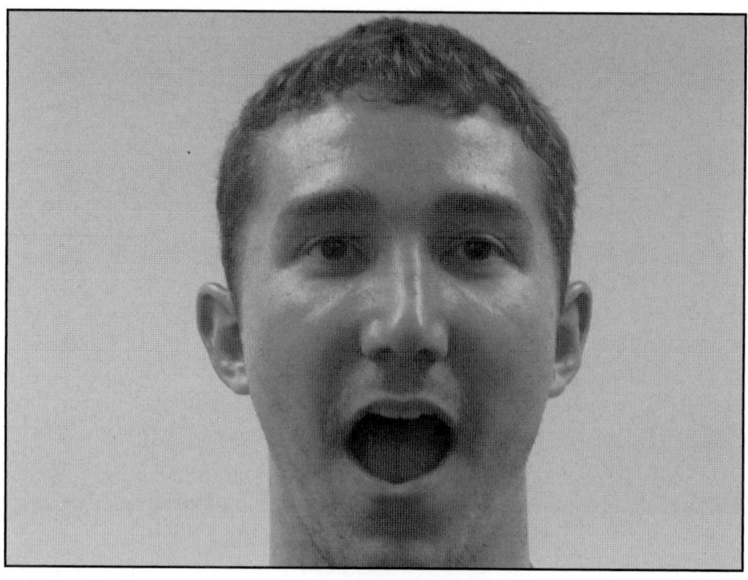

FIGURE 1-12

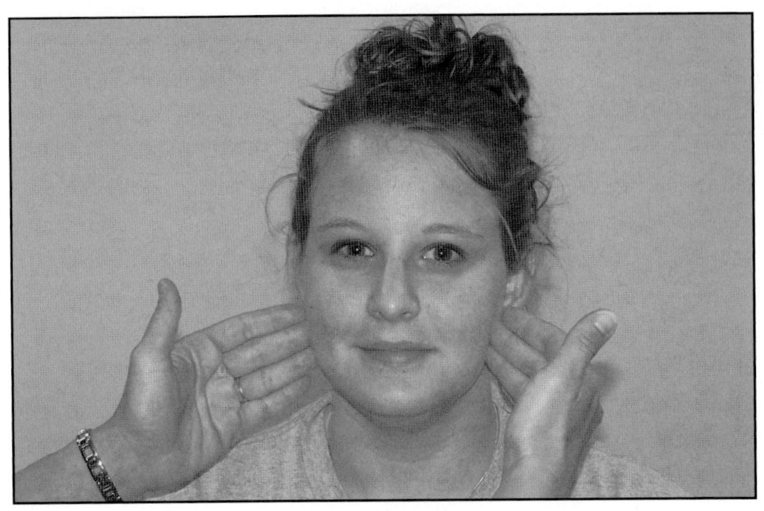

FIGURE 1-13

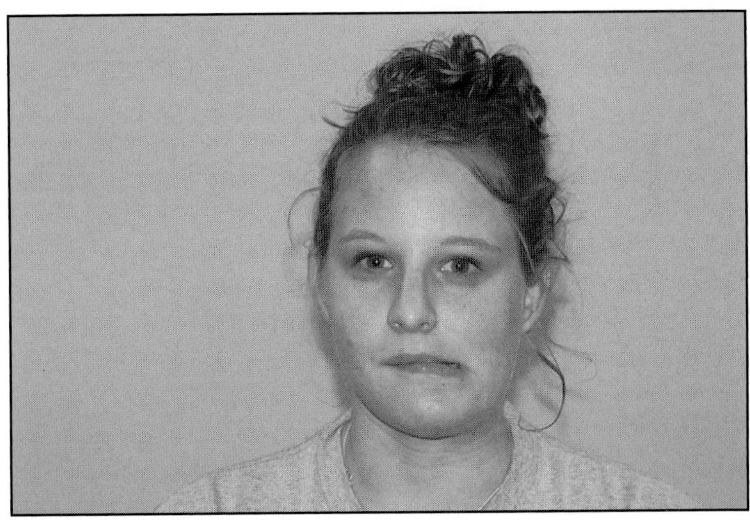

FIGURE 1-14

HEAD

Cranial Nerve VI: Abducens Nerve

Materials Required

None

Cranial Nerve Function

Motor control to the lateral rectus muscle of the eye.

Test Position

The patient is positioned in sitting.

Action

The clinician instructs the patient to abduct the eye (Figure 1-15).

Positive Finding

The patient is unable to abduct the eye.

Special Considerations

End-point nystagmus is a normal finding when assessing this cranial nerve.

References

Magee DJ. *Orthopedic Physical Assessment.* 4th ed. Philadelphia, PA: W.B. Saunders; 2002.

Meadows JTS. *Orthopedic Differential Diagnosis in Physical Therapy.* New York: McGraw-Hill; 1999.

Reese NB. *Muscle and Sensory Testing.* 2nd ed. Philadelphia, PA: W.B. Saunders; 2005.

Starkey C, Ryan JL. *Evaluation of Orthopedic and Athletic Injuries.* 2nd ed. Philadelphia, PA: F.A. Davis; 2002.

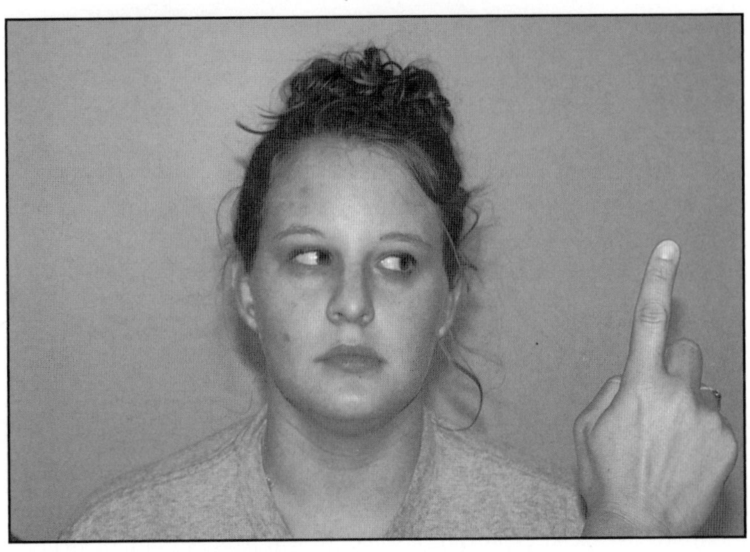

FIGURE 1-15

Cranial Nerve VII: Facial Nerve

Materials Required

A piece of hard candy.

Cranial Nerve Function

Taste to the anterior one-third of the tongue and motor control of the facial muscles.

Test Position

The patient is positioned in sitting.

Action

The clinician instructs the patient to close his or her eyes and stick out his or her tongue. The clinician places a piece of hard candy on the tip of the patient's tongue and asks the patient to identify the object (Figure 1-16). The clinician also instructs the patient to demonstrate the following facial expressions: smile, frown, pout, elevate or depress eyebrows, and puff the cheeks (Figures 1-17 through 1-19).

Positive Finding

The patient is unable to taste with the anterior one-third of the tongue or is unable to identify the taste of the object. The patient may also demonstrate deficits in performing facial expressions on one side of the face.

Special Considerations

Cranial nerve VII is involved in the condition Bell's Palsy.

References

Magee DJ. *Orthopedic Physical Assessment.* 4th ed. Philadelphia, PA: W.B. Saunders; 2002.

Meadows JTS. *Orthopedic Differential Diagnosis in Physical Therapy*. New York: McGraw-Hill; 1999.

Reese NB. *Muscle and Sensory Testing*. 2nd ed. Philadelphia, PA: W.B. Saunders; 2005.

Starkey C, Ryan JL. *Evaluation of Orthopedic and Athletic Injuries*. 2nd ed. Philadelphia, PA: F.A. Davis; 2002.

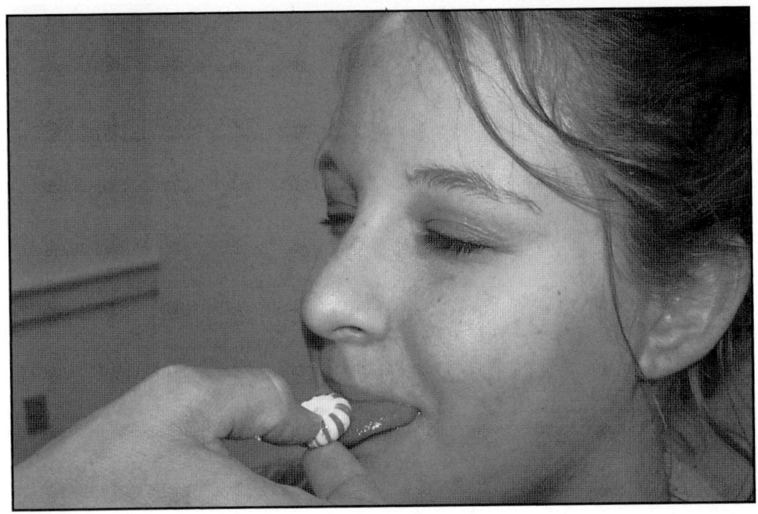

FIGURE 1-16

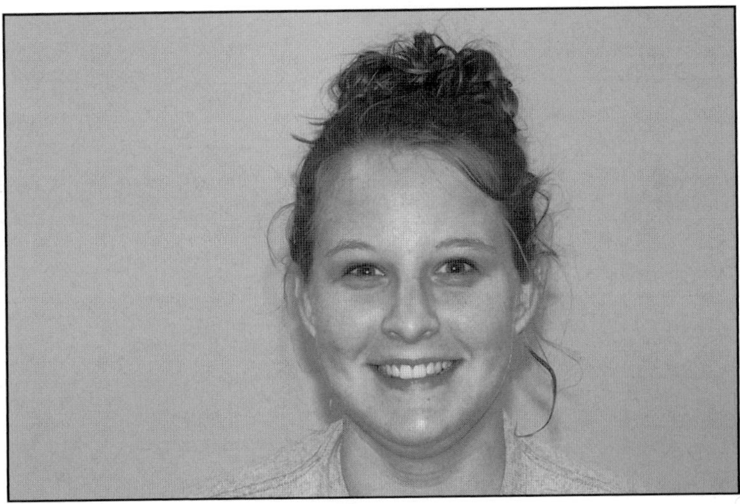

FIGURE 1-17

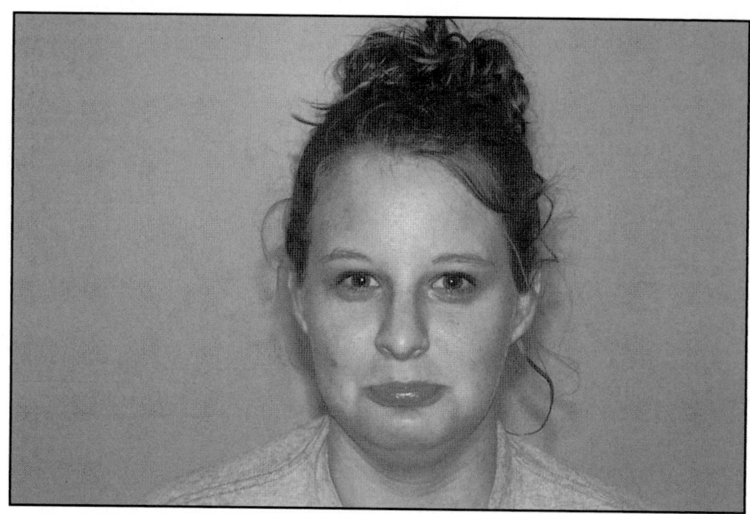

FIGURE 1-18

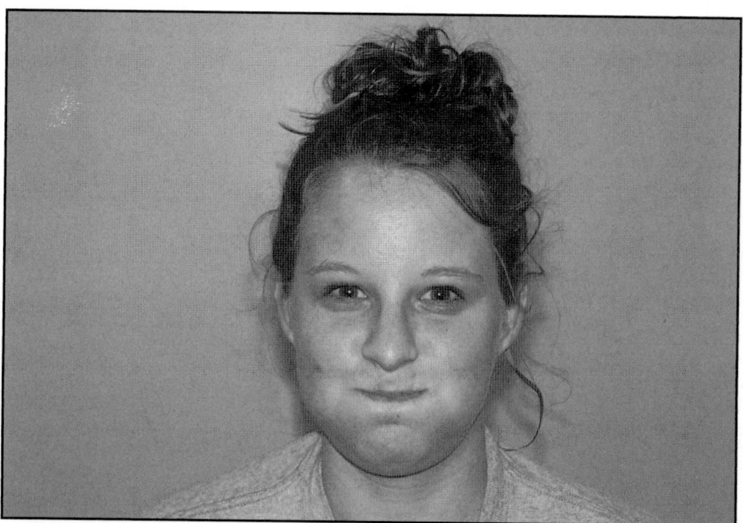

FIGURE 1-19

Cranial Nerve VIII: Acoustic Nerve

Materials Required

A tuning fork.

Cranial Nerve Function

Hearing and balance using the inner ear.

Test Position

The patient is positioned in standing.

Action

The clinician assesses the patient's ability to hear equally in both ears by placing the tuning fork close to the ear or by snapping next to each ear (Figure 1-20). The clinician also instructs the patient to balance on both legs with the eyes closed (Figure 1-21).

Positive Finding

The patient demonstrates a hearing deficit in one ear. The patient is unable to maintain balance with the eyes closed.

Special Considerations

This cranial nerve is also known as the vestibulocochlear nerve and the auditory nerve. The clinician may also assess cranial nerve VIII by performing the Weber Test, the Rhine Test, and the Halpike-Dix Test.

References

Magee DJ. *Orthopedic Physical Assessment.* 4th ed. Philadelphia, PA: W.B. Saunders; 2002.

Meadows JTS. *Orthopedic Differential Diagnosis in Physical Therapy.* New York: McGraw-Hill; 1999.

Reese NB. *Muscle and Sensory Testing.* 2nd ed. Philadelphia, PA: W.B. Saunders; 2005.

Starkey C, Ryan JL. *Evaluation of Orthopedic and Athletic Injuries.* 2nd ed. Philadelphia, PA: F.A. Davis; 2002.

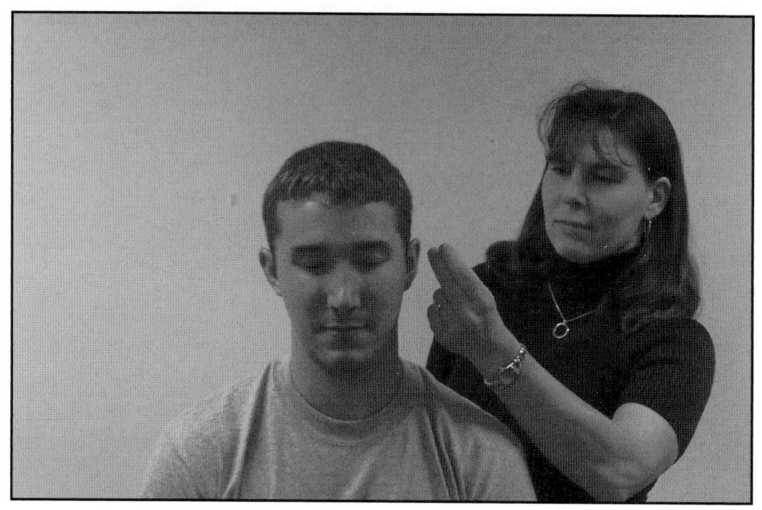

FIGURE 1-20

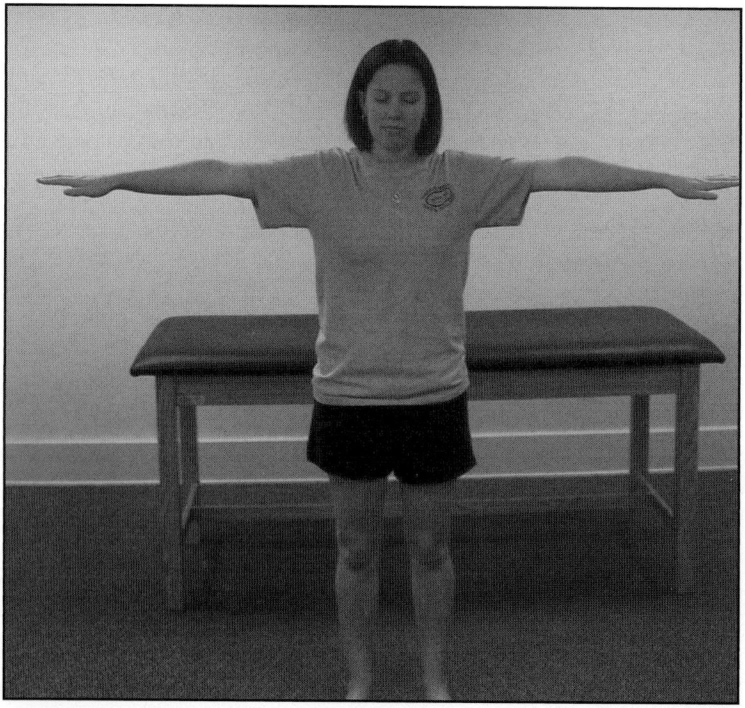

FIGURE 1-21

Cranial Nerve IX: Glossopharyngeal Nerve

Materials Required

A piece of hard candy.

Cranial Nerve Function

Taste to the posterior portion of the tongue and motor control of the pharynx.

Test Position

The patient is positioned in sitting.

Action

The clinician instructs the patient to close his or her eyes and stick out his or her tongue. The clinician places a piece of hard candy on the posterior portion of the patient's tongue and asks the patient to identify the object (Figure 1-22). The clinician also instructs the patient to swallow and say "ahh," assessing for uvula displacement to the strong side (Figure 1-23).

Positive Finding

The patient is unable to taste with the posterior portion of the tongue or is unable to identify the taste of the object. The patient is unable to swallow or the patient demonstrates lateral uvula displacement while saying "ahh."

Special Considerations

The clinician may also assess the patient's gag reflex as a test for cranial nerve IX.

References

Magee DJ. *Orthopedic Physical Assessment.* 4th ed. Philadelphia, PA: W.B. Saunders; 2002.

Meadows JTS. *Orthopedic Differential Diagnosis in Physical Therapy*. New York: McGraw-Hill; 1999.

Reese NB. *Muscle and Sensory Testing*. 2nd ed. Philadelphia, PA: W.B. Saunders; 2005.

Starkey C, Ryan JL. *Evaluation of Orthopedic and Athletic Injuries*. 2nd ed. Philadelphia, PA: F.A. Davis; 2002.

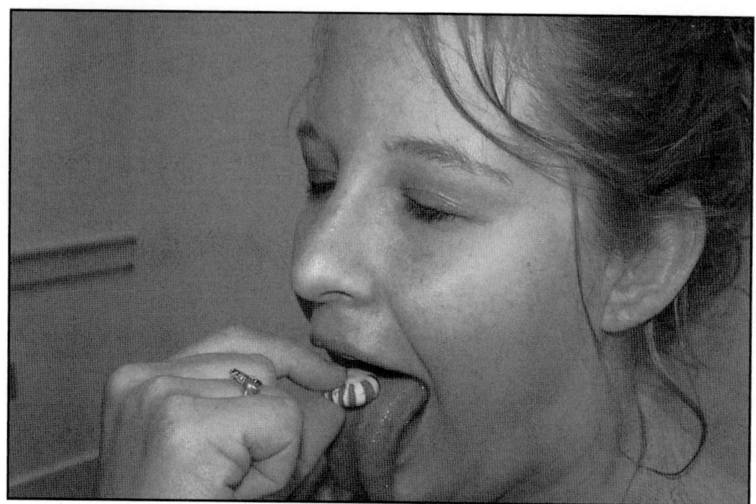

FIGURE 1-22

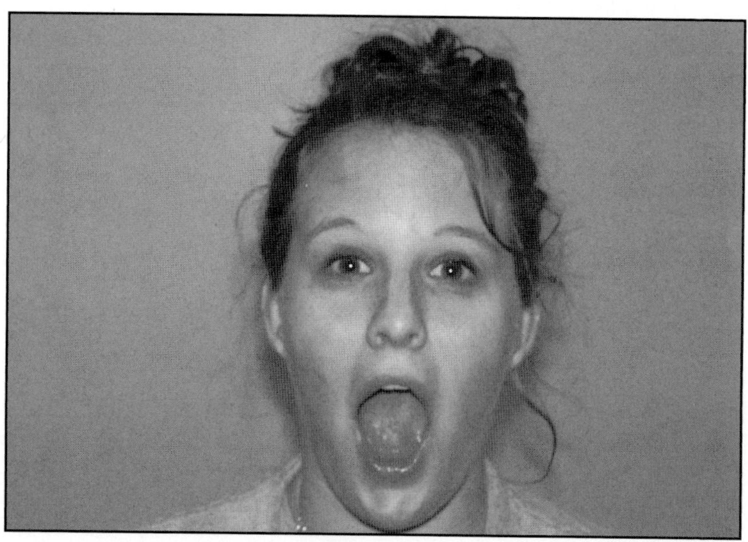

FIGURE 1-23

Cranial Nerve X: Vagus Nerve

Materials Required

A tongue depressor.

Cranial Nerve Function

Sensation and muscles of the pharynx and larynx, autonomic muscle control of thoracic and abdominal viscera.

Test Position

The patient is positioned in sitting or supine.

Action

The clinician instructs the patient to open his or her mouth and say "ahh", assessing for uvula displacement to the strong side (Figure 1-24). The clinician instructs the patient to swallow. The clinician assesses the patient's gag reflex (Figure 1-25).

Positive Finding

The patient demonstrates loss of phonation or the patient's uvula deviates to one side while saying "ahh". The patient may also demonstrate an inability to swallow or the absence of a gag reflex.

Special Considerations

The clinician may also assess the function of the patient's thoracic and abdominal viscera as an assessment of cranial nerve X.

References

Magee DJ. *Orthopedic Physical Assessment*. 4th ed. Philadelphia, PA: W.B. Saunders; 2002.

Meadows JTS. *Orthopedic Differential Diagnosis in Physical Therapy*. New York: McGraw-Hill; 1999.

Reese NB. *Muscle and Sensory Testing*. 2nd ed. Philadelphia, PA: W.B. Saunders; 2005.

Starkey C, Ryan JL. *Evaluation of Orthopedic and Athletic Injuries*. 2nd ed. Philadelphia, PA: F.A. Davis; 2002.

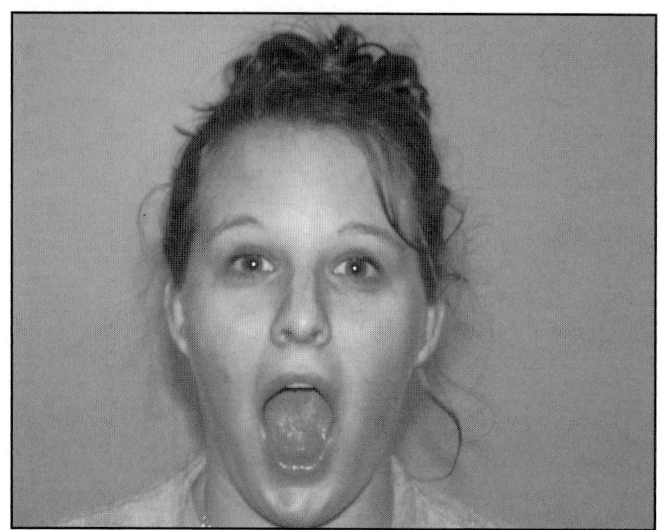

FIGURE 1-24

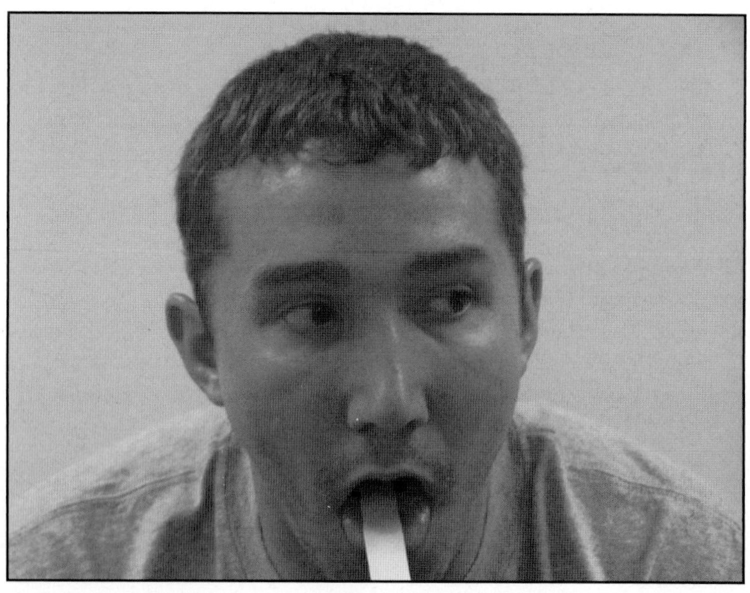

FIGURE 1-25

Cranial Nerve XI: Spinal Accessory Nerve

Materials Required

None

Cranial Nerve Function

Motor control to the trapezius and the sternocleidomastoid muscles.

Test Position

The patient is positioned in sitting.

Action

The clinician instructs the patient to shrug his or her shoulders against the clinician's resistance (Figure 1-26).

Positive Finding

The patient demonstrates unilateral weakness during resisted shoulder shrugs.

Special Considerations

Cranial nerve XI may also be tested by performing a manual muscle test of the upper trapezius and sternocleidomastoid muscles, assessing for unilateral strength deficits.

References

Magee DJ. *Orthopedic Physical Assessment*. 4th ed. Philadelphia, PA: W.B. Saunders; 2002.

Meadows JTS. *Orthopedic Differential Diagnosis in Physical Therapy*. New York: McGraw-Hill; 1999.

Reese NB. *Muscle and Sensory Testing*. 2nd ed. Philadelphia, PA: W.B. Saunders; 2005.

Starkey C, Ryan JL. *Evaluation of Orthopedic and Athletic Injuries*. 2nd ed. Philadelphia, PA: F.A. Davis; 2002.

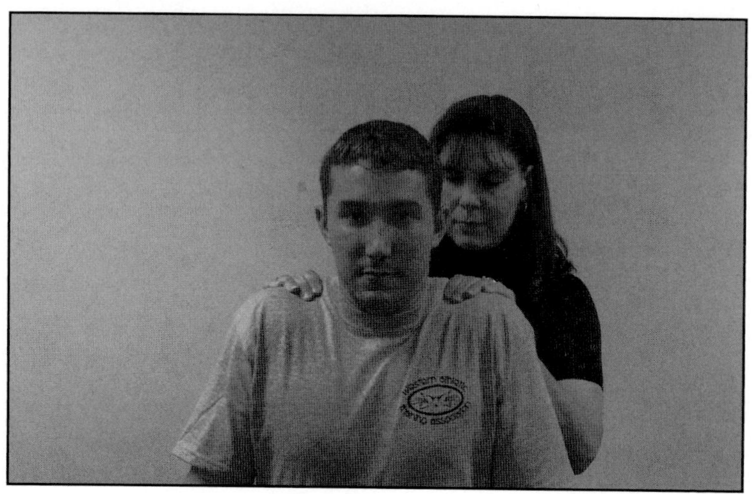

FIGURE 1-26

Cranial Nerve XII: Hypoglossal Nerve

Materials Required

None

Cranial Nerve Function

Motor control of the tongue.

Test Position

The patient is positioned in sitting.

Action

The clinician instructs the patient to stick out his or her tongue, assessing for deviation to the weak side (Figure 1-27). The clinician instructs the patient to move his tongue from side to side (Figures 1-28 and 1-29).

Positive Finding

The patient demonstrates deviation to one side when protruding his or her tongue, or the patient cannot move his or her tongue equally from side to side.

Special Considerations

Slurred speech may also be indicative of cranial nerve XII involvement.

References

Magee DJ. *Orthopedic Physical Assessment.* 4th ed. Philadelphia, PA: W.B. Saunders; 2002.

Meadows JTS. *Orthopedic Differential Diagnosis in Physical Therapy*. New York: McGraw-Hill; 1999.

Reese NB. *Muscle and Sensory Testing*. 2nd ed. Philadelphia, PA: W.B. Saunders; 2005.

Starkey C, Ryan JL. *Evaluation of Orthopedic and Athletic Injuries.* 2nd ed. Philadelphia, PA: F.A. Davis; 2002.

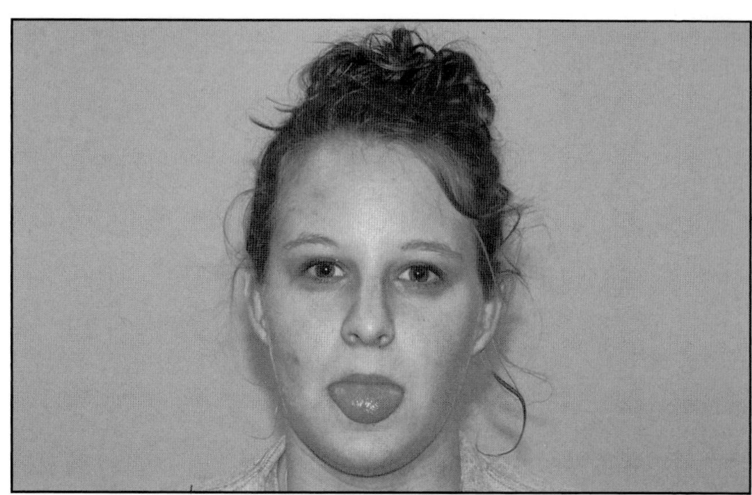

FIGURE 1-27

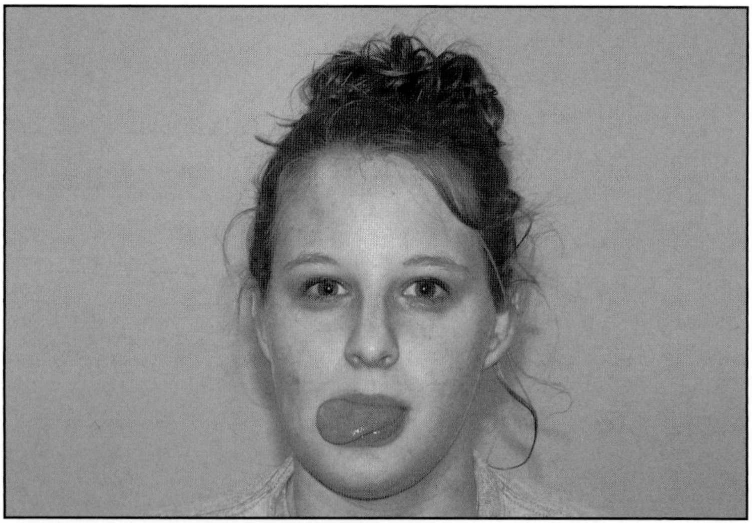

FIGURE 1-28

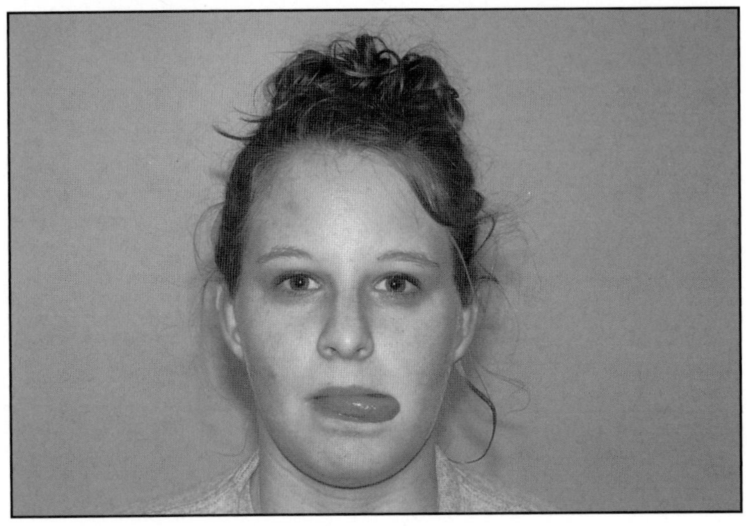

FIGURE 1-29

Chapter

2

Concussion Grading Scales/Coma Scales

Jill A. Manners, MS, LAT, ATC

GLASGOW COMA SCALE

The Glasgow Coma scale is used to assess the level of consciousness following head trauma (Tables 2-1 and 2-2). This scale was originally developed in 1974 by Graham Teasdale and Bryan Jennett and is currently the most widely used Level of Consciousness scale. When using this scale, scores should be assessed immediately after the initial trauma and reassessed frequently during the initial stages of the injury.

Table 2-1

GLASGOW COMA SCALE

Category	*Response*	*Points Allotted*
Eye Opening Response	Eyes open spontaneously	4
	Eyes open to speech or verbal stimuli	3
	Eyes open to painful stimuli	2
	Eyes do not open to stimuli	1
Verbal Response	Oriented and converses appropriately	5
	Converses, but disoriented	4
	Inappropriate words or responses	3
	Incomprehensible sounds	2
	No response	1
Motor Response	Obeys verbal commands for movement (Can you wiggle your toes?)	6
	Localizes painful stimuli (Can the patient identify where the pain is?)	5
	Withdraws due to painful stimulus	4
	Decorticate posturing/rigidity (flexion posturing) due to painful stimulus	3
	Decerebrate posturing/rigidity (extension posturing) due to painful stimulus	2
	No response	1

Table 2-2

GLASGOW COMA SCALE SCORE SUMMARY

Score	*Level of Trauma*
13 – 15	Mild head injury
9 – 12	Moderate head injury
3 – 8	Severe head injury

The total score is obtained by adding the values obtained in each of the three areas: Eye Opening, Verbal Response and Motor Response.

When evaluating a patient using this scale, it is important to differentiate an altered (or lack of) motor response from a musculoskeletal or spinal cord injury. This scale has limited function in infants and very young children (less than 36 months of age) due to the verbal response. There is a pediatric version of the Glasgow Coma Scale available.

REFERENCES

Cooper ER, Ferrara MS, Mrazik M, Castro S. Defining problems in mild head injury epidemiology. *Athletic Therapy Today*. 2001;6(1):6-12.

Drake AI, McDonald EC, Magnus NE, Gray N, Gottshall K. Utility of Glasgow Coma Scale-Extended in symptom prediction following mild traumatic brain injury. *Brain Injury*. 2006;20(5):469-475.

Guskiewicz KM. Concussion in sport: The grading-system dilemma. *Athletic Therapy Today*: 2001;6(1):18-27.

Magee DJ. *Orthopedic Physical Assessment*. 4th ed. Philadelphia, PA: W.B. Saunders; 2002.

Starkey C, Ryan JL. *Evaluation of Orthopedic and Athletic Injuries*. 2nd ed. Philadelphia, PA: F.A. Davis; 2002.

Teasdale G, Jennett B. Assessment of coma and impaired consciousness: A practical scale. *Lancet*. 1974;2:81-84.

Rancho Levels of Cognitive Functioning

The Rancho Levels of Cognitive Functioning, also known as the Rancho Los Amigos Scale of Cognitive Function (RLA), was originally developed in 1968 by Chris Hagen, PhD. This original scale was revised in 1973 by Hagen, Danese Malkmus, MS, and Katherine Stenderup-Bowman at the Rancho Los Amigos National Rehabilitation Center. This scale is primarily used on patients who demonstrate cognitive and memory deficits following a traumatic brain injury (Table 2-3). Today, this scale is very widely used in rehabilitation centers to assess the recovery status of patients. In 1997, this scale was once again revised by the original author, Chris Hagen (Table 2-4). The original RLA scale was designed with eight levels of function; however, the most recently revised RLA scale by Hagen now includes 10 levels. Both scales are currently used, although there are some controversies with the revised scale due to lack of reliability and validity studies. Therefore, the original version seems to be more widely accepted and is described in much greater depth below.

Table 2-3

Rancho Levels of Cognitive Functioning—Original Scale

Level	*Clinical Characteristics*	*Typical Responses*
Level I	Unresponsive	No response to any stimuli.
Level II	Generalized Response	Limited and inconsistent responses to stimuli. Responses may be physiological in nature. Responses are nonspecific to stimuli. Responses may be delayed. Typical first response is to pain.
Level III	Localized Response	Periods of awakening. Slow and inconsistent, but specific reactions to stimuli. Responses are typically related to stimulus presented.

continued

Table 2-3, continued

RANCHO LEVELS OF COGNITIVE FUNCTIONING—ORIGINAL SCALE

Level	*Clinical Characteristics*	*Typical Responses*
		Withdraw from painful stimuli. Turn head towards a sound. Ability to inconsistently follow simple directions such as opening or closing his eyes, or squeezing a hand. Possible recognition of some people.
Level IV	Confused and Agitated	Typically confused, disoriented, frightened, aggressive. May overreact to what he sees, feels, or to emotions. May occasionally recognize family and friends. May be able to perform routine activities. Incoherent words that are typically inappropriate. May react to previous events due to short-term memory loss.
Level V	Confused and Inappropriate	Appears alert. Able to consistently respond to simple commands. May demonstrate short attention span and is easily distracted. May be easily confused and demonstrate agitated behavior with excessive stimuli. Frequently speaks inappropriately.

continued

Table 2-3, continued

RANCHO LEVELS OF COGNITIVE FUNCTIONING—ORIGINAL SCALE

Level	*Clinical Characteristics*	*Typical Responses*
		Confusion regarding past and current events. Can typically perform self-care activities with assistance.
Level VI	Confused and Appropriate	Typical responses to stimuli are appropriate. Consistently follows simple directions. Confused due to memory loss. May remember major points but forget details. Can follow a routine schedule, but is easily confused with variation. Some self-awareness. Can perform self-care activities independently. Consistently oriented to time and place. Attention span typically no longer than 30 minutes. Recognizes family and friends, increased recognition of new acquaintances and rehabilitation staff. Responses typically appropriate to the situation; however, may be delayed or immediate.
Level VII	Automatic and Appropriate	Appropriately oriented to familiar settings.

continued

Table 2-3, continued

RANCHO LEVELS OF COGNITIVE FUNCTIONING—ORIGINAL SCALE

Level	*Clinical Characteristics*	*Typical Responses*
		May appear "robot-like." May be able to follow a set schedule or routine. Has difficulty planning and following through on activities. Minimal problem-solving abilities. Increased short-term memory and demonstrates an ability to carry over new learning. Able to initiate tasks that interest him. Improved attention span unless significant external stimuli. Poor safety awareness. Inflexible and rigid in decisions.
Level VIII	Purposeful and Appropriate	Alert and oriented. Able to recall and differentiate long- and short-term memory. Aware of surroundings. Independent in activities of daily living, within physical limitations. Able to learn and retain new information. May be able to problem solve. May be able to drive. May become confused or have an inability to think clearly in emergency, difficult or stressful situations.

HEAD

Table 2-4

Rancho Levels of Cognitive Functioning—Revised (1997)

Level	*Clinical Characteristics*
Level I	No response: Total Assistance
Level II	Generalized Response: Total Assistance
Level III	Localized Response: Total Assistance
Level IV	Confused/Agitated: Maximal Assistance
Level V	Confused, Inappropriate Non-Agitated: Maximal Assistance
Level VI	Confused, Appropriate: Moderate Assistance
Level VII	Automatic, Appropriate: Minimal Assistance for Daily Living Skills
Level VIII	Purposeful, Appropriate: Stand-By Assistance
Level IX	Purposeful, Appropriate: Stand-By Assistance on Request
Level X	Purposeful, Appropriate: Modified Independent

References

Hagen C. The expert's corner: proper use of the Rancho Levels of Cognitive Functioning. *Re-Learning Times*. 2001;8(1):4-6.

Magee DJ. *Orthopedic Physical Assessment*. 4th ed. Philadelphia, PA: W.B. Saunders; 2002.

The Rancho Los Amigos National Rehabilitation Center Website: www.rancho.org/research_home.htm

Levels of Consciousness

In assessing levels of consciousness, you are typically assessing whether or not the patient is awake, alert, and oriented. Many times you will see this written as Alert and Oriented x 3 or A & O x3. While assessing whether a patient is A & O x3, you are evaluating to see whether the patient knows his or her surroundings.

Awake:	Is the patient responsive to stimuli? Is he or she conscious?
Alert:	Is the patient mentally responsive, reactive, and attentive?
Oriented x 3:	Is the patient oriented to person, place and time? Does the patient know WHO he or she is? Does the patient know WHERE he or she is? Does the patient know WHAT TIME it is?

When assessing the level of consciousness you find that a patient is alert and oriented, but not in all three categories, make sure not to write A & O x 2, as this can be confusing. Clinicians should specifically document to what the patient is oriented. Many concussion tests, such as the Standardized Assessment of Concussion (SAC), assess for A & O x 3 during the evaluation.

References

Almquist J, Broshek D, Erlanger D. Assessment of mild head injuries. *Athletic Therapy Today*. 2001;6(1):13-17.

Cooper ER, Ferrara MS, Mrazik M, Castro S. Defining problems in mild head injury epidemiology. *Athletic Therapy Today*. 2001;6(1):6-12.

Guskiewicz KM. Concussion in sport: The grading-system dilemma. *Athletic Therapy Today*. 2001;6(1):18-27.

Magee DJ. *Orthopedic Physical Assessment*. 4th ed. Philadelphia, PA: W.B. Saunders; 2002.

GALVESTON ORIENTATION AND AMNESIA TEST (GOAT)

The Galveston Orientation and Amnesia Test was developed in 1979 by Levin, O'Donnell, and Grossman to evaluate cognition during the subacute stages of rehabilitation following head trauma. The test was revised in 2000 by Bode, Heinemann, and Semik. The GOAT is used most commonly in acute care and rehabilitation hospital settings.

This test is an oral and written test that evaluates the patient's orientation and memory of events prior to and after the injury. Specific test questions assess the patient's orientation to person, place, and time and assess for antegrade and retrograde amnesia.

A total number of "error points" is determined based on the number of incorrect responses the patient provides. Scoring is then completed on a 0 to 100 scale by subtracting the number of "error points" from 100. Scores of 76 to 100 are considered normal, scores of 66 to 75 are considered borderline, and scores below 65 are considered impaired.

REFERENCES

Levin HS, O'Donnell VM, Grossman RG. The Galveston Orientation and Amnesia Test: A practical scale to assess cognition after head injury. *Journal of Nervous and Mental Diseases*. 1979;167(11):675-684.

Magee DJ. *Orthopedic Physical Assessment*. 4th ed. Philadelphia, PA: W.B. Saunders; 2002.

AMERICAN ACADEMY OF NEUROLOGY (AAN) GRADING SCALE

In 1997, The American Academy of Neurology, under the guidance of lead authors James Kelly, MD and Jay Rosenberg, MD, created the AAN Guidelines based upon the guidelines of the Colorado Medical Society. According to a study conducted by Notebaert and Guskiewicz in 2005, the AAN guidelines are the most frequently used concussion grading scale (Table 2-5) and return to play guidelines (Table 2-6). The AAN also supports the use of a sideline evaluation that includes mental status testing (orientation, concentration, and memory), external provocation testing (physical activity tests), and neurologic testing (pupil evaluation, coordination, and sensation). This sideline evaluation should be used in the evaluation of all three concussion grades.

Table 2-5

AMERICAN ACADEMY OF NEUROLOGY GRADING SCALE

Grade	*Signs and Symptoms*
I (Mild)	No loss of consciousness Transient confusion Symptoms resolve in less than 15 minutes
II (Moderate)	No loss of consciousness Transient confusion Symptoms or mental status abnormalities resolve in more than 15 minutes
III (Severe)	Any loss of consciousness, either brief (seconds) or prolonged (minutes)

Table 2-6

RETURN TO PLAY GUIDELINES

Concussion Grade	*Number of Concussions Suffered*	*Guideline*
Grade I (Mild)	First	Remove immediately from activity Examine immediately and at 5-minute intervals for the development of post concussion symptoms and mental status abnormalities (at rest and exertion). May return to play if symptom-free within 15 minutes.
Grade I (Mild)	Second	May not return to activity that day. May return to activity after asymptomatic for 7 days.
Grade II (Moderate)	First	May not return to activity that day. May return to activity after asymptomatic for 7 days. Physician evaluation. End of season if abnormal diagnostic testing (CT scan or MRI).
Grade II (Moderate)	Second	May not return to activity that day. May return to activity after asymptomatic for 14 days. Physician evaluation. End of season if abnormal diagnostic testing (CT scan or MRI).

continued

Table 2-6, continued

RETURN TO PLAY GUIDELINES

Concussion Grade	*Number of Concussions Suffered*	*Guideline*
Grade III (Severe)	First	May not return to activity that day. Physician referral (treat as cervical spine injury if unconscious). If brief LOC (seconds), return to activity 7 days after asymptomatic. If prolonged LOC (minutes), return to activity 14 days after asymptomatic. End of season if abnormal diagnostic testing (CT scan or MRI).
Grade III (Severe)	Second	May not return to activity that day. Physician referral. May return 1 month after symptom-free. End of season if CT/MRI abnormality.

REFERENCES

Bailes JE, Hudson V. Classification of sport-related head trauma: a spectrum of mild to severe injury. *J Athl Train*. 2001;36(3):236-243.

Cooper ER, Ferrara MS, Mrazik M, Castro S. Defining problems in mild head injury epidemiology. *Athletic Therapy Today*. 2001;6(1):6-12.

Guskiewicz KM. Concussion in sport: The grading-system dilemma. *Athletic Therapy Today*. 2001;6(1):18-27.

Kelly JP, Rosenberg J. Practice parameter: the management of concussion in sports: report of the quality standards committee. *Neurology*. 1997;48:581-585.

Notebaert AJ, Guskiewicz KM. Current trends in athletic training practice for concussion assessment and management. *J Athl Train*. 2005;40(4):320-325.

Cantu Concussion Grading Guidelines

After its introduction in 1986, Dr. Robert Cantu, MD revised his scale in 2001. This scale is considered the Cantu Evidence-Based Grading System for concussion (Tables 2-7 and 2-8). Cantu's scale is one of the most widely known and referred to grading scales and emphasizes post-traumatic amnesia and post-concussive signs and symptoms.

Table 2-7

Cantu Concussion Grading Scale

Grade	*Signs and Symptoms*
I (Mild)	No loss of consciousness. Post-concussion symptoms resolving in less than 24 hours. Post-traumatic amnesia for less than 30 minutes.
II (Moderate)	Loss of consciousness for less than 1 minute. OR Post-traumatic amnesia for more than 30 minutes, but less than 24 hours. OR Post-concussion symptoms for more than 24 hours, but less than 7 days.
III (Severe)	Loss of consciousness for more than 1 minute. OR Post-traumatic amnesia for more than 24 hours. OR Post-concussion symptoms for more than 7 days.

Table 2-8

RETURN TO PLAY GUIDELINES

Concussion Grade	*Number of Concussions Suffered*	*Guideline*
Grade I (Mild)	First	Return to activity if asymptomatic for 7 days.
Grade I (Mild)	Second	May not return to activity that day. May return to activity after asymptomatic for 7 days.
Grade I (Mild)	Third	May not return to activity that day. End of season, return to activity next season if asymptomatic.
Grade II (Moderate)	First	May not return to activity that day. May return to activity after asymptomatic for 7 days.
Grade II (Moderate)	Second	May not return to activity that day. Minimum of 1 month, must be asymptomatic for at least 1 week. Consider end of season.
Grade II (Moderate)	Third	End of season. May return next season if asymptomatic.
Grade III (Severe)	First	May not return to activity that day. Minimum of 1 month after asymptomatic for at least 1 week.
Grade III	Second	May not return to activity that day. End of season. May return next season if asymptomatic.

References

Bailes JE, Hudson V. Classification of sport-related head trauma: a spectrum of mild to severe injury. *J Athl Train*. 2001;36(3):236-243.

Cantu RC. Return to play guidelines after a head injury. *Clin Sports Med*. 1998;17(1):45-60.

Cantu RC. Athletic head injuries. *Clin Sports Med*. 1997;16(3):531-542.

Cantu RC. Minor head injuries in sports. *Adolescent Medicine*. 1991;2(1):141-154.

Cantu RC. Second-impact syndrome. *Clin Sports Med*. 1988;17:37-44.

Cantu RC. Guidelines for return to contact sports after a cerebral concussion. *Phys Sportsmed*. 1984;14(10):75-83.

Cooper ER, Ferrara MS, Mrazik M, Castro S. Defining problems in mild head injury epidemiology. *Athletic Therapy Today*. 2001;6(1):6-12.

Guskiewicz KM. Concussion in sport: the grading-system dilemma. *Athletic Therapy Today*. 2001;6(1):18-27.

Colorado Medical Society Concussion Rating Guidelines

In 1991, the Colorado Medical Society proposed this scale for grading concussions (Tables 2-9 and 2-10). This scale is not commonly utilized in sports medicine.

Table 2-9

Colorado Medical Society Concussion Grading Scale

Grade	*Signs and Symptoms*
I (Mild)	No loss of consciousness Transient confusion No amnesia
II (Moderate)	No loss of consciousness Transient confusion Amnesia
III (Severe)	Any loss of consciousness

Table 2-10

RETURN TO PLAY GUIDELINES

Concussion Grade	*Number of Concussions Suffered*	*Guideline*
Grade I (Mild)	First	Same day return to activity if asymptomatic for 20 minutes.
Grade I (Mild)	Second	Return to activity if asymptomatic for 7 days.
Grade I (Mild)	Third	No return to activity until asymptomatic for 3 months.
Grade II (Moderate)	First	Return to activity when asymptomatic for 7 days.
Grade II (Moderate)	Second	Return to activity if asymptomatic for 1 month.
Grade II (Moderate)	Third	End of season. May return next season if asymptomatic.
Grade III (Severe)	First	Transport to hospital (treat as cervical spine injury). Return to activity after 1 month if asymptomatic for 14 days.
Grade III (Severe)	Second	End of season. Discourage return to activity.

References

Bailes JE, Hudson V. Classification of sport-related head trauma: a spectrum of mild to severe injury. *J Athl Train*. 2001;36(3):236-243.

Colorado Medical Society. Report of the Sports Medicine Committee: Guidelines for the management of concussion in sports (revised). Paper presented at the Colorado Medical Society Meeting, Denver, 1991.

Cooper ER, Ferrara MS, Mrazik M, Castro S. Defining problems in mild head injury epidemiology. *Athletic Therapy Today*. 2001;6(1):6-12.

Guskiewicz KM. Concussion in sport: the grading-system dilemma. *Athletic Therapy Today*. 2001;6(1):18-27.

Torg Concussion Grading Guidelines

In 1982, Joseph Torg, MD created this concussion grading scale guideline (Table 2-11). This was the first presented concussion grading scale and has been the basis for many scales to be created. Torg's scale is not frequently used today for concussion evaluation.

Table 2-11

Torg Concussion Grading Guidelines

Grade	*Signs and Symptoms*
I	"Bell rung" Short-term confusion Unsteady gait Dazed appearance No amnesia
II	Post-traumatic amnesia Vertigo No loss of consciousness
III	Post-traumatic retrograde amnesia Vertigo No loss of consciousness
IV	Immediate, transient loss of consciousness
V	Paralytic coma
VI	Death

REFERENCES

Cooper ER, Ferrara MS, Mrazik M, Castro S. Defining problems in mild head injury epidemiology. *Athletic Therapy Today*. 2001;6(1):6-12.

Guskiewicz KM. Concussion in sport: the grading-system dilemma. *Athletic Therapy Today*. 2001;6(1):18-27.

Torg JS. *Athletic Injuries to the Head, Neck and Face*. St. Louis, MO: C.V. Mosby; 1991.

University of North Carolina Concussion Grading Scale

When using this scale, the "3 C's" are defined as coordination, cognition, and cranial nerves. Balance and proprioceptive tests or skills are evaluated for coordination, while memory and thought processes are evaluated for cognition. The cranial nerves that are evaluated during this scale include the optic (CNII), oculomotor (CN III), trochlear (CN IV), facial (CN VII), and vestibulocochlear (CN VIII).

Athletes returning to activity based on this concussion grading scale ultimately need to be asymptomatic prior to considering a return to activity (Tables 2-12 and 2-13). Once the athlete is asymptomatic, meaning he or she has no current signs or symptoms, he or she may progress through the guidelines based upon the severity of the concussion. According to the University of North Carolina grading scale, any athlete who sustains a second concussion within a 3-month period should rest twice as long as the initial recommendation prior to returning to activity.

Table 2-12

University of North Carolina Concussion Grading Scale

Grade	*Consciousness*	*"3 C's" (Cranial Nerves, Cognition, & Coordination)*	*Headache*
0 (Mild)	No loss of consciousness	Mild confusion, asymptomatic within 10 minutes Passes functional tests without increased signs or symptoms	Possibly develops later
I (Mild)	No loss of consciousness	At least one of the "3 C's" is present: Abnormal cranial nerve function lasting <1 hour Abnormal cognition lasting <1 hour Abnormal coordinaton lasting < 3 days	Probable (10 minutes – 2 days)
II (Moderate)	Brief LOC (10 seconds to 1 minute) OR Altered consciousness lasting <2 minutes	At least one of the "3 C's" is present: Abnormal cranial nerve function lasting >1 hour Abnormal cognition lasting <1 hour Abnormal coordination lasting >3 days	Probable (24 hours – 4 days)
III (Severe)	Altered consciousness lasting >2 minutes	At least 2 of the "3 C's" are abnormal for >24 hours	Likely (greater than 4 days)

Table 2-13

THE UNIVERSITY OF NORTH CAROLINA GUIDELINES FOR RETURN TO ACTIVITY

Concussion Grade	*Return to Activity Guidelines*
Grade 0 (Mild)	The athlete should be removed from activity immediately. Reassess the athlete every 5 minutes for changes in signs or symptoms, including abnormal cranial nerve development, cognition, and coordination. Assess the athlete at rest and during physical exertion. Athlete may return to activity if there are no developing signs or symptoms once he or she has been asymptomatic for at least 20 minutes.
Grade 1 (Mild)	Asymptomatic at rest and during physical exertion for at least 2 days. One additional day of being asymptomatic during modified/restricted activity.
Grade 2 (Moderate)	Immediate removal from activity for that day. Re-evaluation every 5 minutes for developing pathology. Re-examine daily. Asymptomatic at rest and physical exertion for at least 4 days. Return to activity if asymptomatic for at least 2 additional days during modified/restricted activity.
Grade 3 (Severe)	Immediate removal from activity with initial treatment as a cervical spine injury. Daily re-examinations. If asymptomatic within 7 days: No participation until asymptomatic for 10 days at rest and physical exertion.

continued

Table 2-13, continued

THE UNIVERSITY OF NORTH CAROLINA GUIDELINES FOR RETURN TO ACTIVITY

Concussion Grade	*Return to Activity Guidelines*
Grade 3 (Severe)	After 10 days of asymptomatic rest, 3 days of restricted and modified activities.
	Unrestricted activity if still asymptomatic after a total of 13 days of being asymptomatic.
	If asymptomatic after 7 days:
	No participation until asymptomatic for 17 days at rest and physical exertion.
	After 17 days of asymptomatic rest, 3 additional days of restricted and modified activities.
	Unrestricted activity if still asymptomatic after a total of 17 days of being asymptomatic.

REFERENCES

Guskiewicz KM. Concussion in sport: the grading-system dilemma. *Athletic Therapy Today*. 2001;6(1):18-27.

Guskiewicz K, Riemann B, Perrin D, Gansneder B. Alternative approaches to the assessment of mild head injuries in athletes. *Med Sci Sports Exerc*. 1997;29(7):213-221.

Oliaro S, Anderson S, Hooker D. Management of cerebral concussion in sports: The athletic trainer's perspective. *J Athl Train*. 2001;36(3):257-262.

Chapter

3

Concussion Testing

Jill A. Manners, MS, LAT, ATC

Romberg Test

Test Position

The patient is instructed to stand with his or her feet together, arms at his or her sides.

Action

This test is a progressive test that becomes more challenging as the patient moves from one step to the next. The additional steps to this test include:

1. Patient stands with feet together and eyes open.
2. Patient stands with feet together and eyes closed.
3. Patient stands on one foot with eyes open.
4. Patient stands on one foot with eyes closed.
5. Patient stands on one foot with eyes closed and tilts head backwards.
6. Patient stands on one foot with eyes closed and tilts head backward while performing finger-to-nose activity.

The clinician observes the patient's ability to resist loss of balance and coordination when the patient closes his or her eyes (Figures 3-1 through 3-4).

Positive Finding

A positive test is the inability of the patient to remain steady and control his position when his or her eyes are closed. This is indicative of proprioceptive dysfunction. There is debate as to whether this test also assesses for cerebellar dysfunction, expanding intracranial lesion, proprioceptive problems, or cranial nerve X dysfunction (Vagus Nerve).

Special Considerations

It is recommended that the clinician guard the patient while performing this test to ensure that he or she does not fall.

Historical Notes

This test was named for Moritz Heinrich Romberg, a German neurologist in the early 1800s.

Specificity

No data available.

Sensitivity

No data available.

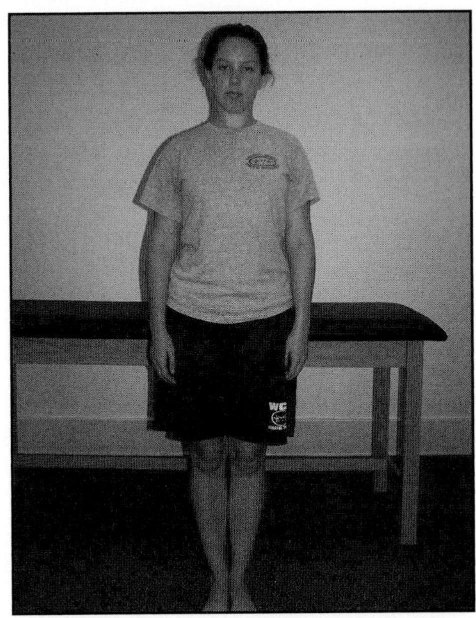

FIGURE 3-1

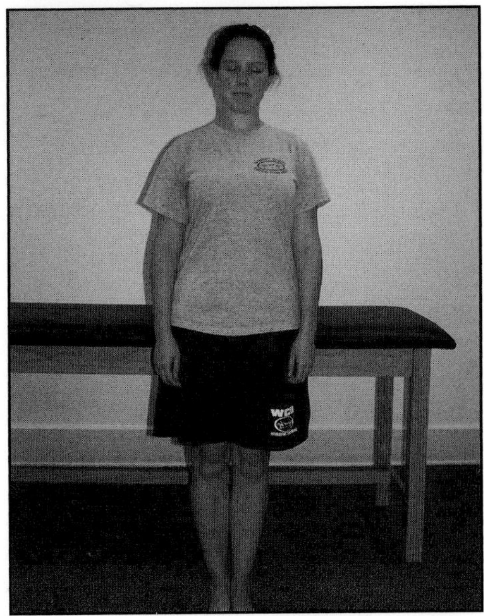

FIGURE 3-2

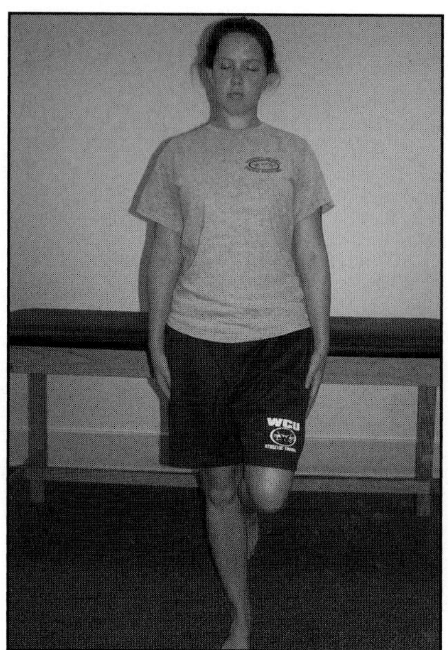

FIGURE 3-3

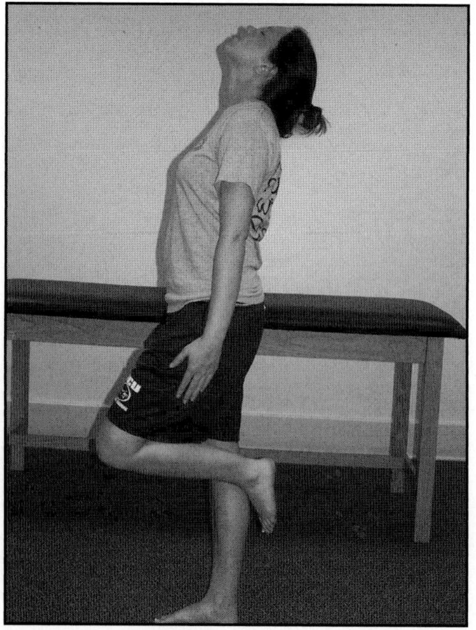

FIGURE 3-4

REFERENCES

Lanska DJ, Goetz CG. Romberg's sign: Development, adoption and adaptation in the 19th century. *Neurology*. 2000;55:1201-6.

Magee DJ. *Orthopedic Physical Assessment.* 4th ed. Philadelphia, PA: W.B. Saunders; 2002.

Starkey C, Ryan JL. *Evaluation of Orthopedic and Athletic Injuries.* 2nd ed. Philadelphia, PA: FA Davis; 2002.

TANDEM TEST

TEST POSITION

Patient is standing with his or her eyes open and feet straddling a line.

ACTION

Patient is asked to place one foot directly in front of the other, with the heel of the foot in front touching the toes of the foot in back. (Standing Tandem Test). The patient is then asked to walk in a straight line, repeatedly placing the heel of the front foot immediately in front of the toes of the rear foot (Figure 3-5).

POSITIVE FINDING

A positive test is the inability of the patient to maintain balance or remain steady. This test assesses for cerebral dysfunction or inner ear dysfunction.

SPECIAL CONSIDERATIONS

This test can be progressed to having the patient return to the starting position walking backwards.

ALTERNATE NAMES

This test is also known as the *Tandem Romberg, the Walking Tandem Test* and the *Standing Tandem Test.*

SPECIFICITY

No data available.

SENSITIVITY

No data available.

REFERENCES

Starkey C, Ryan JL. *Evaluation of Orthopedic and Athletic Injuries.* 2nd ed. Philadelphia, PA: F.A. Davis; 2002.

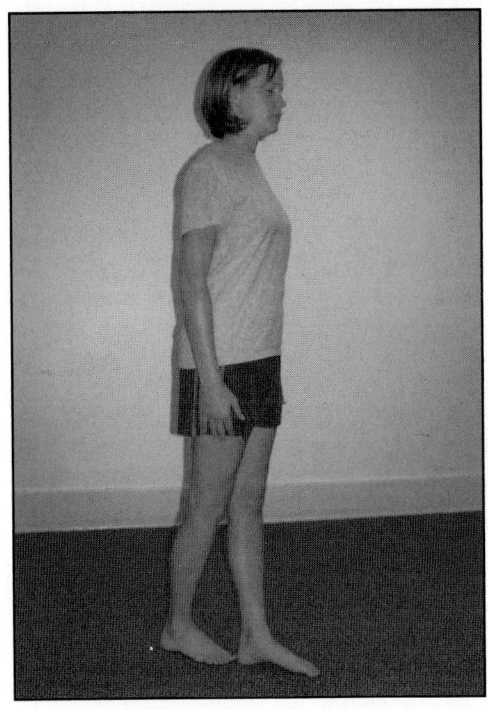

FIGURE 3-5

Finger-to-Nose Test

Test Position

Patient is sitting or standing with his or her eyes open and arms abducted to 90 degrees.

Action

Patient is asked to touch his or her nose with one index finger and return to the starting position. This test is then repeated on the opposite side. Once the test is performed with the eyes open, the test is once again repeated with the eyes closed (Figures 3-6 and 3-7).

Positive Finding

A positive test is the inability of the patient to smoothly and consistently touch the end of his or her nose with his or her index finger. This test indicates cerebellar dysfunction.

Special Considerations

The difficulty of this test can be increased by increasing the speed in which the patient touches his or her nose.

Specificity

No data available.

Sensitivity

No data available.

References

Magee DJ. *Orthopedic Physical Assessment.* 4th ed. Philadelphia, PA: W.B. Saunders; 2002.

Starkey C, Ryan JL. *Evaluation of Orthopedic and Athletic Injuries.* 2nd ed. Philadelphia, PA: F.A. Davis; 2002.

Swaine BR, Desrosiers J, Bourbonnais D, Larochelle JL. Norms for 15 to 34 year-olds for different versions of the finger-to-nose test. *Archives of Physical Medicine and Rehabilitation.* 2005;86(8):1665-1669.

Swaine BR, Lortie E, Gravel, D. The reliability of the time to execute various forms of the finger-to-nose test in healthy subjects. *Physiotherapy Theory and Practice.* 2005;21(4):271-279.

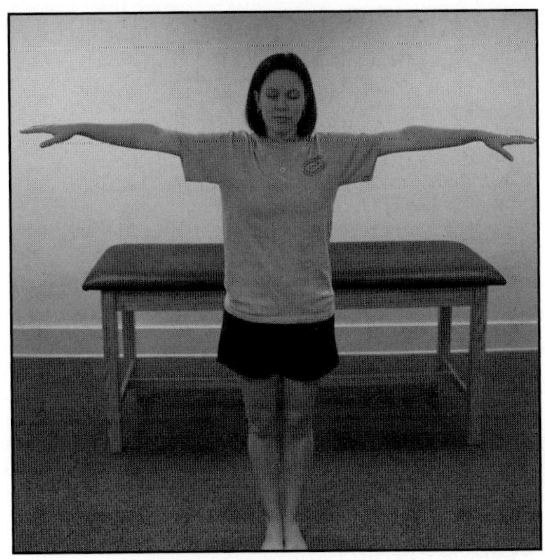

FIGURE 3-6

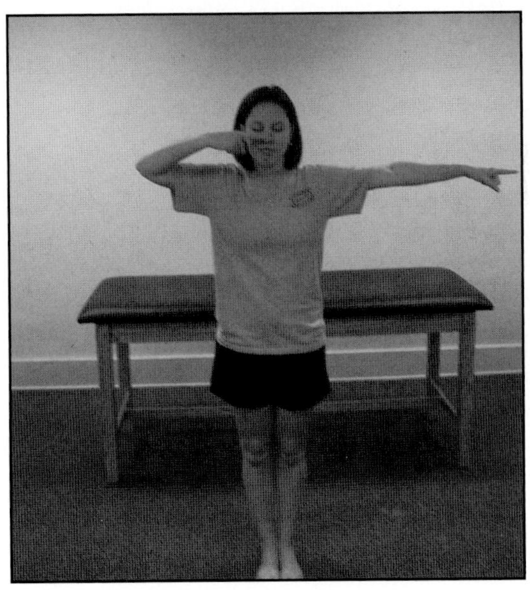

FIGURE 3-7

Proprioceptive Finger-to-Nose Test

Test Position

Patient is sitting or standing with his or her eyes closed and arms abducted to 90 degrees (Figure 3-8).

Action

The clinician touches one of the fingers on the patient's hand. The patient is asked to touch his or her nose with the finger that was identified, and then return to the starting position. This test is then repeated on both sides with multiple fingers (Figure 3-9).

Positive Finding

A positive test is the inability of the patient to smoothly and consistently touch the end of his or her nose with the identified finger. A positive test indicates a loss of proprioceptive sense.

Special Considerations

The difficulty of this test can be increased by increasing the speed at which the test is administered.

Specificity

No data available.

Sensitivity

No data available.

References

Magee DJ. *Orthopedic Physical Assessment.* 4th ed. Philadelphia, PA: W.B. Saunders; 2002.

Starkey C, Ryan JL. *Evaluation of Orthopedic and Athletic Injuries.* 2nd ed. Philadelphia, PA: F.A. Davis; 2002.

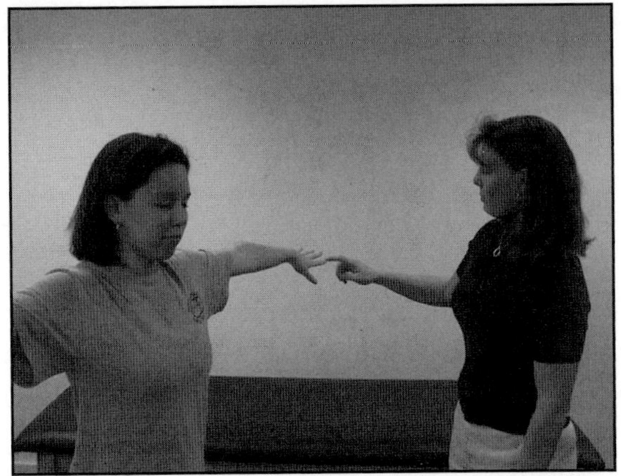

FIGURE 3-8

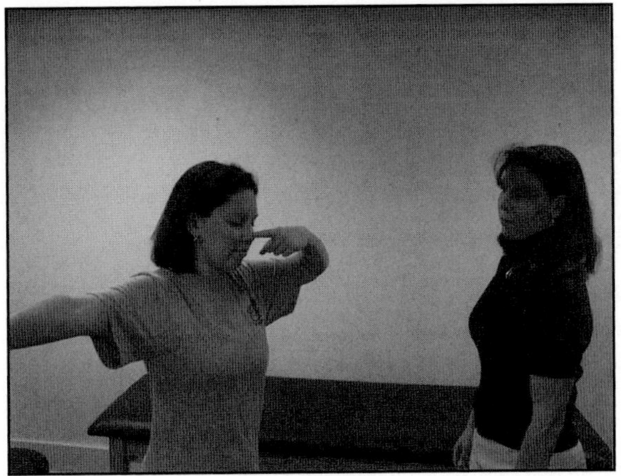

FIGURE 3-9

SERIAL SEVEN TEST

TEST POSITION

The patient is seated or standing.

ACTION

The clinician asks the patient to subtract 7 from 100. The patient is then continually asked to subtract 7 from the result.

POSITIVE FINDING

A positive test is the inability of the patient to be able to accurately answer the questions asked. This test assesses concentration and memory.

SPECIAL CONSIDERATIONS

This test can also be performed by using 3 in place of 7. It has been questioned that the mathematical calculation skills affect the results of this test more highly than the ability of the patient to concentrate. Therefore, if a clinician chooses to use this test, he or she may need to evaluate the process by which the patient determines the answer. It is also a concern that patients may memorize the calculations prior to administration of the exam. This is especially noted in patients who have been repeatedly evaluated.

SPECIFICITY

No data available.

SENSITIVITY

No data available.

REFERENCES

Karzmark P. Validity of the serial seven procedure. *International Journal of Geriatric Psychiatry*. 2000;15(8):677-679.

Magee DJ. *Orthopedic Physical Assessment*. 4th ed. Philadelphia, PA: W.B. Saunders; 2002.

Starkey C, Ryan JL. *Evaluation of Orthopedic and Athletic Injuries*. 2nd ed. Philadelphia, PA: F.A. Davis; 2002.

PAST-POINTING TEST

TEST POSITION

Patient is seated or standing and facing the clinician. The clinician holds both index fingers up in the air, approximately 6 inches apart. The patient holds both arms overhead, with his or her index fingers extended (Figure 3-10).

ACTION

The patient is then asked to bring both index fingers straight down to touch the fingers of the clinician (Figure 3-11). The patient then brings both arms back overhead to the original starting position.

POSITIVE FINDING

A positive test is an inability of the patient to touch the index fingers of the clinician. This test indicates an altered proprioceptive ability and vestibular disease.

SPECIAL CONSIDERATIONS

This test can be repeated with the patient's eyes open while the examiner moves his or her hands to a variety of positions for each individual motion. It is important that the patient return to the starting position after each examiner contact.

SPECIFICITY

No data available.

SENSITIVITY

No data available.

REFERENCES

Magee DJ. *Orthopedic Physical Assessment.* 4th ed. Philadelphia, PA: W.B. Saunders; 2002.

Starkey C, Ryan JL. *Evaluation of Orthopedic and Athletic Injuries.* 2nd ed. Philadelphia, PA: F.A. Davis; 2002.

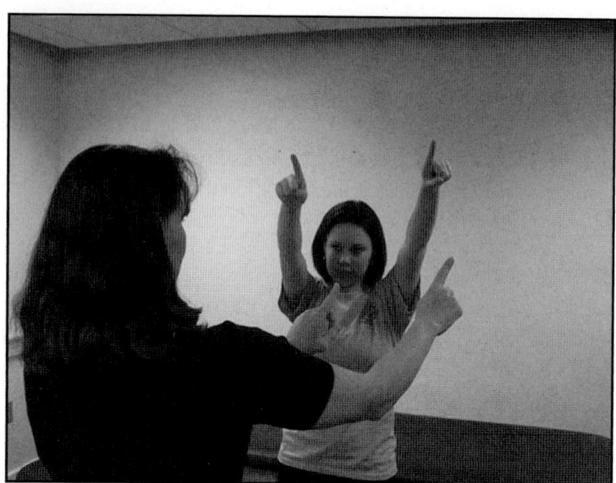

FIGURE 3-10

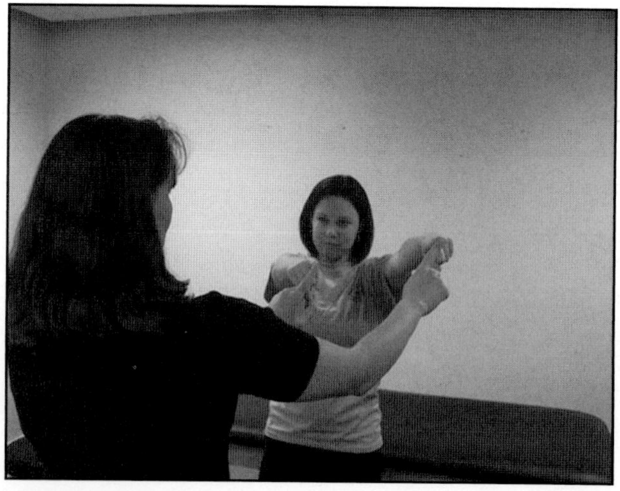

FIGURE 3-11

NEUROLOGICAL CONTROL TEST — UPPER EXTREMITY

TEST POSITION

This test is performed with the patient seated or standing with his or her eyes closed and arms flexed to 90 degrees (Figure 3-12).

ACTION

The patient is asked to hold this position for 30 seconds.

POSITIVE FINDING

A positive test is a drifting of one extremity in an outward and downward direction (Figure 3-13). A positive test is indicative of an expanding intracranial lesion on the side opposite the extremity that has drifted.

SPECIAL CONSIDERATIONS

Patients with an inability to perform this test due to musculoskeletal problems may be able to perform the Neurological Control Test —Lower Extremity.

SPECIFICITY

No data available.

SENSITIVITY

No data available.

REFERENCES

Magee DJ. *Orthopedic Physical Assessment.* 4th ed. Philadelphia, PA: W.B. Saunders; 2002.

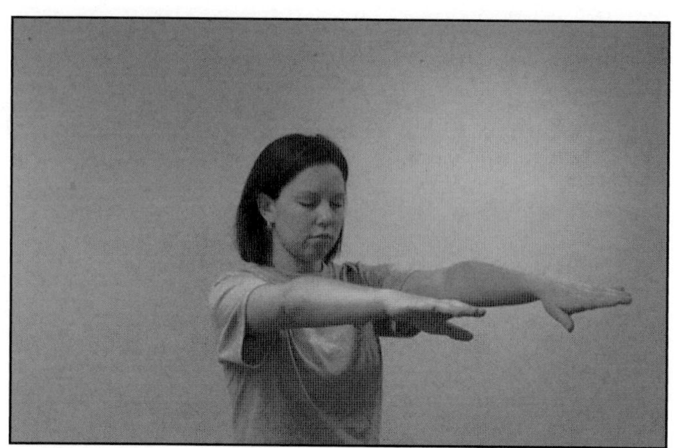

FIGURE 3-12

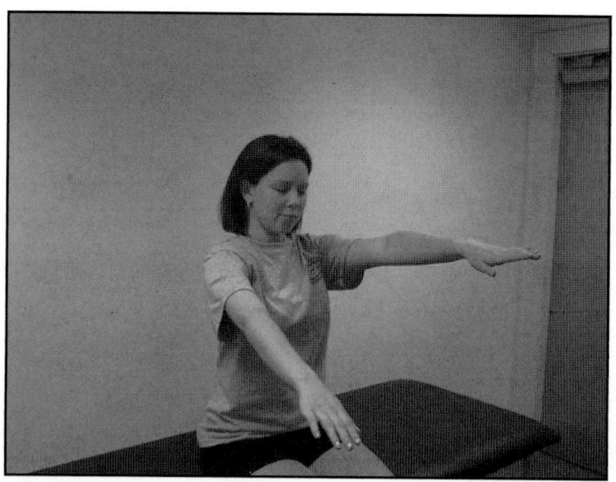

FIGURE 3-13

Neurological Control Test – Lower Extremity

Test Position

This test is performed with the patient seated on the edge of a table with his or her eyes closed and hips flexed to 90 degrees with his or her knees fully extended (Figure 3-14).

Action

The patient is asked to hold this position for 30 seconds.

Positive Finding

A positive test is a drifting of one extremity in an outward and downward direction (Figure 3-15). A positive test is indicative of an expanding intracranial lesion on the side opposite the extremity that has drifted.

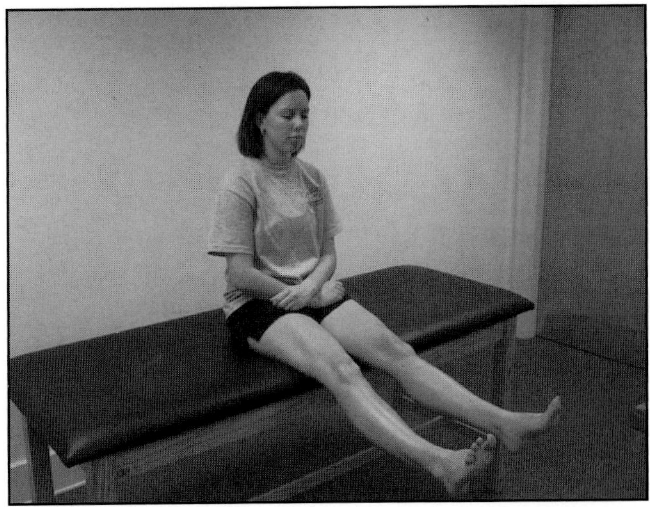

Figure 3-14

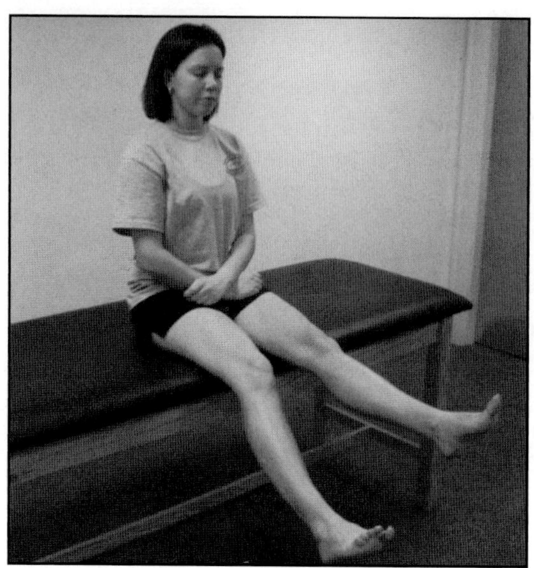

FIGURE 3-15

Balance Error Scoring System (BESS) Test

Test Position

The patient is standing barefoot, with no external support on the foot or ankle. The patient's hands are placed on his or her iliac crests while his or her eyes are closed (Figure 3-16). The clinician stands in front of the patient. A second clinician spots the patient.

Action

This test is performed in stages. Each stage lasts for 20 seconds. The patient progresses through the test as follows:

- Double leg stance with feet together (see Figure 3-16).
- Single leg stance on the non-dominant extremity. The patient's non-weight-bearing hip is flexed to 20 to 30 degrees, and the knee is flexed between 40 and 50 degrees (Figure 3-17).
- Tandem leg stance with the non-dominant leg placed behind the dominant leg while standing heel-to-toe (Figure 3-18).

Once the patient has progressed through each stage, the test is repeated on a foam pad (Figures 3-19 through 3-21). The patient must be able to stand in the testing position in order for the trial to count.

Positive Finding

The patient is scored based upon the number of "errors" that occur during each stance. During this evaluation, one point is awarded for each of the following:

- Lifting the hands off of the iliac crests.
- Opening the eyes.
- Stepping, stumbling, or falling from the test position.
- Moving the weight-bearing hip into more than 30 degrees of flexion or abduction
- Lifting the weight-bearing foot or heel.
- Remaining out of the test position for more than 5 seconds.

While evaluating a patient, a score of 10 is assigned in the event that he or she is unable to hold the testing position for more than 5 seconds. Additionally, in the event that more than one error occurs at a time, only one error is recorded.

A positive test is a score that is 25% above the patient's baseline score and indicates cerebral dysfunction.

Special Considerations

It is important that clinicians obtain baseline scores to evaluate a patient in the event of a head trauma. It is also important to understand that the evaluation of this patient is completely subjective. It is recommended that more than one clinician count the errors that occur during any one patient's evaluation. The BESS test has been shown to demonstrate a significant learning effect with serial testing. Therefore, the clinician should expect repeat testing scores to be improved (fewer total balance errors) with repeated BESS testing. This effect has been demonstrated immediately upon retesting and when retesting is administered up to 60 days after initial test administration.

Alternate Names

This test is commonly referred to as the *BESS Test*.

Specificity

No data available.

Sensitivity

No data available.

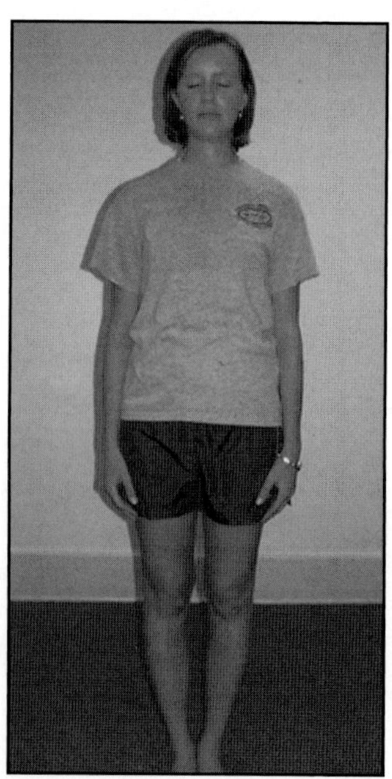

Figure 3-16

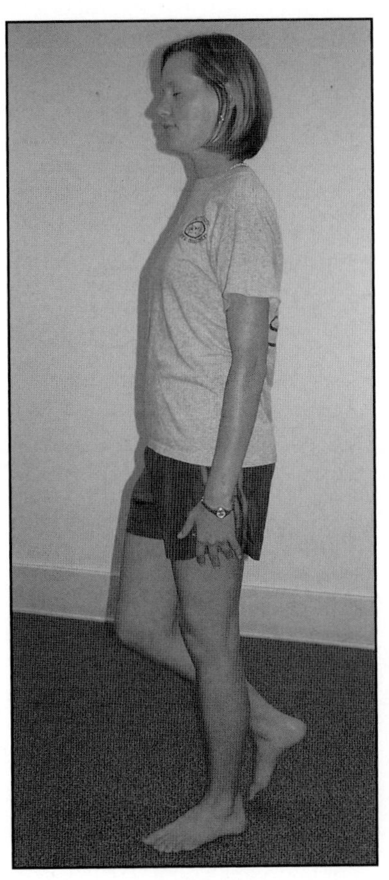

Figure 3-17

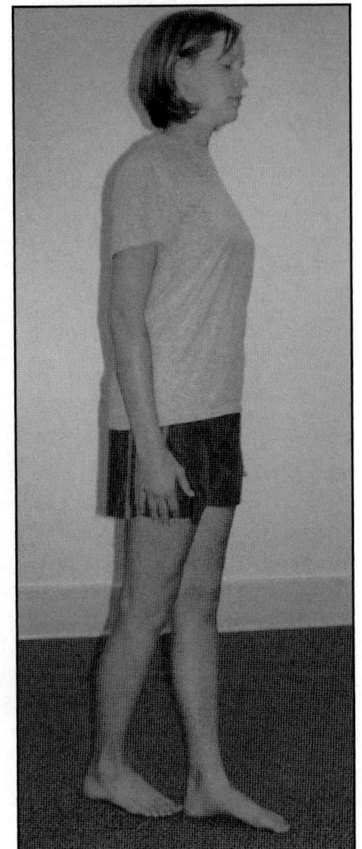

Figure 3-18

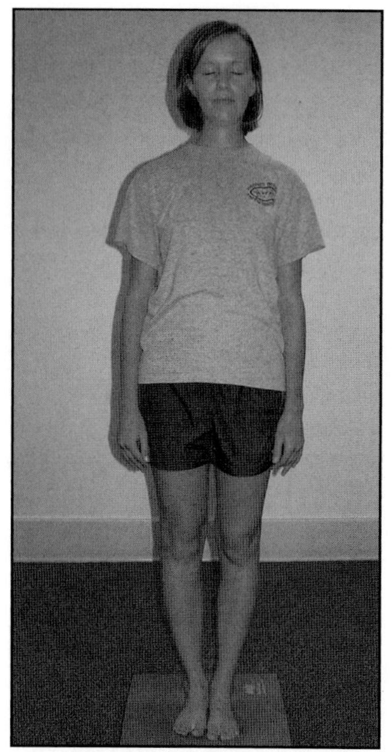

FIGURE 3-19

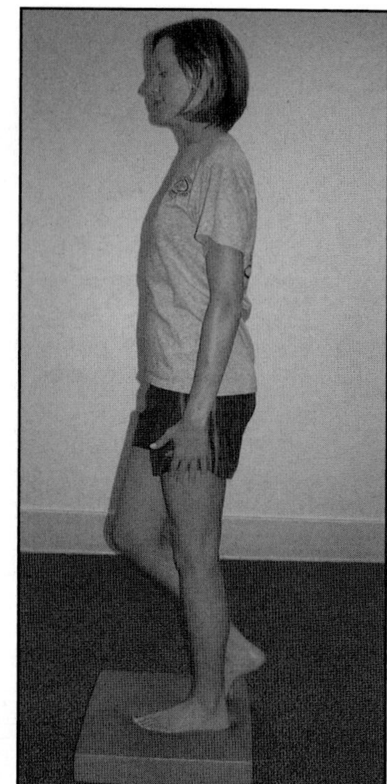

FIGURE 3-20

REFERENCES

Docherty CL, Valovich-McLeod TC, Schultz SJ. Postural control deficits in participants with functional ankle instability as measured by the balance error scoring system. *Clinical Journal of Sport Medicine*. 2006;16(3):203-208.

Guskiewicz KM. Concussion in sport: The grading-system dilemma. *Athletic Therapy Today*. 2001;6(1):18-27.

Guskiewicz K, Perrin D, Gansneder B. Effect of mild head injury on postural sway. *J Athl Train*. 1996;31(4):300-306.

Guskiewicz KM, Ross SE, Marshall SW. Postural stability and neuropsychological deficits after concussion in collegiate athletes. *J Athl Train*. 2001;36(3):263–273.

McLeod TCV, Perrin DH, Guskiewicz KM, Schultz SJ, Diamond R, Gansneder BM. Serial administration of clinical concussion assessments and learning effects in healthy young athletes. *Clinical Journal of Sports Medicine*. 2004;14(5):287-295.

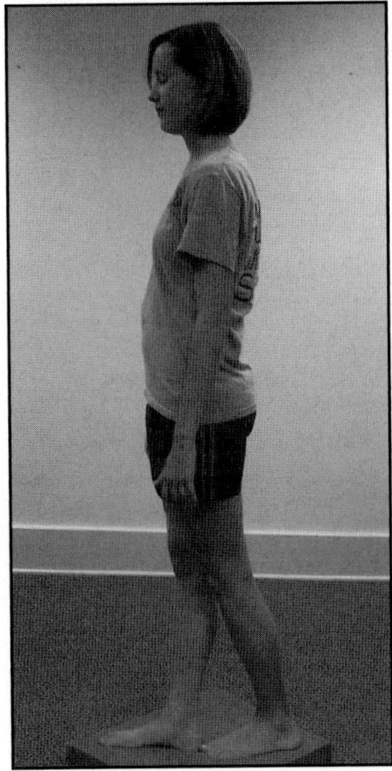

FIGURE 3-21

Oliaro S, Anderson S, Hooker D. Management of cerebral concussion in sports: The athletic trainer's perspective. *J Athl Train*. 2001;36(3):257-262.

Riemann BL, Guskiewicz KM. Effects of mild head injury on postural stability as measured through clinical balance testing. *J Athl Train*. 2000;35(1):19-25.

Starkey C, Ryan JL. *Evaluation of Orthopedic and Athletic Injuries*. 2nd ed. Philadelphia, PA: F.A. Davis; 2002.

Valovich TC, Perrin DH, Gansneder BM. Repeat administration elicits a practice effect with the Balance Error Scoring System but not with the Standardized Assessment of Concussion in high school athletes. *J Athl Train*. 2003;38(1):51-56.

Valovich-McLeod TC, Barr WB, McCrea M, Guskiewicz KM. Psychometric and measurement properties of concussion assessment tools in youth sports. *J Athl Train*. 2006;41(4):399-408.

Valovich-McLeod, TC, Perrin DH, Guskiewicz KM, Schultz SJ, Diamond R, Gansneder BM. Serial administration of clinical concussion assessments and learning effects in healthy young athletes. *Clinical Journal of Sport Medicine*. 2004;14(5):287-295.

Chapter

4

Neuropsychological Tests

HEAD

Computerized Assessments

ImPACT

Immediate Post Concussion Assessment and Cognitive Testing or ImPACT™ is a computer-based system that offers the clinician an individualized concussion management system. ImPACT has been specifically designed for the assessment and management of sports-related concussions. The system is used to perform neurocognitive testing of patients prior to concussion in order to gather objective baseline data. This initial data can then be used to determine the degree of recovery and appropriate return to play guidelines for patients post-concussion.

The system is Windows-based and requires minimal training to initiate. Because it is computer-based testing, ImPACT allows for both individualized and group administration.

ImPACT testing includes a measure of the patient's symptoms, attention, memory, processing speed, and reaction time, to .01 of a second. Testing involves 10 separate modules that allow for assessment of patient fatigue. The program measures multiple aspects of cognitive functioning in patients, including word discrimination, design and working memory, visual attention span, symbol matching and color matching, sustained and selective attention time, non-verbal problem solving, and reaction time. "Practice effects" are minimized by the large variety of test batteries available in the program. This feature is a significant improvement over pencil-and-paper neuropsychological testing.

Testing requires approximately 20 to 30 minutes to complete. The program produces a comprehensive report that includes a detailed past medical history, current patient symptoms, and information regarding the current mechanism of injury. Results can be e-mailed or faxed for consultation. Data is automatically stored for reference and comparisons during repeat testing.

References

Almquist J, Broshek D, Erlanger D. Assessment of mild head injuries. *Athletic Therapy Today*. 2001;6(1):13-17.

Erlanger DM, Saliba E, Barth J, Almquist J, Weberight W, Freeman J. Monitoring resolution of post-concussion symptoms in athletes: preliminary results of a web-based neuropsychological test protocol. *J Athl Train*. 2001;36(3):280-287.

Guskiewicz KM, Bruce SL, Cantu RC, et al. National Athletic Trainers' Association position statement: Management of sport-related concussion. *J*

Athl Train. 2004;39(3):280-297.

Schatz P, Pardini JE, Lovell MR, Collins MW, Podell K. Sensitivity and specificity of the ImPACT test battery for concussion in athletes. *Arch Clin Neuropsychol*. 2006;21(1):91-9.

HeadMinder

HeadMinder™ has developed the Concussion Management System and Concussion Resolution Index (CRI) as a key component in the assessment of sports-related concussions. The system is used to perform neurocognitive testing of patients prior to concussion in order to gather objective baseline data. This initial data can then be used to determine the degree of recovery and appropriate return to play guidelines for patients post-concussion.

HeadMinder's Concussion Management System measures simple and complex reaction time, memory, and processing speed. Test results include patient medical history, detailed mechanism of injury, and details regarding patient symptomology. Follow-up test results give the clinician a comparison to previous tests to assess for symptom resolution. Practice effects are minimized through the use of normative statistics gathered from over 600 subjects.

Testing requires 25 to 30 minutes to complete. The system is Internet based, allowing for testing to occur on any computer with an Internet connection. Unique features of HeadMinder include the ability to complete sideline testing using Standardized Assessment of Concussion (SAC) testing on a PDA. Sideline testing can later be synchronized with a desktop and the data entered into the patient's record.

References

Almquist J, Broshek D, Erlanger D. Assessment of mild head injuries. *Athletic Therapy Today*. 2001;6(1):13-17.

Erlanger DM, Saliba E, Barth J, Almquist J, Weberight W, Freeman J. Monitoring resolution of post-concussion symptoms in athletes: preliminary results of a web-based neuropsychological test protocol. *J Athl Train*. 2001;36(3):280-287.

CogSport

CogState features computerized cognitive testing to measure reaction time, attention, visual memory, visual learning, social cognition, verbal memory, verbal learning, planning and problem solving. Their sports concussion testing and management system is called CogState Sport. The system is used to perform neurocognitive testing of patients prior to concussion in order to gather objective baseline data. This initial data can then be used to determine the degree of recovery and appropriate return to play guidelines for patients post-concussion.

Testing requires 15 minutes to complete and report forms include baseline and post-injury data. The company features separate testing systems for professional/elite athletes and amateur athletes.

References

Guskiewicz KM, Bruce SL, Cantu RC, et al. National Athletic Trainers' Association position statement: management of sport-related concussion. *J Athl Train*. 2004;39(3):280-297.

Moriarity J, Collie A, Olson D, et al. A prospective controlled study of cognitive function during an amateur boxing tournament. *Neurology*. 2004;62(9):1462-1463.

Pencil-and-Paper Tests

Standard Assessment of Concussion (SAC) Test

The Standardized Assessment of Concussion (SAC) Test was developed as a method for performing objective, reliable on-field assessment of concussions. The system is used to perform a quick neurocognitive testing of patients prior to concussion in order to gather objective baseline data. This initial data can then be used to determine the degree of recovery and appropriate return to play guidelines for patients post-concussion.

The test involves four neurocognitive tests that assess orientation, immediate memory, concentration, and delayed recall. In the orientation section, patients are asked to identify month, date, day of the week, year, and approximate time. For immediate memory testing, the patient is given five words and is asked to repeat them back to the clinician. The concentration area includes a section using reverse digits and a section for months of the year in reverse order. Finally, the patient is asked to recall the same five words from the immediate recall section at the conclusion of testing.

Each of the four test areas is scored based on the number of correct responses provided by the patient. The total score is calculated, with a maximum score of 30 points possible. After testing, the clinician can compare the patient's baseline test score to his post-injury score as a measure of readiness for return to play.

The examination procedure also includes an area for neurologic screening (retrograde amnesia assessment, strength assessment, sensation assessment and coordination assessment) as well as exertional testing (40 yard sprint, sit-ups, push-ups, and knee bends).

The test can be administered in less than 5 minutes. The test can be easily administered as a pencil-and-paper test for baseline and post-injury testing in athletes. The test is easy to administer and can be completed in isolation or as part of a test battery.

The SAC test features three different versions to minimize the "practice effect." Each of these three versions has been shown to be reliable and valid as a concussion assessment tool. Research demonstrates that repeated SAC testing does not demonstrate a practice effect.

References

Daniel JC, Nassiri JD, Wilckens J, Land BC. The implementation and use of the Standardized Assessment of Concussion at the U.S. Naval Academy. *Military Medicine*. 2002;167(10):873-876.

McCrea M. Standardized mental status testing on the sideline after sport-related concussion. *J Athl Train*. 2001;36(3):274-279.

McCrea M, Kelly JP, Kluge J, Ackley B, Randolph C. Standardized assessment of concussion in football players. *Neurology*. 1997;48:586–588.

McCrea M, Kelly JP, Randolph C, et al. Standardized Assessment of Concussion (SAC): onsite mental status evaluation of the athlete. *Journal of Head Trauma Rehabilitation*. 1998;13(2):27–35.

McLeod TCV, Perrin DH, Guskiewicz KM, Schultz SJ, Diamond R, Gansneder BM. Serial administration of clinical concussion assessments and learning effects in healthy young athletes. *Clinical Journal of Sports Medicine*. 2004;14(5):287-295.

Oliaro S, Anderson S, Hooker D. Management of cerebral concussion in sports: the athletic trainer's perspective. *J Athl Train*. 2001;36(3):257–262.

Starkey C, Ryan JL. *Evaluation of Orthopedic and Athletic Injuries*. 2nd ed. Philadelphia, PA: F.A. Davis; 2002.

Valovich TC, Perrin DH, Gansneder BM. Repeat administration elicits a practice effect with the Balance Error Scoring System but not with the Standardized Assessment of Concussion in high school athletes. *J Athl Train*. 2003;38(1):51-56.

Valovich-McLeod TC, Barr WB, McCrea M, Guskiewicz KM. Psychometric and measurement properties of concussion assessment tools in youth sports. *J Athl Train*. 2006;41(4): 399-408.

Trail Making Test

The Trail Making Test is an easily-administered two-part neurocognitive test that requires the patient to complete two timed tests. The test is designed to assess visual conceptual function and visuomotor tracking speed and attention. The first test, known as Trail Making Test Part A, requires the patient to draw a line connecting numbers from 1 to 25 in order (Figure 4-1). The second test, known as Trail Making Test Part B, requires the patient to draw a line connecting numbers and letters in an alternating pattern. The patient is instructed to draw a line from the number one to the letter A, from the letter A to the number 2, from the number 2 to the letter B, and so on (Figure 4-2). The test includes 13 numbers and 12 letters.

Each test is timed for speed and scored for accuracy, recording the number of errors. The tests are designed to be used together; however, Part B is often performed in isolation due to its increased complexity. The test can be easily administered as a pencil-and-paper test for baseline and post-injury testing in athletes. The test is easy to administer and can be completed in isolation or as part of a test battery.

REFERENCES

Barr WB. Methodologic issues in neuropsychological testing. *J Athl Train.* 2001;36(3):297-302.

Guskiewicz KM. Concussion in sport: The grading-system dilemma. *Athletic Therapy Today.* 2001;6(1):18-27.

Guskiewicz KM, Bruce SL, Cantu RC, et al. National Athletic Trainers' Association position statement: Management of sport-related concussion. *J Athl Train.* 2004;39(3):280-297.

McCaffrey RJ, Krahula MM, Heimberg RG, Keller KE, Purcell MJ. A comparison of the trail making test, symbol digit modalities test and the Hooper Visual Organization Test in an inpatient substance abuse population. *Arch Clin Neuropsychol.* 1988;3(2):181-187.

Valovich McLeod TC, Barr WB, McCrea M, Guskiewicz KM. Psychometric and measurement properties of concussion assessment tools in youth sports. *J Athl Train.* 2006;41(4):399-408.

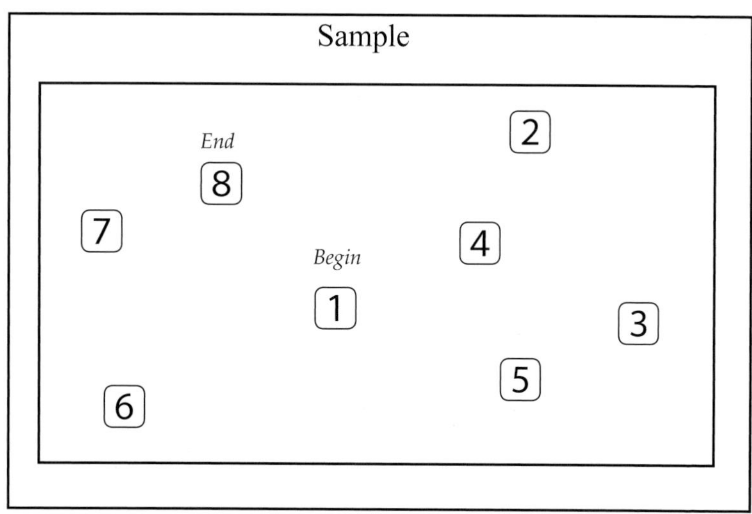

FIGURE 4-1. TRAIL MAKING TEST PART A.

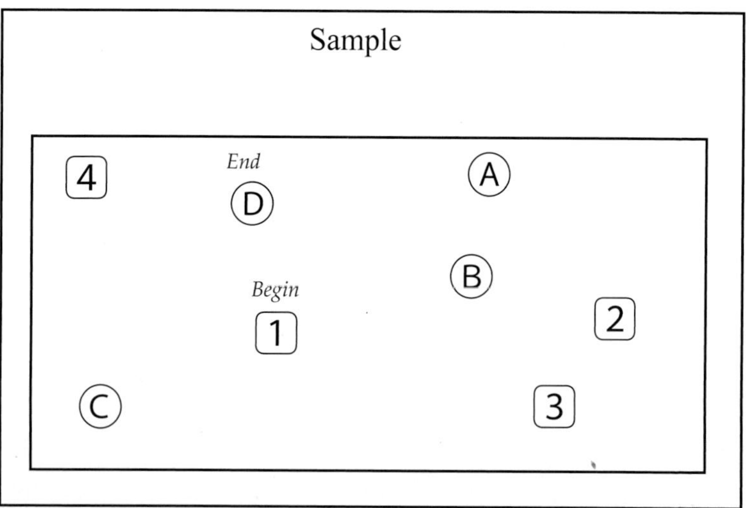

FIGURE 4-2. TRAIL MAKING TEST PART B.

Symbol Digit Modalities Test

The Symbol Digit Modality Test, developed by Dr. Aaron Smith, is designed to measure concentration, rapid decision making, and visual-motor speed. The test requires a simple substitution task using a reference key. The clinician provides the patient with a list of specific numbers and geometrical shapes. The patient has 90 seconds to match as many numbers to the geometric shapes as possible.

The test can be administered in less than 5 minutes. Scoring is based on the number of correct responses. The test can be easily administered as a pencil-and-paper test for baseline and post-injury testing in athletes. The test is easy to administer and can be completed in isolation or as part of a test battery.

Responses are typically provided in writing, but responses can also be given orally. The test is similar in format to the Wechsler Intelligence Scale. Normative data is available for a variety of ages.

References

Barr WB. Methodologic issues in neuropsychological testing. *J Athl Train*. 2001;36(3):297-302.

Guskiewicz KM, Bruce SL, Cantu RC, et al. National Athletic Trainers' Association position statement: Management of sport-related concussion. *J Athl Train*. 2004;39(3):280-297.

Guskiewicz KM. Concussion in sport: The grading-system dilemma. *Athletic Therapy Today*. 2001;6(1):18-27.

McCaffrey RJ, Krahula MM, Heimberg RG, Keller KE, Purcell MJ. A comparison of the trail making test, symbol digit modalities test and the Hooper Visual Organization Test in an inpatient substance abuse population. *Arch Clin Neuropsychol*. 1988;3(2):181-187.

Sheridan LK, Fitzgerald HE, Adams KM, et al. Normative symbol digit modalities test performance in a community-based sample. *Arch Clin Neuropsychol*. 2006;21(1):23-28.

Valovich McLeod TC, Barr WB, McCrea M, Guskiewicz KM. Psychometric and measurement properties of concussion assessment tools in youth sports. *J Athl Train*. 2006;41(4):399-408.

Stroop Color and Word Test

The Stroop Color and Word Test was developed almost 75 years ago to measure cognitive processing The test endures as one of the most commonly administered neuropsychological tests performed. Testing provides valuable diagnostic information regarding cognitive function and pathology.

The test is designed based on the observation that an individual can read words faster than he or she can identify and name colors. The timed test creates an environment that challenges the patient to cope with cognitive stress and process complex input. Testing yields three scores based on the number of items correctly completed in the assigned test time. Scores can be used to analyze a patient's cognitive flexibility, creativity, and reaction to cognitive pressures.

The test is easy to administer and can be completed in isolation or as part of a test battery. The test can be easily administered as a pencil-and-paper test for baseline and post-injury testing in athletes. Normative data is available for patients aged 15 to 90. There is also a great deal of literature regarding the validity and reliability of this examination procedure.

References

Barr WB. Methodologic issues in neuropsychological testing. *J Athl Train*. 2001;36(3):297-302.

Guskiewicz KM. Concussion in sport: The grading-system dilemma. *Athletic Therapy Today*. 2001;6(1):18-27.

Guskiewicz KM, Bruce SL, Cantu RC, et al. National Athletic Trainers' Association position statement: Management of sport-related concussion. *J Athl Train*. 2004;39(3):280-297.

Uttl B, Graf P. Color-Word Stroop test performance across the adult life span. *Journal of Clinical Exp Neuropsychology*. 1997;19(3):405-420.

Chapter

5

Special Tests for Central Nervous System Involvement

HOFFMANN'S SIGN

TEST POSITION

The patient is positioned in sitting with the forearm pronated and the wrist slightly flexed. The upper extremity on the test side should be supported by the clinician.

ACTION

The clinician forcibly "flicks" the patient's middle finger at the fingernail in the direction of flexion (Figure 5-1).

POSITIVE FINDING

A positive finding is a reflexive flexion of the distal phalanx (twitching) of the ipsilateral thumb in response to the middle finger being struck. A positive test is indicative of an upper motor neuron lesion.

SPECIAL CONSIDERATIONS

This test is often considered the upper extremity equivalent of Babinski's Test.

HISTORICAL NOTES

This test was described in the teachings of Johann Hoffmann and was used clinically prior to 1900. However, the test is first described in medical literature by Hans Curshmann in 1911.

ALTERNATE NAMES

This test is also commonly referred to as the *Digital Reflex*, *Finger Flexor Reflex* or *Hoffmann's Reflex*.

SPECIFICITY

.78

SENSITIVITY

.58

POSITIVE PREDICTIVE VALUE

.62

NEGATIVE PREDICTIVE VALUE

.75

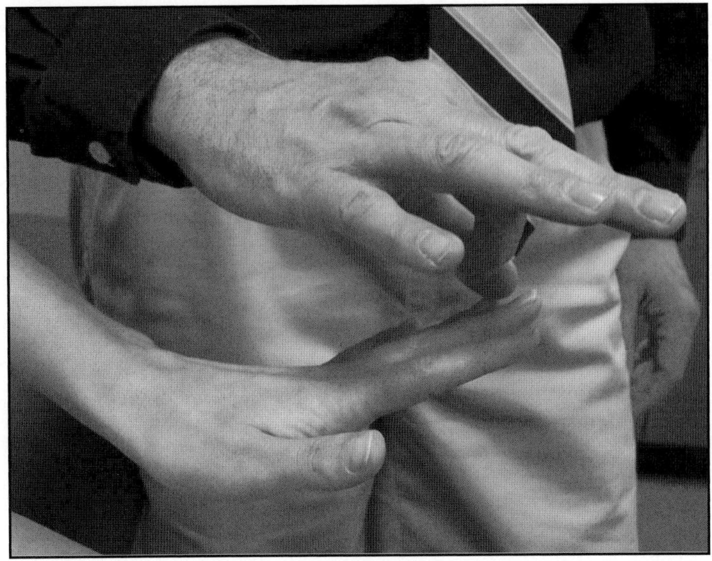

FIGURE 5-1

REFERENCES

Denno JJ, Meadows GR. Early diagnosis of cervical spondylotic myelopathy: a useful clinical sign. *Spine*. 1991;16:1353-1355.

Glaser JA, Cure JK, Bailey KL, Morrow DL. Cervical spinal cord compression and the Hoffmann sign. *Iowa Orthopedic Journal*. 2001;21:49-52.

Magee DJ. *Orthopedic Physical Assessment*. 4th ed. Philadelphia, PA: W.B. Saunders; 2002.

Malanga GA, Landes P, Nadler SF. Provocative tests in cervical spine examination: Historical basis and scientific analyses. *Pain Physician*. 2003;6(2):199-205.

Meadows JTS. *Orthopedic Differential Diagnosis in Physical Therapy*. New York: McGraw-Hill; 1999.

Babinski's Test

Test Position

The patient is positioned in sitting or long sitting.

Action

The clinician firmly strokes the plantar surface of the foot, beginning at the heel, moving to the lateral portion of the foot, and ending medially at the metatarsal pads using the end of a reflex hammer or another blunt object (Figures 5-2 through 5-4).

Positive Finding

A positive test is extension of the great toe and splaying of the other four toes, indicating an upper motor neuron lesion (Figure 5-5).

Special Considerations

A positive test is considered normal in children under age 2.

Historical Notes

This finding was first described in 1846 by Felix Alfred Vulpian and again by Ernst Julius Remak in 1849. However, it was Joseph Babinski's research in 1896 and 1903 that identified the clinical importance of the finding.

Alternate Names

This test is also known as *Babinski's Sign, Babinski's Reflex,* and the *Plantar Reflex.*

Specificity

No data available.

Sensitivity

No data available.

References

Dommisse GF, Grobler L. Arteries and veins of the lumbar nerve roots and cauda equina. *Clinical Orthopedics.* 1976;115:22-29.

Magee DJ. *Orthopedic Physical Assessment.* 4th ed. Philadelphia, PA: W.B. Saunders; 2002.

Miller TM, Johnston SC. Should the Babinski sign be part of the routine neurologic exam? *Neurology.* 2005;65:1165-1168.

Starkey C, Ryan JL. *Evaluation of Orthopedic and Athletic Injuries.* 2nd ed. Philadelphia, PA: F.A. Davis; 2002.

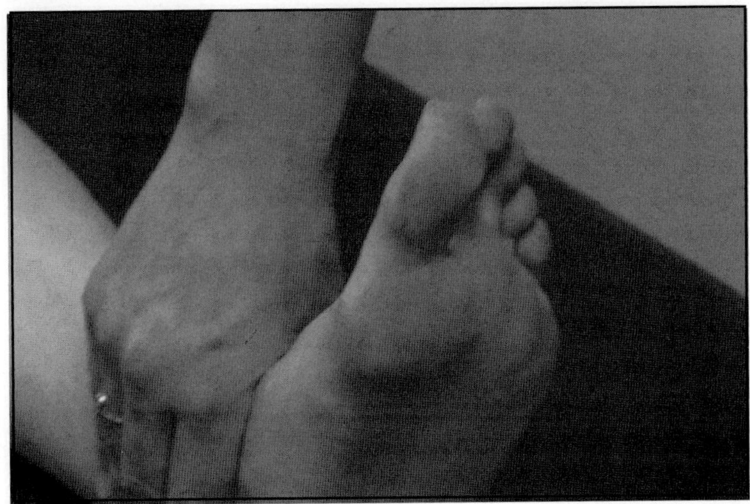

FIGURE 5-2

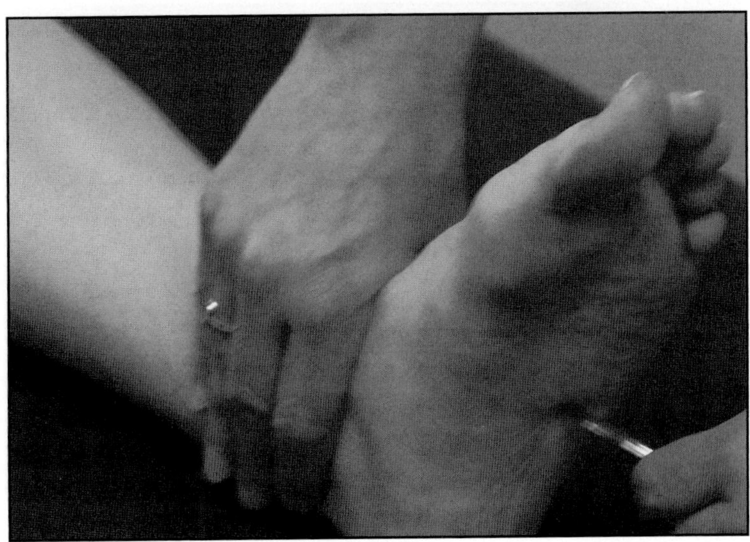

FIGURE 5-3

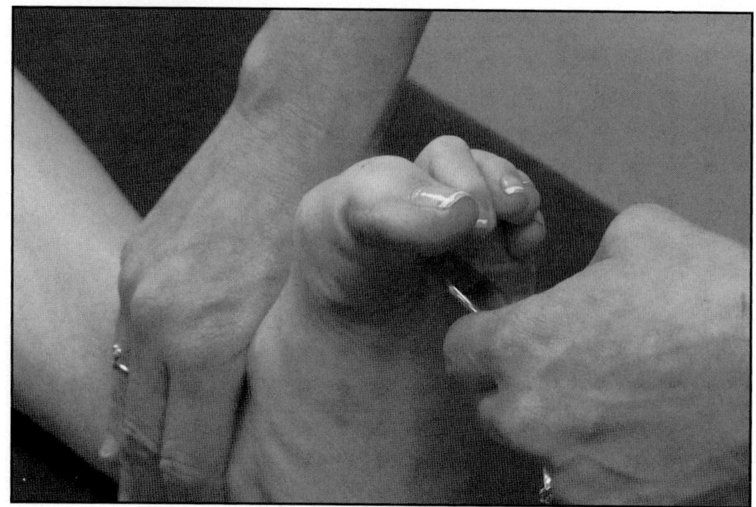

FIGURE 5-4

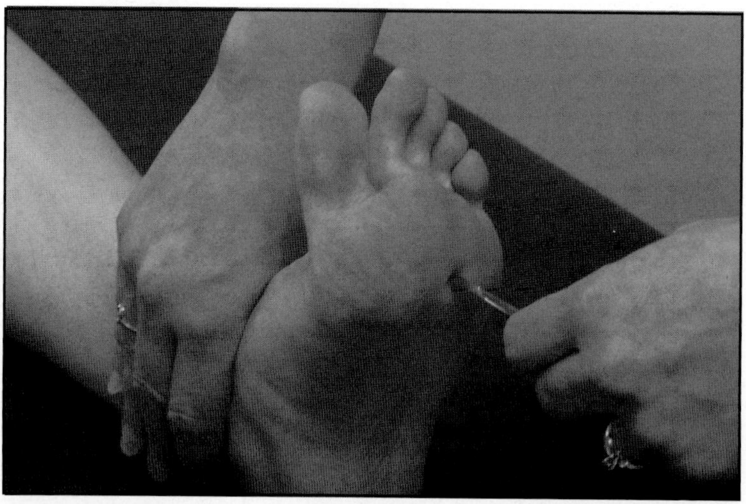

FIGURE 5-5

OPPENHEIM'S TEST

TEST POSITION

The patient is positioned in supine.

ACTION

The clinician firmly strokes inferiorly on the medial aspect of the tibia using the end of a reflex hammer or another blunt object (Figure 5-6).

POSITIVE FINDING

A positive finding is extension of the great toe, indicating upper motor neuron lesion (Figure 5-7).

SPECIAL CONSIDERATIONS

The findings of this test often correlate to the findings of Babinski's Test.

HISTORICAL NOTES

This test was initially described by Hermann Oppenheim in 1902.

ALTERNATE NAMES

This test is also known as *Oppenheim's Foot Reflex* and *Oppenheim's Sign*.

SPECIFICITY

No data available.

SENSITIVITY

No data available.

REFERENCES

Dommisse GF, Grobler L. Arteries and veins of the lumbar nerve roots and cauda equina. *Clinical Orthopedics*. 1976;115:22-29.

Magee DJ. *Orthopedic Physical Assessment*. 4th ed. Philadelphia, PA: W.B. Saunders; 2002.

Starkey C, Ryan JL. *Evaluation of Orthopedic and Athletic Injuries*. 2nd ed. Philadelphia, PA: F.A. Davis; 2002.

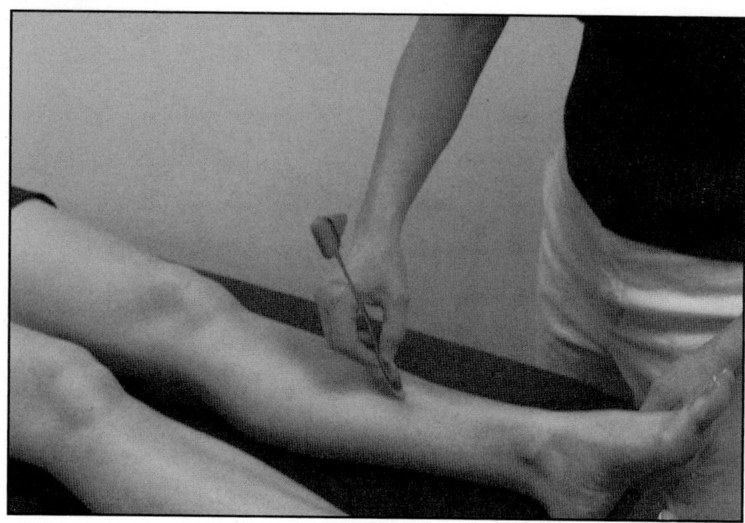

FIGURE 5-6

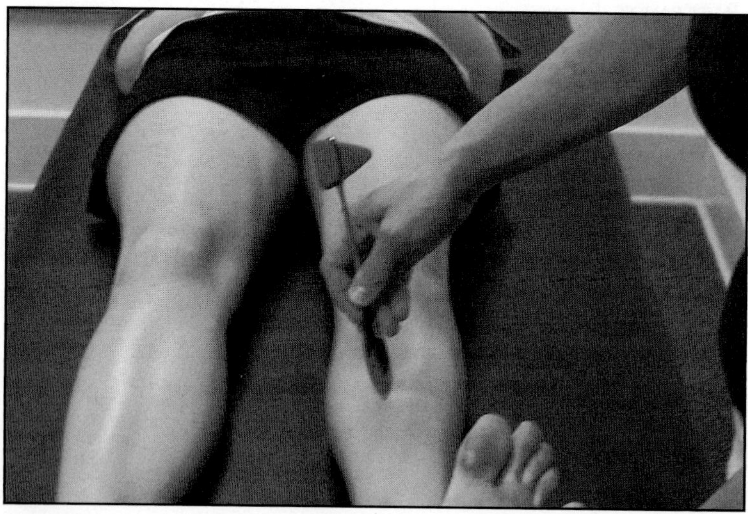

FIGURE 5-7

Chvostek's Sign

Test Position

The patient can be seated or standing.

Action

The clinician taps over the masseter muscle and the parotid gland at the angle of the jaw (Figure 5-8).

Positive Finding

A positive finding is twitching of the ipsilateral facial musculature (most notably the masseter muscle), indicating facial nerve pathology.

Special Considerations

A positive test may be the result of hypocalcemia or respiratory alkalosis (in the presence of hyperventilation).

Historical Notes

This test was first described in 1876 by Austrian physician Frantisek Chvostek.

Alternate Names

This test is also known as *Weiss' Sign*.

Specificity

No data available.

Sensitivity

No data available.

References

Konin JG, Wiksten DL, Isear JA, Brader H. *Special Tests for Orthopedic Examination*. 3rd ed. Thorofare, NJ: SLACK Incorporated; 2006.

Magee DJ. *Orthopedic Physical Assessment*. 4th ed. Philadelphia, PA: W.B. Saunders; 2002.

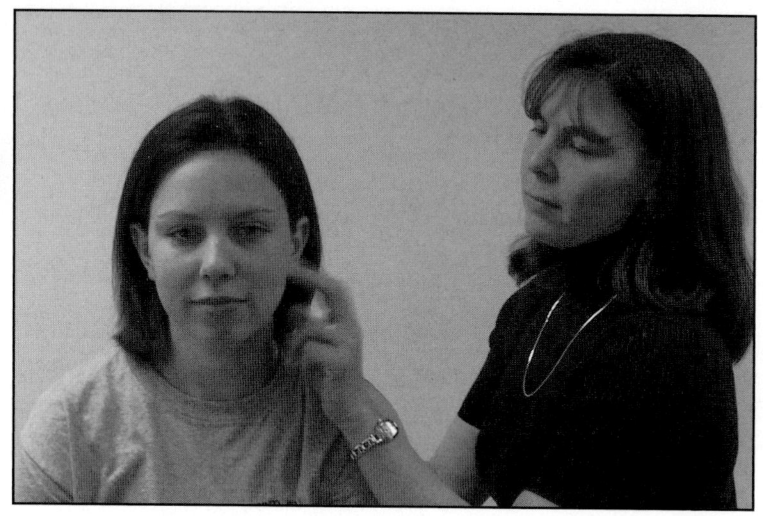

FIGURE 5-8

WEBER TEST

TEST POSITION

The patient is positioned in sitting.

ACTION

The clinician places the base of a vibrating tuning fork on the center of the patient's forehead (Figure 5-9). The patient is asked if he or she can hear the sound equally in both ears or if the sound is louder in one ear than the other, known as "lateralization of sound."

POSITIVE FINDING

In the presence of conductive hearing loss, a positive finding is the sound being louder on the side of conductive loss. In the presence of a sensorineural loss, the sound will be louder on the uninvolved side.

HISTORICAL NOTES

This test was initially described by Ernst Heinrich Weber.

SPECIAL CONSIDERATIONS

A 256 Hz tuning fork is the preferred tool used in performing this test. Research has also been completed using either a 128 or 512 Hz tuning fork.

ALTERNATE NAMES

This test is also known as the *Bing Test* when it is performed with one ear occluded by the clinician's finger. The Bing Test should reveal a louder sound in the occluded ear, indicating an occlusive hearing loss.

SPECIFICITY

No data available.

SENSITIVITY

No data available.

REFERENCES

Blakley BW, Siddique S. A qualitative explanation of the Weber test. *Otolaryngology*. 1999;120(1):1-4.

Golabek W, Stephens SD. Some tuning fork tests revisited. *Clin Otolaryngol Allied Sci*. 1979;4(6):421-430.

Huizing EH. The early descriptions of so-called tuning fork tests of Weber, Rinne, Schwabach and Bing. *Journal of Oto-Rhino-Laryngology and its Related Specialties*. 1975;37(2):88-91.

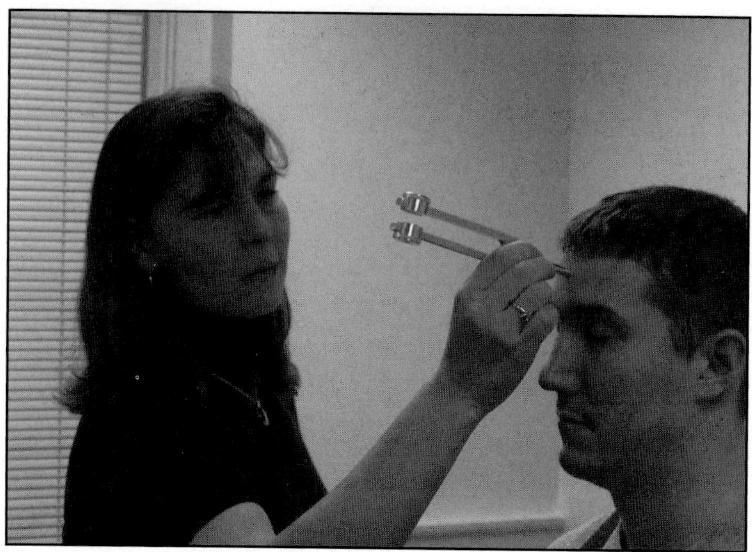

FIGURE 5-9

Magee DJ. *Orthopedic Physical Assessment*. 4th ed. Philadelphia, PA: W.B. Saunders; 2002.

Reese NB. *Muscle and Sensory Testing*. 2nd ed. Philadelphia, PA: W.B. Saunders; 2005.

Sichel JY, Eliashar R, Dano I. Explaining the Weber test. *Otolaryngology*. 2000;122(3):465-466.

Swan IR, Browning GG. The Bing test in the detection of conductive hearing impairment. *Clin Otolaryngol Allied Sci*. 1989;14(6):539-543.

RINNE TEST

TEST POSITION

The patient is positioned in sitting.

ACTION

The clinician places the base of a vibrating tuning fork on the patient's mastoid process (Figure 5-10). The patient is asked to tell the clinician when he or she can no longer hear the sound of the vibrating tuning fork. This time is recorded by the examiner. The clinician then rapidly relocates the still vibrating tuning fork 1 cm to 2 cm from the patient's auditory canal. The patient is asked to tell the clinician when he or she can no longer hear the sound of the vibrating tuning fork. This time is recorded by the examiner.

POSITIVE FINDING

A variation in time between bone conduction and air conduction is noted by the clinician. Air conduction sound should be heard twice as long as bone conduction sound. An air conduction time shorter than twice the bone conduction time indicates a sensorineural hearing loss, while air conduction time greater than twice bone conduction time indicates a conductive hearing loss.

HISTORICAL NOTES

This test was initially described by German otologist, Heinrich Adolf Rinne.

SPECIAL CONSIDERATIONS

The Rinne Test should always be accompanied by the Weber Test to confirm the cause of the hearing loss. A 256 Hz tuning fork is the preferred tool used in performing this test. Research has also been completed using either a 128 or 512 Hz tuning fork.

SPECIFICITY

No data available.

SENSITIVITY

No data available.

REFERENCES

Browning GG, Swan IR, Chew KK. Clinical role of informal tests of hearing. *Journal of Laryngology and Otology*. 1989;103(1):7-11.

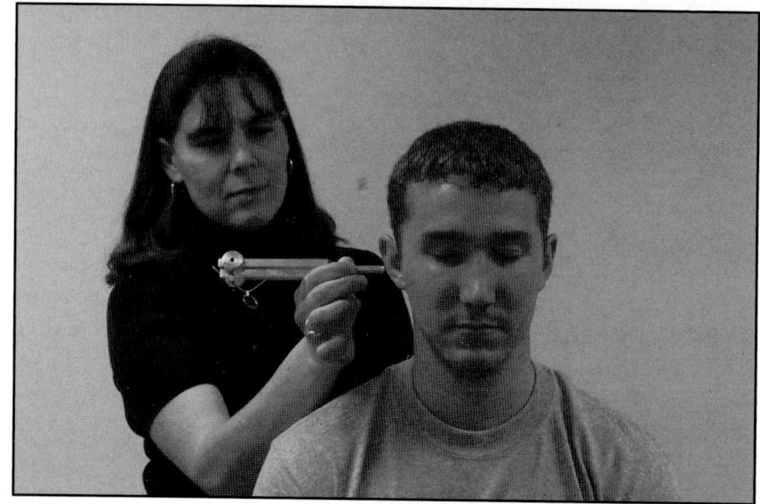

FIGURE 5-10

Golabek W, Stephens SD. Some tuning fork tests revisited. *Clin Otolaryngol Allied Sci*. 1979;4(6):421-430.

Huizing EH. The early descriptions of so-called tuning fork tests of Weber, Rinne, Schwabach and Bing. *Journal of Oto-Rhino-Laryngology and its Related Specialties*. 1975;37(2):88-91.

Johnston DF. A new modification of the Rinne Test. *Clin Otolaryngol Allied Sci*. 1992;17(4):322-326.

Magee DJ. *Orthopedic Physical Assessment*. 4th ed. Philadelphia, PA: W.B. Saunders; 2002.

Reese NB. *Muscle and Sensory Testing*. 2nd ed. Philadelphia, PA: W.B. Saunders; 2005.

Swan IR, Browning GG. The Bing test in the detection of conductive hearing impairment. *Clin Otolaryngol Allied Sci*. 1989;14(6):539-543.

CLONUS

CLINICAL FINDINGS

Clonus is a series of repetitive, rhythmic, involuntary muscle contractions that occur as a result of a sudden stretch of the involved muscles.

POSITIVE FINDING

A finding of clonus is indicative of a neurologic condition, most commonly associated with an upper motor neuron lesion. Clonus is commonly observed in patients suffering from stroke, spinal cord injury, or multiple sclerosis.

SPECIAL CONSIDERATIONS

Clonus can be differentiated from fasciculations—small, spontaneous twitching of muscles indicative of lower motor neuron lesions—by the size of the movements. Clonus causes large muscular response that is initiated by stretching.

REFERENCES

Magee DJ. *Orthopedic Physical Assessment.* 4th ed. Philadelphia, PA: W.B. Saunders; 2002.

Decerebrate Posturing

Clinical Findings

Decerebrate posturing is an abnormal body posture characterized by rigid extension of the upper and lower extremities. The posture also involves plantarflexion of the ankles and extension and retraction of the head and neck (Figure 5-11).

Positive Finding

Decerebrate posture is indicative of severe injury to the brain, typically at the brain stem.

Special Considerations

Decerebrate posture may occur unilaterally or bilaterally. This posture may also alternate with decorticate posture or the patient may demonstrate decerebrate posture on one side of the body and decorticate posture on the opposite side. Opisthotonos, severe muscle spasm of the spine musculature, may accompany decerebrate posture in severe cases.

Alternate Names

This finding is also referred to as *Decerebrate Response*.

References

Magee DJ. *Orthopedic Physical Assessment.* 4th ed. Philadelphia, PA: W.B. Saunders; 2002.

Starkey C, Ryan JL. *Evaluation of Orthopedic and Athletic Injuries*. 2nd ed. Philadelphia, PA: F.A. Davis; 2002.

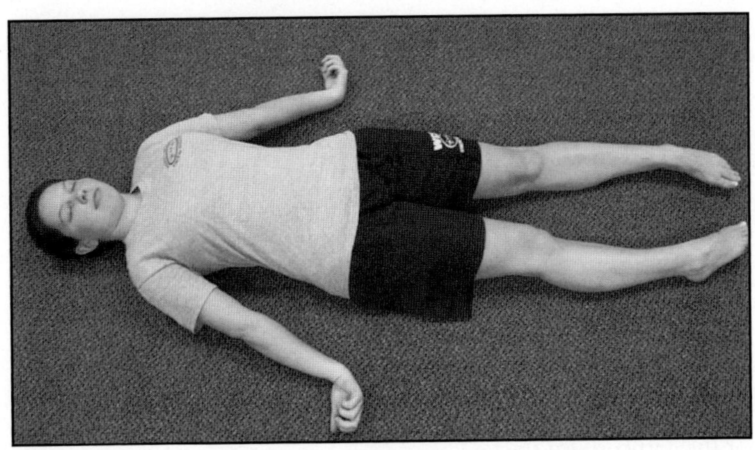

FIGURE 5-11

Decorticate Posturing

Test Position

Decortiate posturing is an abnormal body posture characterized by flexion of the upper extremity and extension of the lower extremity. In this posture, the elbows and wrists are flexed and the fists are clenched. The upper extremities are drawn in toward the midline of the trunk. The lower extremities are extended, with the ankles in a position of plantarflexion (Figure 5-12).

Positive Finding

Decorticate posture is indicative of severe injury to the brain above the level of the brain stem, typically involving the mesencephalic region or the corticospinal tract.

Special Considerations

Decorticate posturing, though serious, indicates a less severe brain injury than decerebrate posturing. Decorticate posture may occur unilaterally or bilaterally and may progress to or alternate with decerebrate posture.

Alternate Names

This finding is also referred to as *Decorticate Response*.

References

Magee DJ. *Orthopedic Physical Assessment.* 4th ed. Philadelphia, PA: W.B. Saunders; 2002.

Starkey C, Ryan JL. *Evaluation of Orthopedic and Athletic Injuries.* 2nd ed. Philadelphia, PA: F.A. Davis; 2002.

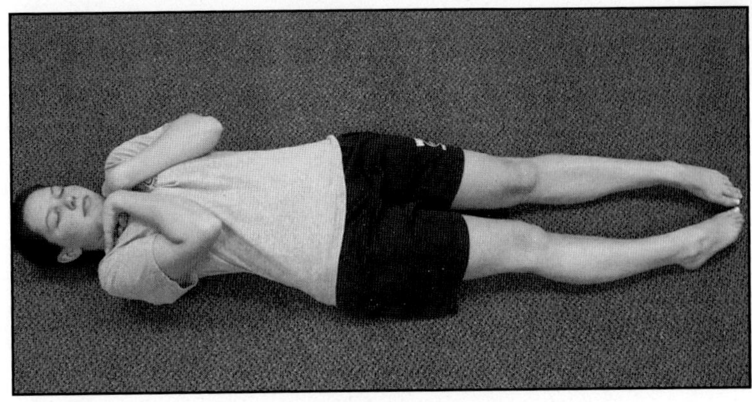

FIGURE 5-12

Section

Two

Cervical Spine

Chapter

6

Dermatome Testing

The following chart presents an overview of dermatome testing location for dermatomes C1 – T1 (Table 6-1). Dermatome testing is most commonly assessed by testing light touch sensation over the desired region. Testing is always performed bilaterally for comparative purposes. Additional tests that may be employed include sharp-dull sensation, two-point discrimination, and temperature sensation. Each of these test procedures will be described in greater detail in this chapter.

The most common positive test finding during dermatome testing is a loss or a decrease in sensation, indicating injury to a spinal nerve root or a peripheral nerve. However, increased sensitivity during sensory testing, known as hyperesthesia, can also be a positive finding. Hyperesthesia can present in several forms. Extreme sensitivity to pain is known as hyperpathia. Neuralgia is described as "shock-like" sensations throughout a dermatome or peripheral nerve distribution, while paresthesia (also known as dysesthesia) is described as burning, numbness, and tingling in a dermatome or peripheral nerve distribution in the absence of external stimulus application.

References

Hoppenfeld S. *Orthopaedic Neurology*. Baltimore, MD: Lippincott-Raven; 1997.

Hoppenfeld S. *Physical Examination of the Spine and Extremities*. East Norwalk, CT: Appleton-Century-Crofts; 1976.

Magee DJ. *Orthopedic Physical Assessment*. 4th ed. Philadelphia, PA: W.B. Saunders; 2002.

Meadows JTS. *Orthopedic Differential Diagnosis in Physical Therapy*. New York: McGraw-Hill; 1999.

Reese NB. *Muscle and Sensory Testing*. 2nd ed. Philadelphia, PA: W.B. Saunders; 2005.

Table 6-1

CERVICAL DERMATOMES

Nerve Root	*Dermatome*
C1	Superior portion of the head
C2	Occipital region of the head
C3	Lateral aspect of the neck
C4	Upper trapezius and superior aspect of the shoulders
C5	Lateral aspect of upper arm
C6	Lateral aspect of forearm, thenar eminence, thumb, and index finger
C7	Middle finger and middle of hand
C8	Ring finger, little finger, hypothenar eminence, medial aspect of forearm
T1	Medial aspect of upper arm to the axilla

Sensory Testing: Light Touch

Test Position

The patient may be positioned in supine or sitting.

Materials Required

Light touch sensation is assessed using a cotton wisp or a cotton-tip applicator, Buck Reflex Hammer.

Action

The clinician should explain the procedure to the patient prior to testing, being sure the patient understands what is expected of him or her during the testing. The patient is instructed to close his eyes prior to initiating the test. The clinician will randomly alternate touching or not touching the patient (in the desired dermatome or region) (Figure 6-1) with the cotton wisp. Each time the patient is asked to respond with a "yes" (meaning he or she is being touched) or a "no" (meaning he or she is not being touched) response when instructed by the clinician. Testing 10 sites within the test area will allow the clinician to quantify the degree of sensation that is intact (eg, 7/10 or 70%) for a given dermatome or region. The test should be performed bilaterally for comparison to determine if deficits exist unilaterally or bilaterally (Figures 6-2 and 6-3).

Positive Finding

A positive finding is decreased sensation in one or more dermatomes, indicating sensory nerve involvement in the region of impaired or absent sensation. The clinician should carefully map areas of normal, impaired, and absent sensation to determine if the loss is due to spinal nerve root (dermatome pattern loss) or peripheral nerve injury. Bilateral deficits may be indicative of a central nervous system lesion.

Special Considerations

The clinician should simply touch the cotton wisp gently to the skin and should avoid any stroking or wiping motion. Additionally, the clinician should not apply a force with the cotton that might stimulate the mechanoreceptors. In cases where the patient appears confused or the test findings appear inappropriate, the clinician should reeducate the patient and repeat the testing procedure, beginning in an area of intact sensation to assess for patient comprehension.

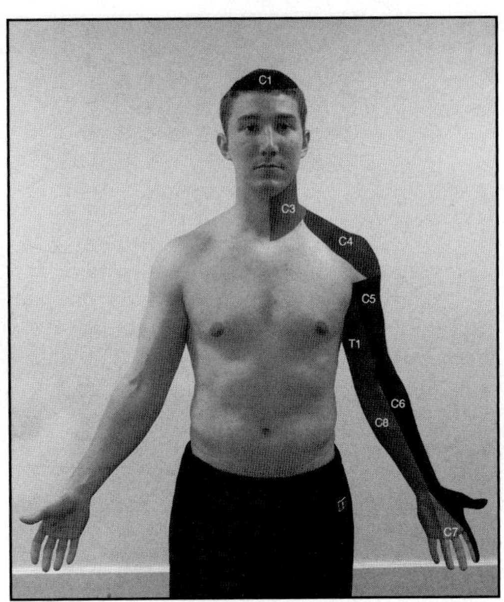

FIGURE 6-1

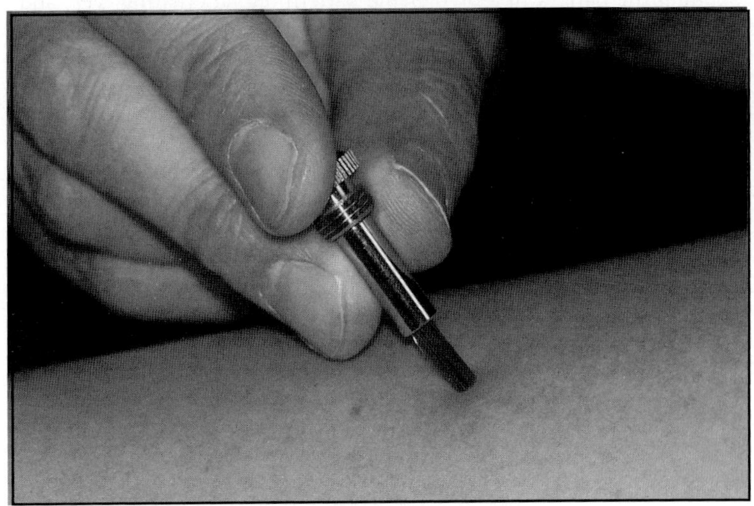

FIGURE 6-2

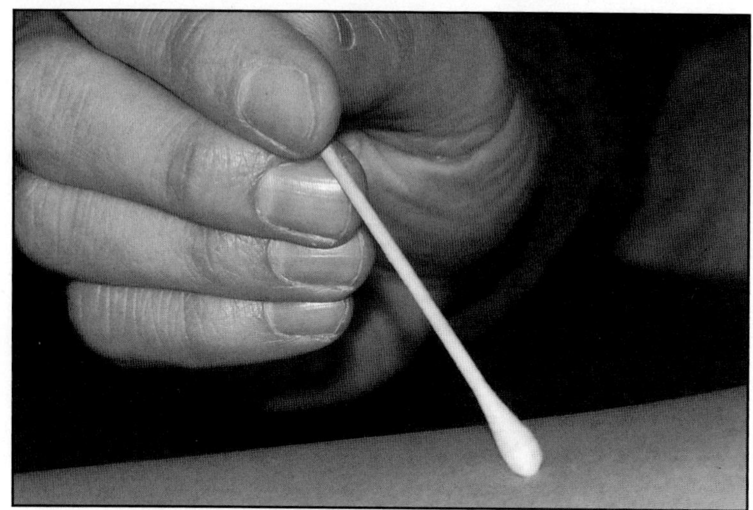

FIGURE 6-3

TESTING ERRORS

The clinician should avoid alternating between touching and not touching the patient in a predictable pattern (eg, alternating "yes" and "no" responses repeatedly or completing five consecutive "yes" responses followed by five consecutive "no" responses). The clinician should also be careful to avoid asking leading questions that might assist the patient in determining the proper response.

REFERENCES

Magee DJ. *Orthopedic Physical Assessment*. 4th ed. Philadelphia, PA: W.B. Saunders; 2002.

Reese NB. *Muscle and Sensory Testing*. 2nd ed. Philadelphia, PA: W.B. Saunders; 2005.

Starkey C, Ryan JL. *Evaluation of Orthopedic and Athletic Injuries*. 2nd ed. Philadelphia, PA: F.A. Davis; 2002.

Sensory Testing: Sharp-Dull

Test Position

The patient may be positioned in supine or sitting.

Materials Required

Sharp-dull sensation is tested using a sterile, broken cotton-tip applicator (to allow for a sharp test), a clean, unused safety pin or a Buck Reflex Hammer with screw-in pointed tip and retractable brush (Figure 6-4).

Action

The clinician should explain the procedure to the patient prior to testing to ensure the patient understands what is expected of him or her during the testing. The patient is instructed to close his or her eyes prior to initiating the test. The clinician will randomly alternate applying a sharp or dull stimulus to the patient (in the desired dermatome or region) using an appropriate testing instrument. Each time, the patient is asked to respond with either a "sharp" or "dull" response when instructed by the clinician. Testing 10 sites within the test area will allow the clinician to quantify the degree of sensation that is intact (eg, 8/10 or 80%) for a given dermatome or region. The test should be performed bilaterally for comparison to determine if deficits exist unilaterally or bilaterally (Figures 6-5 through 6-8).

Positive Finding

A positive finding is decreased ability to differentiate sharp-dull sensation in one or more dermatomes, indicating sensory nerve (pain receptor) involvement in the region of impaired or absent sensation. The clinician should carefully map areas of normal, impaired, and absent sensation to determine if the loss is due to spinal nerve root (dermatome pattern loss) or peripheral nerve injury. Bilateral deficits may be indicative of a central nervous system lesion.

Special Considerations

Prior to having the patient close his or her eyes, the clinician should review the desired responses with the patient to ensure that the patient can differentiate sharp and dull in an area of the body that has intact sensation. This will also allow the clinician to determine if the patient understands the testing procedure. The force used by the clinician for sharp-dull testing should be sufficient to dimple, but not break the skin.

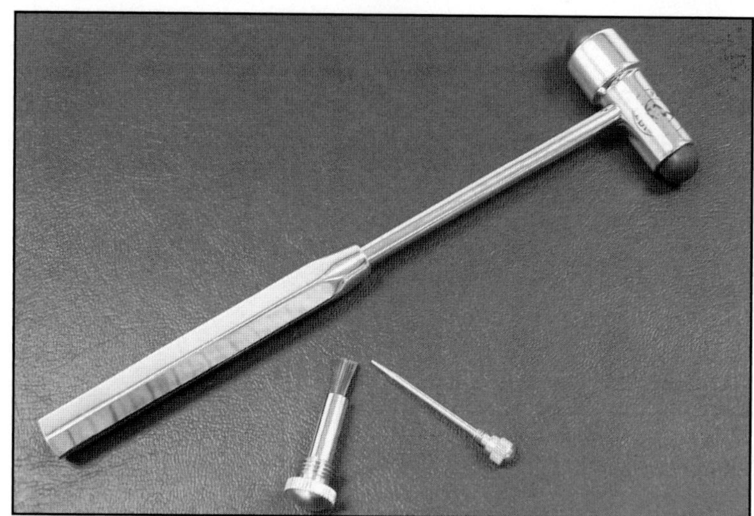

FIGURE 6-4

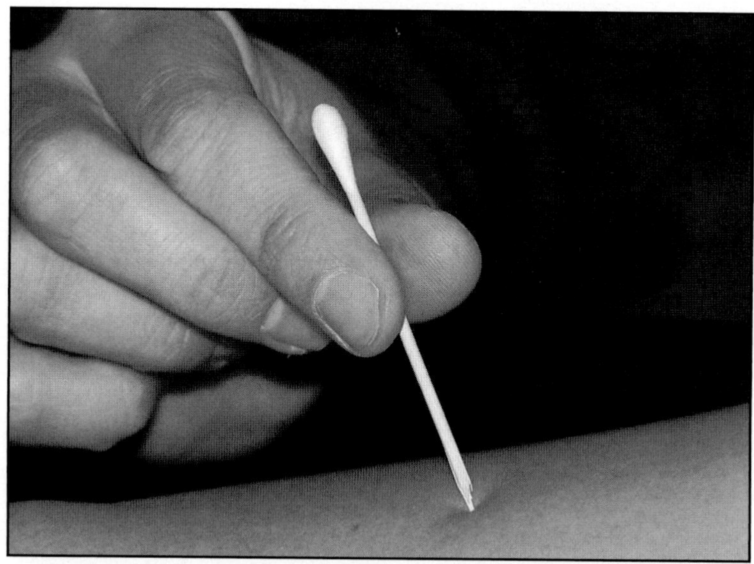

FIGURE 6-5

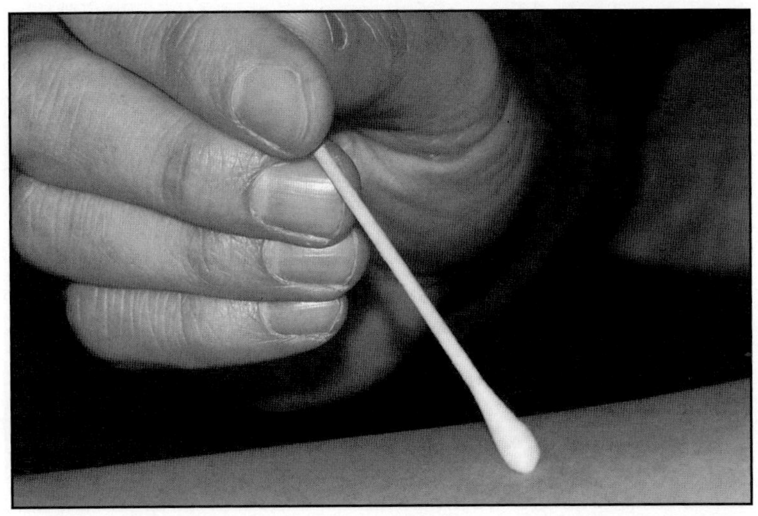

FIGURE 6-6

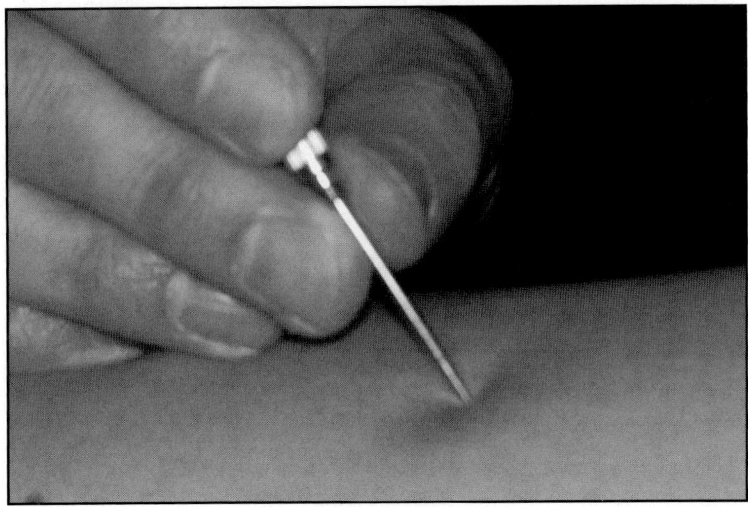

FIGURE 6-7

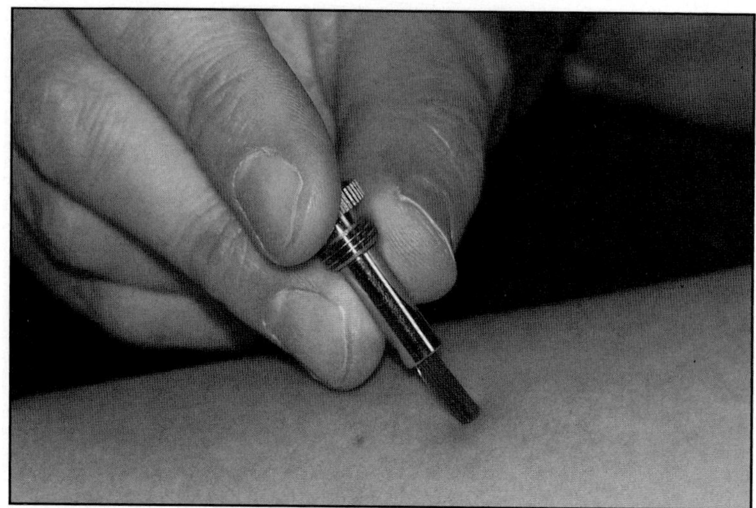

FIGURE 6-8

In cases where the patient appears confused or the test findings appear inappropriate, the clinician should reeducate the patient and repeat the testing procedure, beginning in an area of intact sensation to assess for patient comprehension. After sharp-dull testing is complete, the test instrument should be cleaned (Buck Reflex Hammer) or disposed of in a sharps container (safety pin or cotton-tip applicator).

TESTING ERRORS

The clinician should avoid alternating between sharp and dull testing in a predictable pattern (eg, alternating between sharp and dull responses repeatedly or completing five consecutive sharp tests followed by five consecutive dull tests). The clinician should also be careful to avoid asking leading questions that might assist the patient in determining the proper response.

SENSITIVITY

Sensitivity for pin-prick sensory testing of dermatomes C5–T1 has been found to range from .12 to .29.

SPECIFICITY

Specificity for pin-prick sensory testing of dermatomes C5–T1 has been found to range from .66 to .86.

Positive Likelihood Ratio

The positive likelihood ratio for pin-prick sensory testing of dermatomes C5–T1 has been found to range from .82 to 1.16.

Negative Likelihood Ratio

The negative likelihood ratio for pin-prick sensory testing of dermatomes C5–T1 has been found to range from .61 to 2.1.

References

Magee DJ. *Orthopedic Physical Assessment.* 4th ed. Philadelphia, PA: W.B. Saunders; 2002.

Reese NB. *Muscle and Sensory Testing.* 2nd ed. Philadelphia, PA: W.B. Saunders; 2005.

Starkey C, Ryan JL. *Evaluation of Orthopedic and Athletic Injuries.* 2nd ed. Philadelphia, PA: F.A. Davis; 2002.

Wainner R, Fritz J, Irrgang J, Boninger M, Delito A, Allison S. Reliability and diagnostic accuracy of the clinical examination and patient self-report measures for cervical radiculopathy. *Spine.* 2003;28:52-62.

Sensory Testing: Temperature

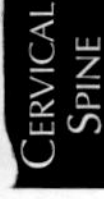

Test Position

The patient may be positioned in supine or sitting.

Materials Required

Two glass containers will be needed for testing. One container is filled with ice water while the second container is filled with hot water (Figure 6-9).

Action

The clinician should explain the procedure to the patient prior to testing to ensure the patient understands what is expected of him or her during the testing. The patient is instructed to close his or her eyes prior to initiating the test. The clinician will randomly alternate applying a cold or hot stimulus to the patient (in the desired dermatome or region) using the glass containers. Each stimulus should be maintained for a minimum of 2 seconds. Each time, the patient is asked to respond with either a "hot" or "cold" response when instructed by the clinician. Testing 10 sites within the test area will allow the clinician to quantify the degree of sensation that is intact (eg, 9/10 or 90%) for a given dermatome or region. The test should be performed bilaterally for comparison to determine if deficits exist unilaterally or bilaterally (Figure 6-10).

Positive Finding

A positive finding is decreased ability to differentiate hot and cold sensation in one or more dermatomes, indicating sensory nerve (thermal receptor) involvement in the region of impaired or absent sensation. The clinician should carefully map areas of normal, impaired, and absent sensation to determine if the loss is due to spinal nerve root (dermatome pattern loss) or peripheral nerve injury. Bilateral deficits may be indicative of a central nervous system lesion.

Special Considerations

Prior to having the patient close his or her eyes, the clinician should review the desired responses with the patient to ensure that the patient can differentiate hot and cold in an area of the body that has intact sensation. This will also allow the clinician to determine if the patient understands the testing procedure. The temperature of the hot water should not exceed 45 degrees Celsius in order to prevent burns to the patient. Additionally, stimulation at too high a temperature will likely invoke a response from pain receptors rather than temperature receptors. In cases where the patient appears confused or the test findings appear inappropriate, the clinician should reeducate the patient and repeat the testing procedure, beginning in an area of intact sensation to assess for patient comprehension.

Testing Errors

The clinician should avoid alternating between hot and cold testing in a predictable pattern (eg, alternating between hot and cold responses repeatedly or completing five consecutive hot tests followed by five consecutive cold tests). The clinician should also be careful to avoid asking leading questions that might assist the patient in determining the proper response.

References

Magee DJ. *Orthopedic Physical Assessment*. 4th ed. Philadelphia, PA: W.B. Saunders; 2002.

Reese NB. *Muscle and Sensory Testing*. 2nd ed. Philadelphia, PA: W.B. Saunders; 2005.

Starkey C, Ryan JL. *Evaluation of Orthopedic and Athletic Injuries*. 2nd ed. Philadelphia, PA: F.A. Davis; 2002.

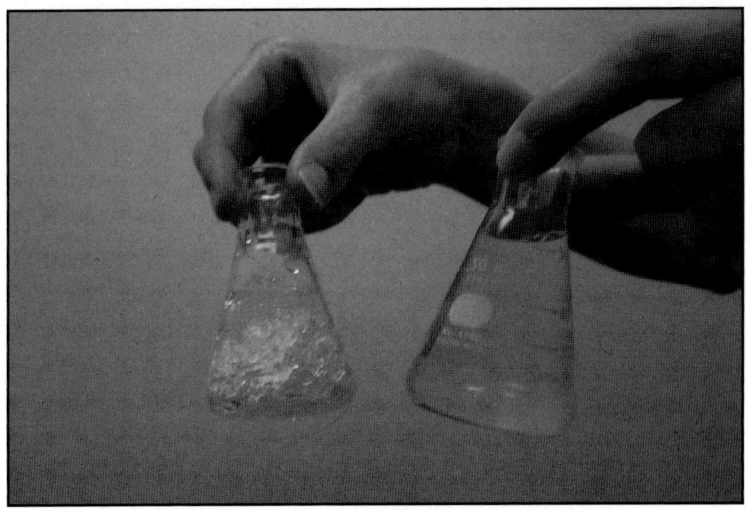

Figure 6-9

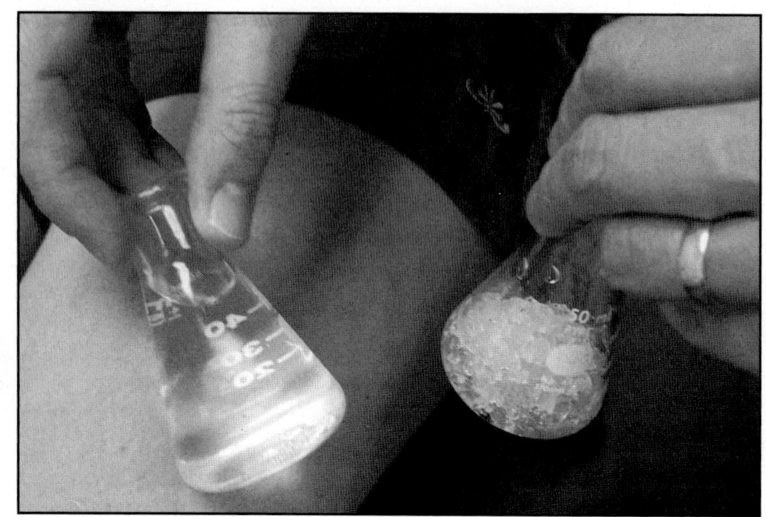

FIGURE 6-10

Sensory Testing: Two-Point Discrimination

Test Position

The patient may be positioned in supine or sitting.

Materials Required

Two-point discriminator, two-point esthesiometer, and caliper or clean, unused paperclip (Figure 6-11).

Action

The clinician should explain the procedure to the patient prior to testing to ensure the patient understands what is expected of him or her during the testing. The patient is instructed to close his or her eyes prior to initiating the test. The clinician begins testing with the two points separated to a distance that allows the patient to easily distinguish the presence of both points. The clinician then gradually decreases the distance between the points, making sure both points contact the skin simultaneously, until the patient can no longer distinguish the presence of two separate points during testing. The minimal distance at which the patient can distinguish the two points is called the threshold for discrimination. This distance is recorded and the process is repeated in another region of the dermatome or in another area of the body. The test should be performed bilaterally for comparison to determine if deficits exist unilaterally or bilaterally (Figures 6-12 and 6-13).

Positive Finding

A positive finding is an inability to discriminate between one and two points during testing or threshold for discrimination that is greater on the involved side than the uninvolved side. Typical thresholds for discrimination have been identified for different zones of the palm. These average values may prove helpful to the clinician in cases of bilateral neurologic involvement. The clinician should carefully map areas of normal, impaired, and absent two-point discrimination to determine if the loss is due to spinal nerve root (dermatome pattern loss) or peripheral nerve injury. Bilateral deficits may be indicative of a central nervous system lesion.

Special Considerations

Prior to having the patient close his or her eyes, the clinician should review the desired responses with the patient to ensure that the patient can differentiate between one and two points in an area of the body that has intact sensation. This will also allow the clinician to determine if the patient understands the testing procedure. The clinician should apply only light force when performing this test. The skin should not dimple or blanch during testing. In cases where the patient appears confused or the test findings appear inappropriate, the clinician should reeducate the patient and repeat the testing procedure, beginning in an area of intact sensation to assess for patient comprehension. After two-point discrimination testing is complete, the test instrument should be cleaned (two-point discriminator, two-point esthesiometer, or caliper) or disposed of in a sharps container (paperclip).

Testing Modifications

If the clinician desires, he or she may alternate between one and two points and ask the patient to respond with the word "one" or "two" corresponding to the number of points contacting the skin. The clinician completes a minimum of 10 repetitions in each test area before changing the distance between the two points. The patient is required to answer correctly 8 out of 10 times in order to narrow the distance between the two points. This technique requires more time to complete but allows for a more objective assessment than the test described above.

References

Magee, DJ. *Orthopedic Physical Assessment.* 4th ed. Philadelphia, PA: W.B. Saunders; 2002.

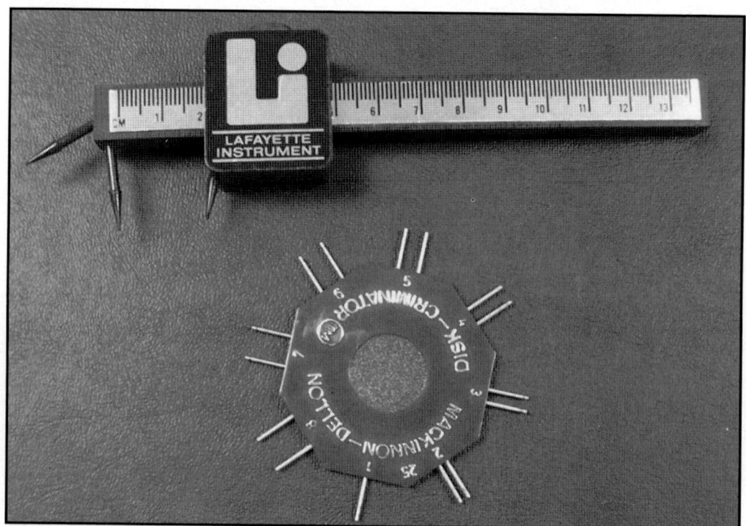

Figure 6-11

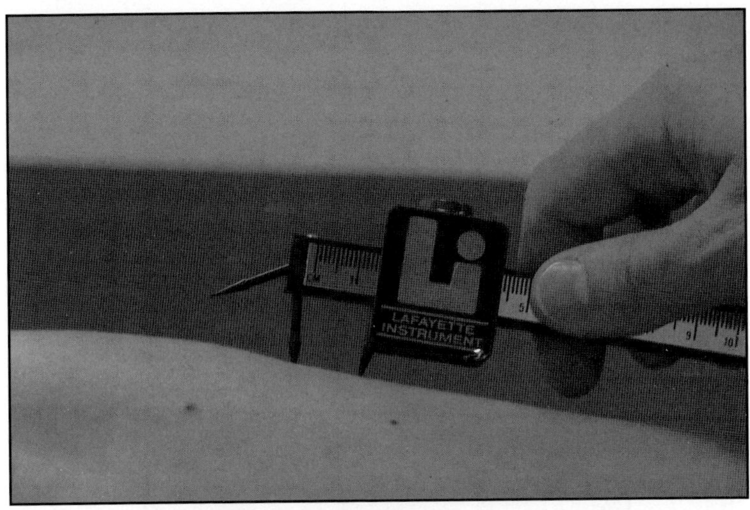

FIGURE 6-12

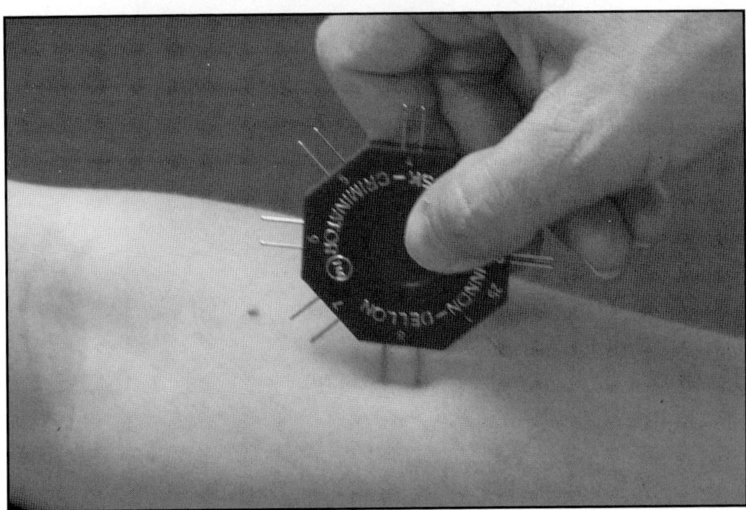

FIGURE 6-13

Individual dermatome locations

See Figures 6-14 through 6-21.

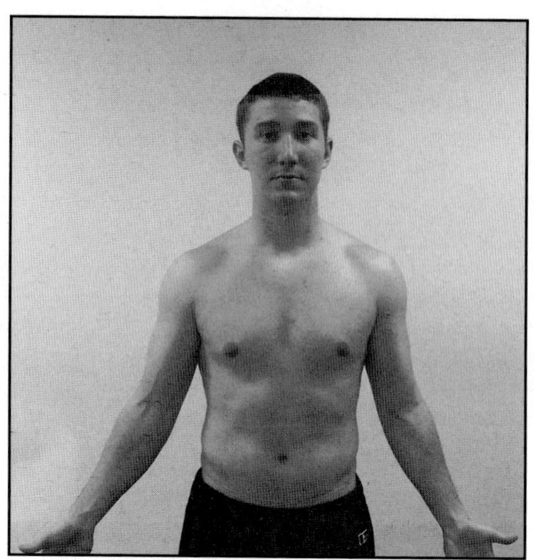

Figure 6-14

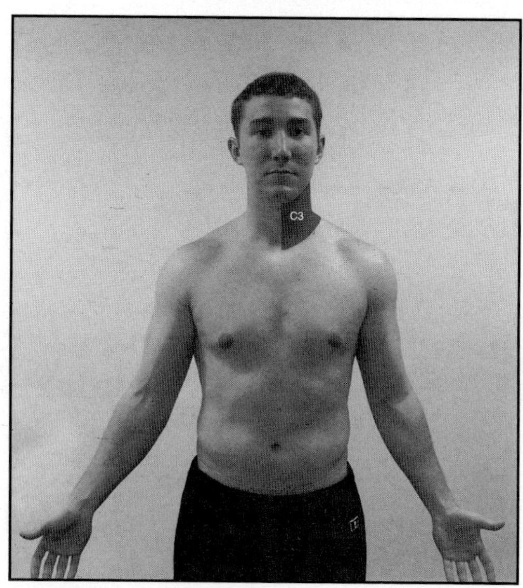

Figure 6-15

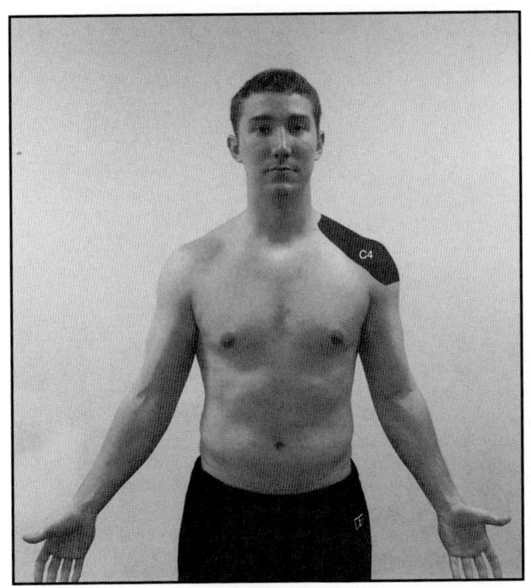

FIGURE 6-16

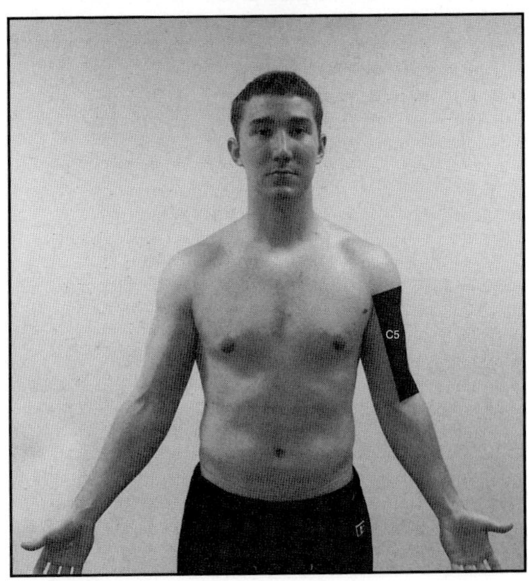

FIGURE 6-17

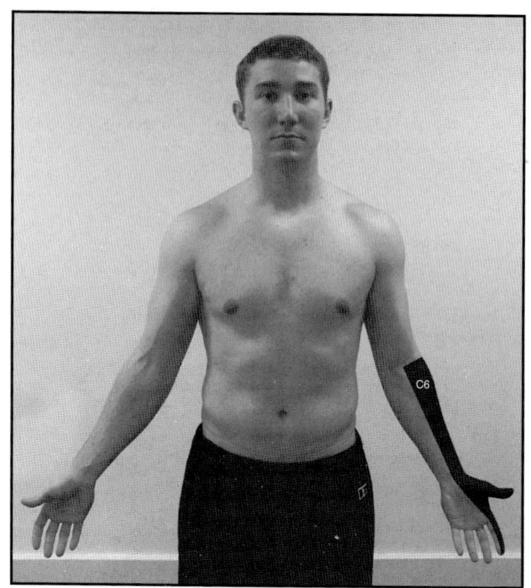

Figure 6-18

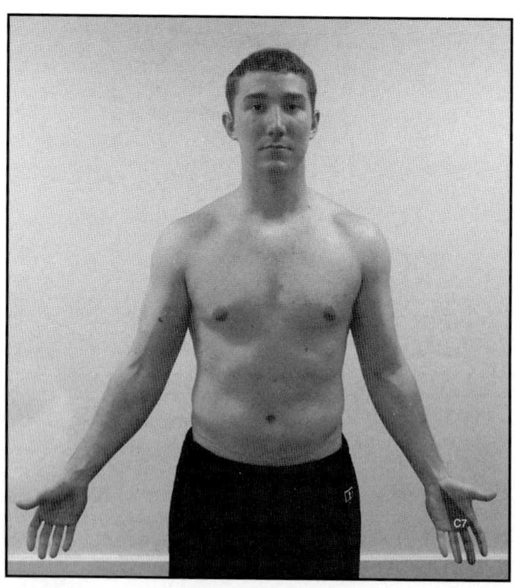

Figure 6-19

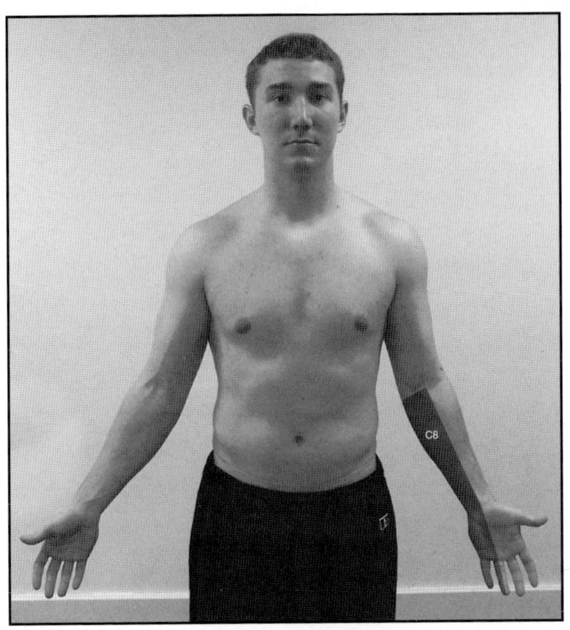

Figure 6-20

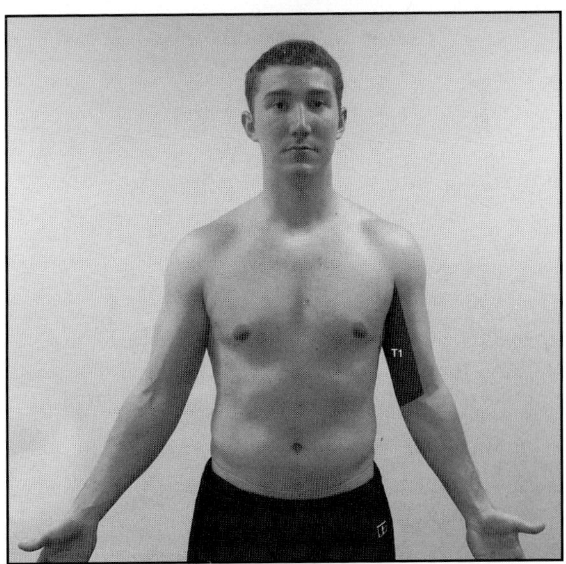

Figure 6-21

Chapter 7

Myotome Testing

The following chart presents an overview of myotome testing for spinal nerve roots C1–T1. Myotome testing involves the performance of "break tests" to assess muscle strength for a given motion. Myotome testing is not intended to be diagnostic for individual muscle weakness—this is accomplished through the application of specific manual muscle testing—but rather to identify weakness of a group of muscles corresponding to a single joint motion. Patterns of muscle weakness can then be related to a single spinal nerve root level. Each of these test procedures will be described in greater detail in this chapter.

References

Hoppenfeld S. *Orthopaedic Neurology*. Baltimore, MD: Lippincott-Raven; 1997.

Hoppenfeld S. *Physical Examination of the Spine and Extremities*. East Norwalk, CT: Appleton-Century-Crofts; 1976.

Magee DJ. *Orthopedic Physical Assessment*. 4th ed. Philadelphia, PA: W.B. Saunders; 2002.

Meadows JTS. *Orthopedic Differential Diagnosis in Physical Therapy*. New York: McGraw-Hill; 1999.

Table 7-1

CERVICAL SPINE MYOTOMES

Nerve Root	*Dermatome*
C1	Cervical spine flexion
C2	Cervical spine flexion
C3	Cervical spine lateral flexion
C4	Scapular elevation or shoulder shrugs
C5	Shoulder abduction
	Elbow flexion
C6	Elbow flexion
	Wrist extension
C7	Elbow extension
	Wrist flexion
	Finger extension
C8	Finger flexion
	Thumb flexion
	Thumb extension
T1	Finger adduction
	Finger abduction

C1 and C2 Myotome Test

Test Position

The patient is positioned in sitting.

Action

The clinician instructs the patient to flex his or her cervical spine approximately 45 degrees. The clinician then instructs the patient to hold his or her head in this position while the clinician applies resistance. The clinician places the stabilization hand on the posterior, inferior portion of the cervical spine and places the resistance hand over the patient's forehead. The clinician applies a force in the direction of cervical spine extension while instructing the patient to hold against the resistance (Figure 7-1).

Positive Finding

A positive finding is weakness; the patient is unable to withstand the clinician's resistance, indicating possible involvement of the C1 or C2 spinal nerve root. Bilateral strength deficits could be indicative of a central nervous system lesion or simply of weakness of the test muscle group.

Special Considerations

The clinician should apply the resistance in a slow, controlled manner, progressing in intensity as tolerated by the patient. A finding of pain or pain and weakness is more indicative of contractile tissue involvement (muscle, tendon, or bony insertion of tendon) and is not indicative of spinal nerve root involvement.

References

Hoppenfeld S. *Orthopaedic Neurology*. Baltimore, MD: Lippincott-Raven; 1997.

Hoppenfeld S. *Physical Examination of the Spine and Extremities*. East Norwalk, CT: Appleton-Century-Crofts; 1976.

Magee DJ. *Orthopedic Physical Assessment*. 4th ed. Philadelphia, PA: W.B. Saunders; 2002.

Meadows JTS. *Orthopedic Differential Diagnosis in Physical Therapy*. New York: McGraw-Hill; 1999.

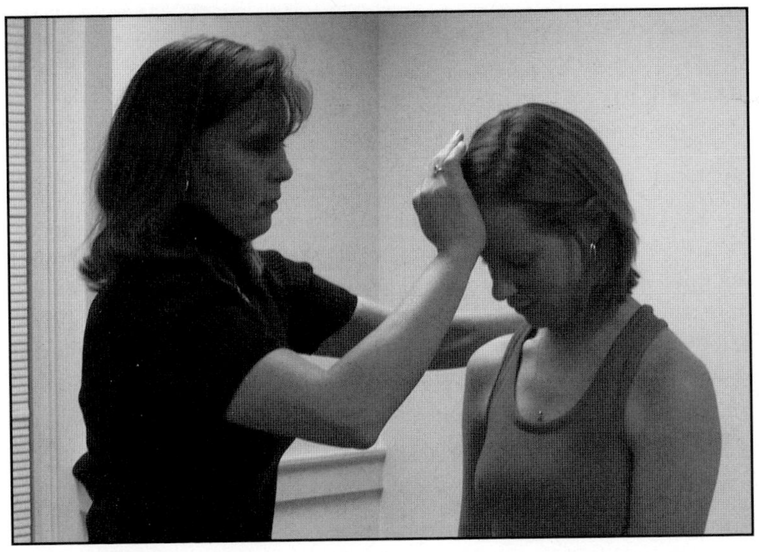

FIGURE 7-1

C3 Myotome Test

Test Position

The patient is positioned in sitting.

Action

The clinician instructs the patient to laterally flex or sidebend his or her cervical spine to end-range. The clinician then instructs the patient to hold his or her head in this position while the clinician applies resistance. The clinician places the stabilization hand on the superior shoulder on the side of movement and the resistance hand on the lateral aspect of the head on the ipsilateral side. The clinician applies a force in the direction of cervical spine lateral flexion to the contralateral side while instructing the patient to hold against the resistance (Figure 7-2).

Positive Finding

A positive finding is weakness; the patient is unable to withstand the clinician's resistance, indicating possible involvement of the C3 spinal nerve root. Bilateral strength deficits could be indicative of a central nervous system lesion or simply of weakness of the test muscle group.

Special Considerations

Perform the test bilaterally to allow for strength comparisons. The clinician should apply the resistance in a slow, controlled manner, progressing in intensity as tolerated by the patient. A finding of pain or pain and weakness is more indicative of contractile tissue involvement (muscle, tendon, or bony insertion of tendon) and is not indicative of spinal nerve root involvement.

References

Hoppenfeld S. *Orthopaedic Neurology*. Baltimore, MD: Lippincott-Raven; 1997.

Hoppenfeld S. *Physical Examination of the Spine and Extremities*. East Norwalk, CT: Appleton-Century-Crofts; 1976.

Magee DJ. *Orthopedic Physical Assessment*. 4th ed. Philadelphia, PA: W.B. Saunders; 2002.

Meadows JTS. *Orthopedic Differential Diagnosis in Physical Therapy*. New York: McGraw-Hill; 1999.

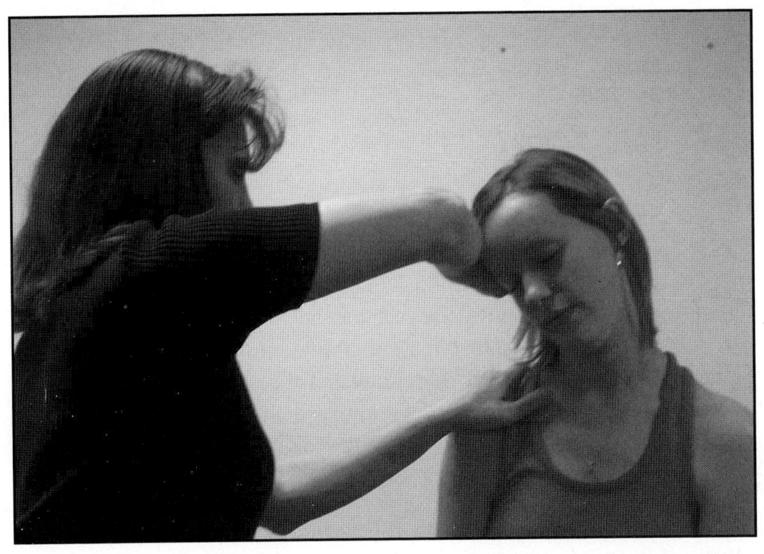

FIGURE 7-2

C4 Myotome Test

Test Position

The patient is positioned in sitting.

Action

The clinician instructs the patient to shrug his shoulders (scapular elevation) bilaterally. The clinician then instructs the patient to hold his or her shoulders in this position while the clinician applies resistance. The clinician places the resistance hand on the superior aspect of one or both shoulders. Resistance may be applied unilaterally or bilaterally as desired by the clinician. The clinician applies a downward force on the shoulder(s) in the direction of scapular depression while instructing the patient to hold against the resistance (Figure 7-3).

Positive Finding

A positive finding is weakness; the patient is unable to withstand the clinician's resistance, indicating possible involvement of the C4 spinal nerve root. Bilateral strength deficits could be indicative of a central nervous system lesion or simply of weakness of the trapezius and levator scapulae muscles.

Special Considerations

Perform the test bilaterally to allow for strength comparisons. The clinician should apply the resistance in a slow, controlled manner, progressing in intensity as tolerated by the patient. A finding of pain or pain and weakness is more indicative of contractile tissue involvement (muscle, tendon, or bony insertion of tendon) and is not indicative of spinal nerve root involvement.

References

Hoppenfeld S. *Orthopaedic Neurology*. Baltimore, MD: Lippincott-Raven; 1997.

Hoppenfeld S. *Physical Examination of the Spine and Extremities*. East Norwalk, CT: Appleton-Century-Crofts; 1976.

Magee DJ. *Orthopedic Physical Assessment*. 4th ed. Philadelphia, PA: W.B. Saunders; 2002.

Meadows JTS. *Orthopedic Differential Diagnosis in Physical Therapy*. New York: McGraw-Hill; 1999.

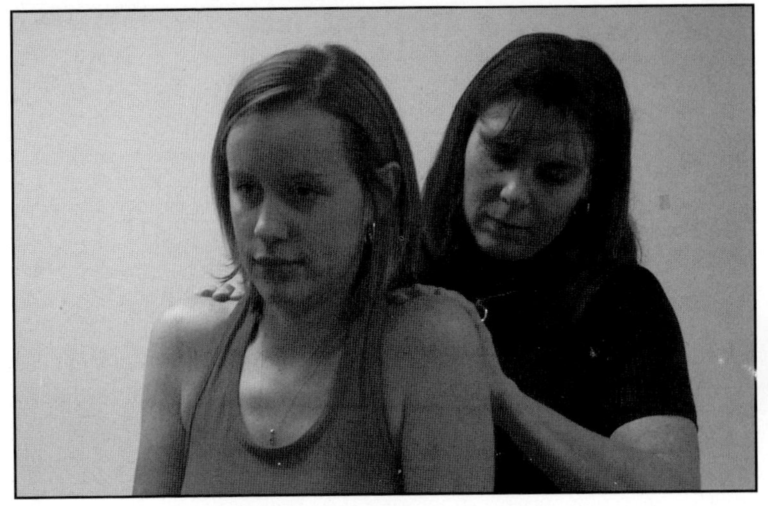

FIGURE 7-3

C5 Myotome Test

Test Position

The patient is positioned in sitting.

Action

The clinician instructs the patient to abduct his or her shoulder 90 degrees. The clinician then instructs the patient to hold his or her shoulder in this position while the clinician applies resistance. The clinician places the stabilization hand on the superior aspect of the test shoulder and the resistance hand just proximal to the elbow of the test shoulder. The clinician applies a force in the direction of shoulder adduction while instructing the patient to hold against the resistance (Figure 7-4).

Positive Finding

A positive finding is weakness; the patient is unable to withstand the clinician's resistance, indicating possible involvement of the C5 spinal nerve root. A complementary finding of weakness in elbow flexion increases the likelihood of C5 nerve root involvement. Bilateral strength deficits could be indicative of a central nervous system lesion or simply of weakness of the deltoid muscles.

Special Considerations

Perform the test bilaterally to allow for strength comparisons. The clinician should apply the resistance in a slow, controlled manner, progressing in intensity as tolerated by the patient. A finding of pain or pain and weakness is more indicative of contractile tissue involvement (muscle, tendon, or bony insertion of tendon) and is not indicative of spinal nerve root involvement.

References

Hoppenfeld S. *Orthopaedic Neurology*. Baltimore, MD: Lippincott-Raven; 1997.

Hoppenfeld S. *Physical Examination of the Spine and Extremities*. East Norwalk, CT: Appleton-Century-Crofts; 1976.

Magee DJ. *Orthopedic Physical Assessment*. 4th ed. Philadelphia, PA: W.B. Saunders; 2002.

Meadows JTS. *Orthopedic Differential Diagnosis in Physical Therapy*. New York: McGraw-Hill; 1999.

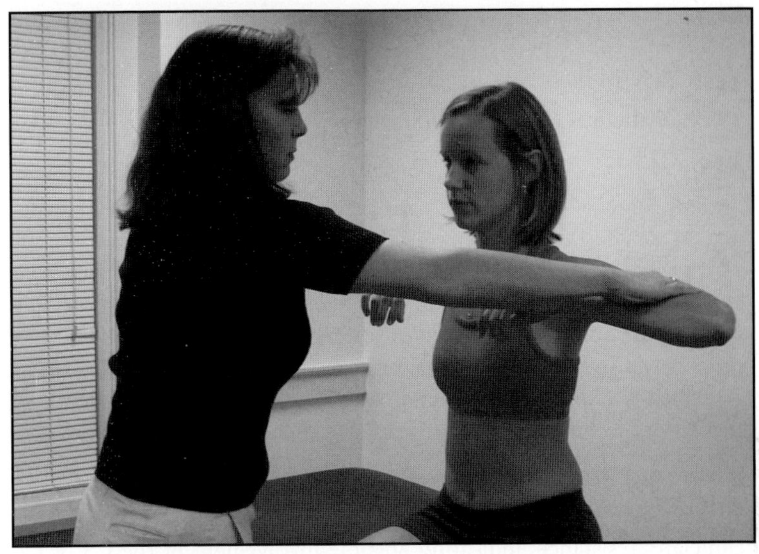

FIGURE 7-4

C5/C6 Myotome Test: Elbow Flexion

Test Position

The patient is positioned in sitting.

Action

The clinician instructs the patient to flex his or her elbow approximately 90 degrees. The clinician then instructs the patient to hold his or her elbow in this position while the clinician applies resistance. The clinician places the stabilization hand on the anterior aspect of the shoulder on the ipsilateral side of testing and the resistance hand just proximal to the wrist (palmar aspect) on the side of testing. The clinician applies a force in the direction of elbow extension while instructing the patient to hold against the resistance (Figure 7-5).

Positive Finding

A positive finding is weakness; the patient is unable to withstand the clinician's resistance, indicating possible involvement of the C5 or C6 spinal nerve root. A complementary finding of weakness in shoulder abduction increases the likelihood of C5 nerve root involvement. A complementary finding of weakness in wrist extension increases the likelihood of C6 nerve root involvement. Bilateral strength deficits could be indicative of a central nervous system lesion or simply of weakness of the biceps brachii, brachialis, or brachioradialis musclature.

Special Considerations

Perform the test bilaterally to allow for strength comparisons. The clinician should apply the resistance in a slow, controlled manner, progressing in intensity as tolerated by the patient. A finding of pain or pain and weakness is more indicative of contractile tissue involvement (muscle, tendon, or bony insertion of tendon) and is not indicative of spinal nerve root involvement.

References

Hoppenfeld S. *Orthopaedic Neurology*. Baltimore, MD: Lippincott-Raven; 1997.

Hoppenfeld S. *Physical Examination of the Spine and Extremities*. East Norwalk, CT: Appleton-Century-Crofts; 1976.

Magee DJ. *Orthopedic Physical Assessment.* 4th ed. Philadelphia, PA: W.B. Saunders; 2002.

Meadows JTS. *Orthopedic Differential Diagnosis in Physical Therapy*. New York: McGraw-Hill; 1999.

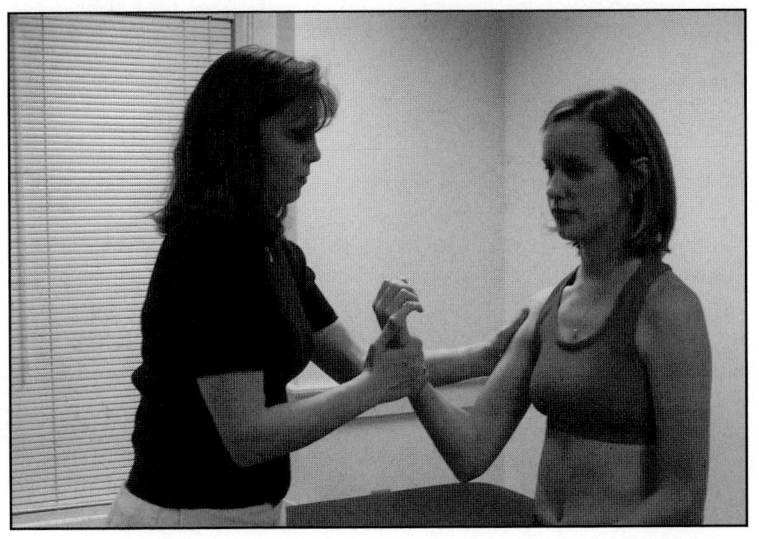

Figure 7-5

C6 Myotome Test: Wrist Extension

Test Position

The patient is positioned in sitting.

Action

The clinician instructs the patient to extend his or her wrist to end-range. The clinician then instructs the patient to hold his or her wrist in this position while the clinician applies resistance. The clinician places the stabilization hand just proximal to the wrist and the resistance hand just proximal to the MCP joints (dorsal side) on the side of testing. The clinician applies a force in the direction of wrist flexion while instructing the patient to hold against the resistance (Figure 7-6).

Positive Finding

A positive finding is weakness; the patient is unable to withstand the clinician's resistance, indicating possible involvement of the C6 spinal nerve root. A complementary finding of weakness in elbow flexion increases the likelihood of C6 nerve root involvement. Bilateral strength deficits could be indicative of a central nervous system lesion or simply of weakness of the extensor carpi ulnaris, extensor carpi radialis longus, and extensor carpi radialis brevis muscles.

Special Considerations

Perform the test bilaterally to allow for strength comparisons. The clinician should apply the resistance in a slow, controlled manner, progressing in intensity as tolerated by the patient. A finding of pain or pain and weakness is more indicative of contractile tissue involvement (muscle, tendon, or bony insertion of tendon) and is not indicative of spinal nerve root involvement.

References

Hoppenfeld S. *Orthopaedic Neurology*. Baltimore, MD: Lippincott-Raven; 1997.

Hoppenfeld S. *Physical Examination of the Spine and Extremities*. East Norwalk, CT: Appleton-Century-Crofts; 1976.

Magee DJ. *Orthopedic Physical Assessment*. 4th ed. Philadelphia, PA: W.B. Saunders; 2002.

Meadows JTS. *Orthopedic Differential Diagnosis in Physical Therapy*. New York: McGraw-Hill; 1999.

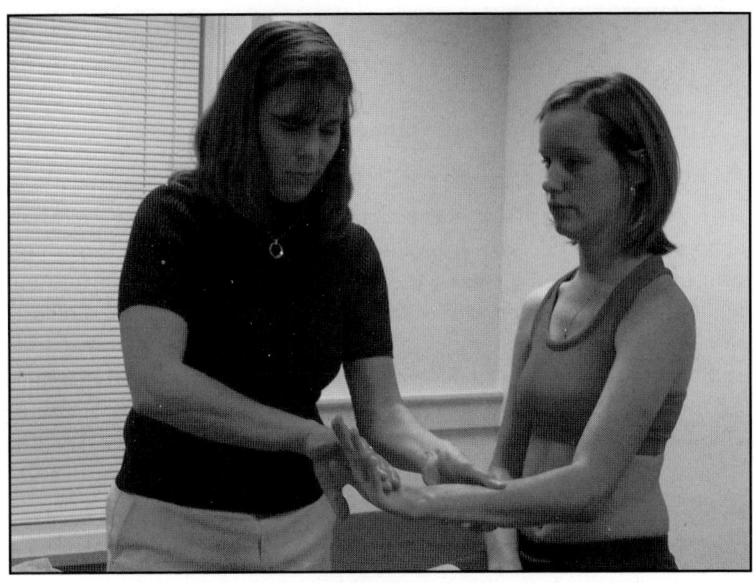

FIGURE 7-6

C7 Myotome Test: Elbow Extension

Test Position

The patient is positioned in sitting.

Action

The clinician instructs the patient to extend his or her elbow to approximately 10 degrees from full extension (-10 degrees). The clinician then instructs the patient to hold his or her elbow in this position while the clinician applies resistance. The clinician places the stabilization hand on the anterior aspect of the shoulder on the ipsilateral side of testing and the resistance hand just proximal to the wrist (dorsal aspect) on the side of testing. The clinician applies a force in the direction of elbow flexion while instructing the patient to hold against the resistance (Figure 7-7).

Positive Finding

A positive finding is weakness; the patient is unable to withstand the clinician's resistance, indicating possible involvement of the C7 spinal nerve root. Complementary findings of weakness in wrist flexion and/or finger extension increases the likelihood of C7 nerve root involvement. Bilateral strength deficits could be indicative of a central nervous system lesion or simply of weakness of the triceps brachii and anconeus muscles.

Special Considerations

Perform the test bilaterally to allow for strength comparisons. The clinician should apply the resistance in a slow, controlled manner, progressing in intensity as tolerated by the patient. A finding of pain or pain and weakness is more indicative of contractile tissue involvement (muscle, tendon, or bony insertion of tendon) and is not indicative of spinal nerve root involvement.

References

Hoppenfeld S. *Orthopaedic Neurology*. Baltimore, MD: Lippincott-Raven; 1997.

Hoppenfeld S. *Physical Examination of the Spine and Extremities*. East Norwalk, CT: Appleton-Century-Crofts; 1976.

Magee DJ. *Orthopedic Physical Assessment*. 4th ed. Philadelphia, PA: W.B. Saunders; 2002.

Meadows JTS. *Orthopedic Differential Diagnosis in Physical Therapy*. New York: McGraw-Hill; 1999.

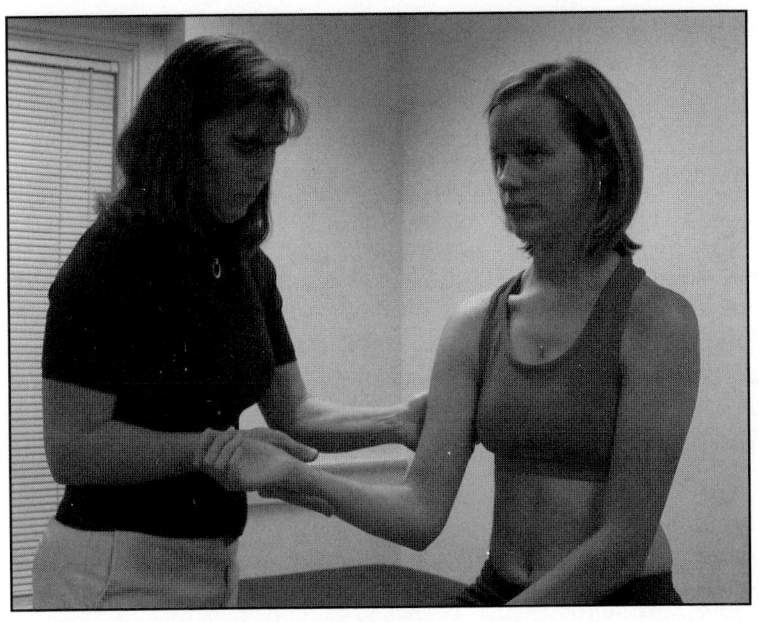

FIGURE 7-7

C7 Myotome Test: Wrist Flexion

Test Position

The patient is positioned in sitting.

Action

The clinician instructs the patient to flex his or her wrist to end-range. The clinician then instructs the patient to hold his or her wrist in this position while the clinician applies resistance. The clinician places the stabilization hand just proximal to the wrist and the resistance hand just proximal to the MCP joints (palmar aspect) on the side of testing. The clinician applies a force in the direction of wrist extension while instructing the patient to hold against the resistance (Figure 7-8).

Positive Finding

A positive finding is weakness; the patient is unable to withstand the clinician's resistance, indicating possible involvement of the C7 spinal nerve root. Complementary findings of weakness in elbow extension and/or finger extension increases the likelihood of C7 nerve root involvement. Bilateral strength deficits could be indicative of a central nervous system lesion or simply of weakness of the flexor carpi ulnaris and flexor carpi radialis muscles.

Special Considerations

Perform the test bilaterally to allow for strength comparisons. The clinician should apply the resistance in a slow, controlled manner, progressing in intensity as tolerated by the patient. A finding of pain or pain and weakness is more indicative of contractile tissue involvement (muscle, tendon, or bony insertion of tendon) and is not indicative of spinal nerve root involvement.

References

Hoppenfeld S. *Orthopaedic Neurology*. Baltimore, MD: Lippincott-Raven; 1997.

Hoppenfeld S. *Physical Examination of the Spine and Extremities*. East Norwalk, CT: Appleton-Century-Crofts; 1976.

Magee DJ. *Orthopedic Physical Assessment*. 4th ed. Philadelphia, PA: W.B. Saunders; 2002.

Meadows JTS. *Orthopedic Differential Diagnosis in Physical Therapy*. New York: McGraw-Hill; 1999.

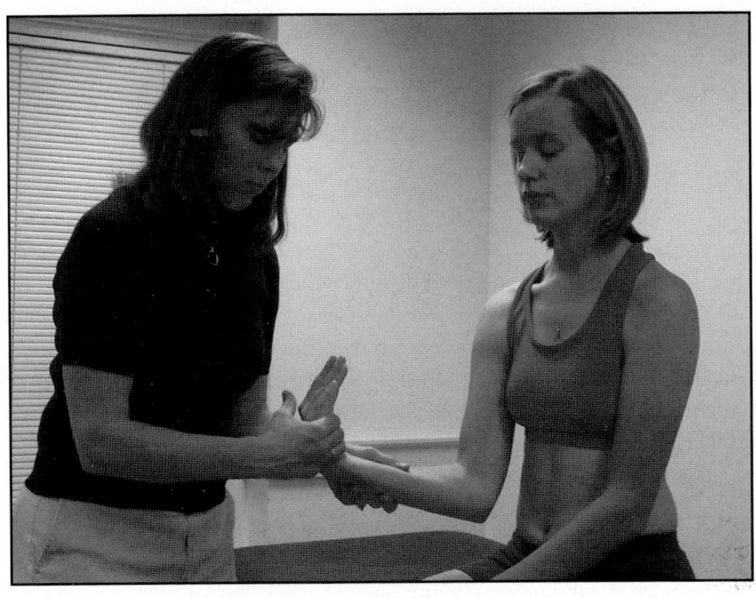

FIGURE 7-8

C7 Myotome Test: Finger Extension

Test Position

The patient is positioned in sitting.

Action

The clinician instructs the patient to extend his or her MCP joints to end-range. The clinician then instructs the patient to hold his or her fingers in this position while the clinician applies resistance. The clinician places the stabilization hand just proximal to the MCP joints (dorsal side) and the resistance hand over the dorsal aspect of the fingers on the side of testing. The clinician applies a force in the direction of finger flexion while instructing the patient to hold against the resistance (Figure 7-9).

Positive Finding

A positive finding is weakness; the patient is unable to withstand the clinician's resistance, indicating possible involvement of the C7 spinal nerve root. Complementary findings of weakness in elbow extension and/or wrist flexion increases the likelihood of C7 nerve root involvement. Bilateral strength deficits could be indicative of a central nervous system lesion or simply of weakness of the finger extensor muscles.

Special Considerations

Perform the test bilaterally to allow for strength comparisons. The clinician may test finger extension individually or as a group. The resistance applied by the clinician should match the number of fingers being tested. For example, the clinician should apply resistance using one finger if testing fingers individually or the clinician can apply resistance using all four fingers when testing finger strength as a group. The clinician should apply the resistance in a slow, controlled manner, progressing in intensity as tolerated by the patient. A finding of pain or pain and weakness is more indicative of contractile tissue involvement (muscle, tendon, or bony insertion of tendon) and is not indicative of spinal nerve root involvement.

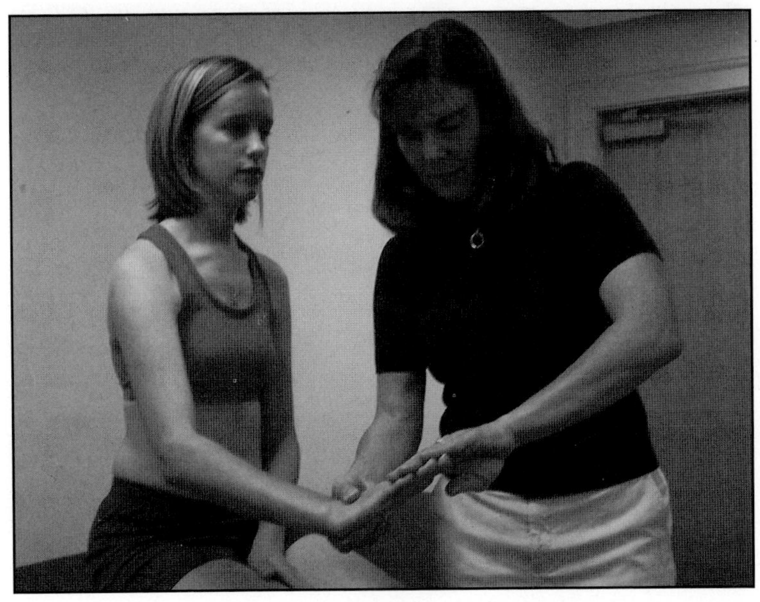

FIGURE 7-9

REFERENCES

Hoppenfeld S. *Orthopaedic Neurology*. Baltimore, MD: Lippincott-Raven; 1997.

Hoppenfeld S. *Physical Examination of the Spine and Extremities*. East Norwalk, CT: Appleton-Century-Crofts; 1976.

Magee DJ. *Orthopedic Physical Assessment*. 4th ed. Philadelphia, PA: W.B. Saunders; 2002.

Meadows JTS. *Orthopedic Differential Diagnosis in Physical Therapy*. New York: McGraw-Hill; 1999.

C8 Myotome Test: Finger Flexion

Test Position

The patient is positioned in sitting.

Action

The clinician instructs the patient to flex his or her MCP joints approximately 90 degrees. The clinician then instructs the patient to hold his or her fingers in this position while the clinician applies resistance. The clinician places the stabilization hand just proximal to the wrist and the resistance finger(s) over the palmar aspect of the fingers on the side of testing. The clinician applies a force in the direction of finger extension while instructing the patient to hold against the resistance (Figure 7-10).

Positive Finding

A positive finding is weakness; the patient is unable to withstand the clinician's resistance, indicating possible involvement of the C8 spinal nerve root. Complementary findings of weakness in thumb flexion and/or extension increases the likelihood of C8 nerve root involvement. Bilateral strength deficits could be indicative of a central nervous system lesion or simply of weakness of the finger flexor muscles.

Special Considerations

Perform the test bilaterally to allow for strength comparisons. The clinician may test finger flexion individually or as a group. The resistance applied by the clinician should match the number of fingers being tested. For example, the clinician should apply resistance using one finger if testing fingers individually or the clinician can apply resistance using all four fingers when testing finger strength as a group. The clinician should apply the resistance in a slow, controlled manner, progressing in intensity as tolerated by the patient. A finding of pain or pain and weakness is more indicative of contractile tissue involvement (muscle, tendon, or bony insertion of tendon) and is not indicative of spinal nerve root involvement.

References

Hoppenfeld S. *Orthopaedic Neurology*. Baltimore, MD: Lippincott-Raven; 1997.

Hoppenfeld S. *Physical Examination of the Spine and Extremities*. East Norwalk, CT: Appleton-Century-Crofts; 1976.

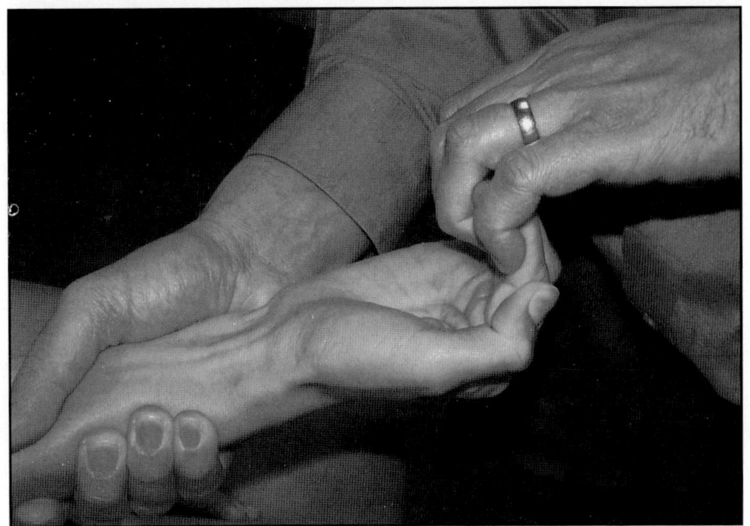

FIGURE 7-10

Magee DJ. *Orthopedic Physical Assessment.* 4th ed. Philadelphia, PA: W.B. Saunders; 2002.

Meadows JTS. *Orthopedic Differential Diagnosis in Physical Therapy*. New York: McGraw-Hill; 1999.

C8 Myotome Test: Thumb Flexion

Test Position

The patient is positioned in sitting.

Action

The clinician instructs the patient to flex his or her second digit and thumb to make a circle (Figure 7-11). The clinician then instructs the patient to hold his or her finger and thumb in this position while the clinician applies resistance by attempting to pull the patient's hands apart. The clinician may also place his or her finger inside the circle and applies resistance, forcing the patient's finger and thumb in the direction of extension while instructing the patient to hold against the resistance (Figure 7-12).

Positive Finding

A positive finding is weakness; the patient is unable to withstand the clinician's resistance, indicating possible involvement of the C8 spinal nerve root. A complementary finding of weakness in thumb extension increases the likelihood of C8 nerve root involvement. Bilateral strength deficits could be indicative of a central nervous system lesion or simply of weakness of the thumb and finger flexor muscles.

Special Considerations

Perform the test bilaterally to allow for strength comparisons. The clinician should apply the resistance in a slow, controlled manner, progressing in intensity as tolerated by the patient. A finding of pain or pain and weakness is more indicative of contractile tissue involvement (muscle, tendon, or bony insertion of tendon) and is not indicative of spinal nerve root involvement.

References

Hoppenfeld S. *Orthopaedic Neurology*. Baltimore, MD: Lippincott-Raven; 1997.

Hoppenfeld S. *Physical Examination of the Spine and Extremities*. East Norwalk, CT: Appleton-Century-Crofts; 1976.

Magee DJ. *Orthopedic Physical Assessment*. 4th ed. Philadelphia, PA: W.B. Saunders; 2002.

Meadows JTS. *Orthopedic Differential Diagnosis in Physical Therapy*. New York: McGraw-Hill; 1999.

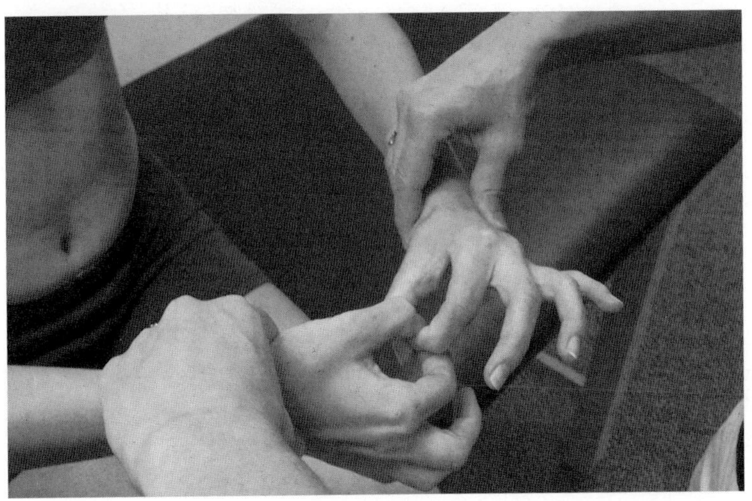

Figure 7-11

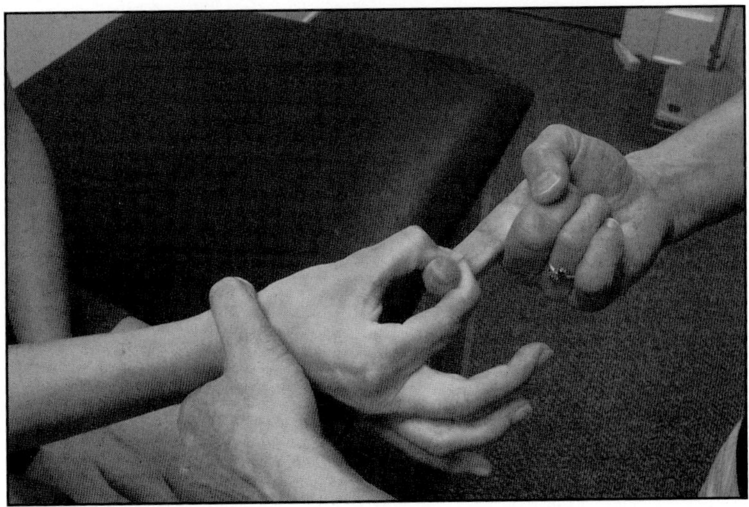

Figure 7-12

C8 Myotome Test: Thumb Extension

Test Position

The patient is positioned in sitting.

Action

The clinician instructs the patient to extend the MCP joint of his or her thumb to end-range. The clinician then instructs the patient to hold his or her thumb in this position while the clinician applies resistance. The clinician places the stabilization hand just proximal to the MCP joint of the thumb (dorsal side) and the resistance finger just proximal to the IP joint of the thumb (dorsal side). The clinician applies a force in the direction of thumb flexion while instructing the patient to hold against the resistance (Figure 7-13).

Positive Finding

A positive finding is weakness; the patient is unable to withstand the clinician's resistance, indicating possible involvement of the C8 spinal nerve root. Complementary findings of weakness in finger flexion and/or thumb flexion increases the likelihood of C8 nerve root involvement. Bilateral strength deficits could be indicative of a central nervous system lesion or simply of weakness of the extensor pollicis longus and extensor pollicis brevis muscles.

Special Considerations

Perform the test bilaterally to allow for strength comparisons. The clinician should apply resistance to the thumb using a single finger. The clinician should apply the resistance in a slow, controlled manner, progressing in intensity as tolerated by the patient. A finding of pain or pain and weakness is more indicative of contractile tissue involvement (muscle, tendon, or bony insertion of tendon) and is not indicative of spinal nerve root involvement.

References

Hoppenfeld S. *Orthopaedic Neurology*. Baltimore, MD: Lippincott-Raven; 1997.

Hoppenfeld S. *Physical Examination of the Spine and Extremities*. East Norwalk, CT: Appleton-Century-Crofts; 1976.

Magee DJ. *Orthopedic Physical Assessment*. 4th ed. Philadelphia, PA: W.B. Saunders; 2002.

Meadows JTS. *Orthopedic Differential Diagnosis in Physical Therapy*. New York: McGraw-Hill; 1999.

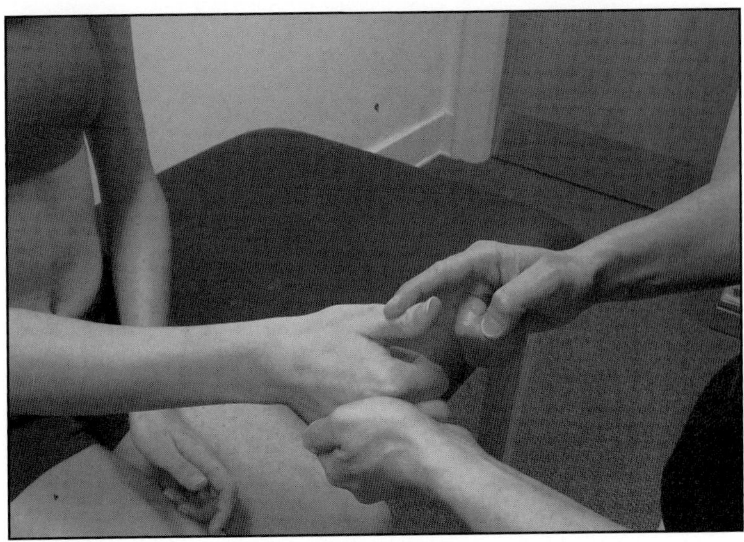

FIGURE 7-13

T1 Myotome Test: Finger Abduction

Test Position

The patient is positioned in sitting.

Action

The clinician instructs the patient to abduct his or her fingers to end-range. The clinician then instructs the patient to hold his or her fingers in this position while the clinician applies resistance. Resistance is applied to two fingers at a time. The clinician applies a force in the direction of finger adduction while instructing the patient to hold against the resistance (Figure 7-14).

Positive Finding

A positive finding is weakness; the patient is unable to withstand the clinician's resistance, indicating possible involvement of the T1 spinal nerve root. A complementary finding of weakness in finger adduction increases the likelihood of T1 nerve root involvement. Bilateral strength deficits could be indicative of a central nervous system lesion or simply of weakness of the dorsal interossei muscles.

Special Considerations

False-positive findings of weakness are not unusual when testing the T1 myotomes due to the mechanical disadvantage of the muscles being tested. The clinician should carefully perform the test bilaterally to allow for strength comparisons. The clinician should apply resistance using a single finger and the thumb on each side of the test fingers. The clinician should apply the resistance in a slow, controlled manner, progressing in intensity as tolerated by the patient. A finding of pain or pain and weakness is more indicative of contractile tissue involvement (muscle, tendon, or bony insertion of tendon) and is not indicative of spinal nerve root involvement.

References

Hoppenfeld S. *Orthopaedic Neurology*. Baltimore, MD: Lippincott-Raven; 1997.

Hoppenfeld S. *Physical Examination of the Spine and Extremities*. East Norwalk, CT: Appleton-Century-Crofts; 1976.

Magee DJ. *Orthopedic Physical Assessment*. 4th ed. Philadelphia, PA: W.B. Saunders; 2002.

Meadows JTS. *Orthopedic Differential Diagnosis in Physical Therapy*. New York: McGraw-Hill; 1999.

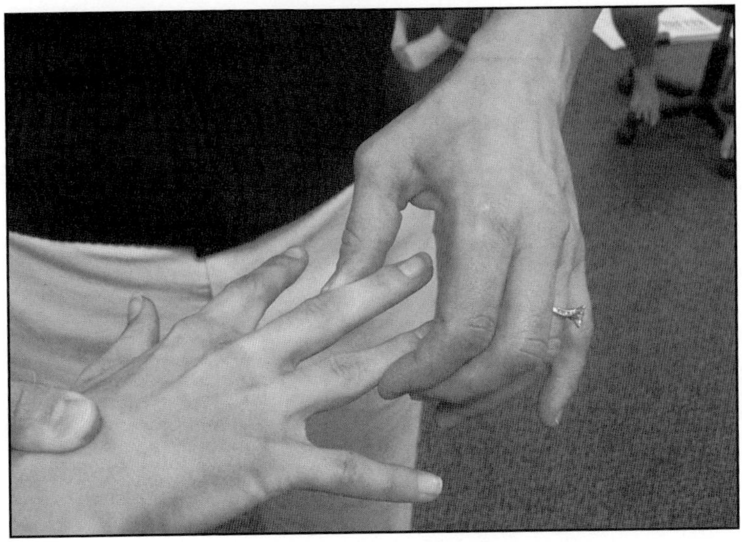

FIGURE 7-14

T1 Myotome Test: Finger Adduction

Test Position

The patient is positioned in sitting.

Action

The clinician instructs the patient to adduct his or her fingers in order to hold a playing card or piece of paper tightly between his or her fingers. The clinician then instructs the patient to hold the object tightly between his or her fingers while the clinician attempts to remove the object by pulling distally (Figure 7-15).

Positive Finding

A positive finding is the inability of the patient to hold the object between his or her fingers, indicating possible involvement of the T1 spinal nerve root. A complementary finding of weakness in finger abduction increases the likelihood of T1 nerve root involvement. Bilateral strength deficits could be indicative of a central nervous system lesion or simply of weakness of the palmar interossei muscles.

Special Considerations

False-positive findings of weakness are not unusual when testing the T1 myotomes due to the mechanical disadvantage of the muscles being tested. The clinician should carefully perform the test bilaterally to allow for strength comparisons. The clinician should attempt to remove the object in a slow, controlled manner, progressing in intensity as tolerated by the patient.

References

Hoppenfeld S. *Orthopaedic Neurology*. Baltimore, MD: Lippincott-Raven; 1997.

Hoppenfeld S. *Physical Examination of the Spine and Extremities*. East Norwalk, CT: Appleton-Century-Crofts; 1976.

Magee DJ. *Orthopedic Physical Assessment*. 4th ed. Philadelphia, PA: W.B. Saunders; 2002.

Meadows JTS. *Orthopedic Differential Diagnosis in Physical Therapy*. New York: McGraw-Hill; 1999.

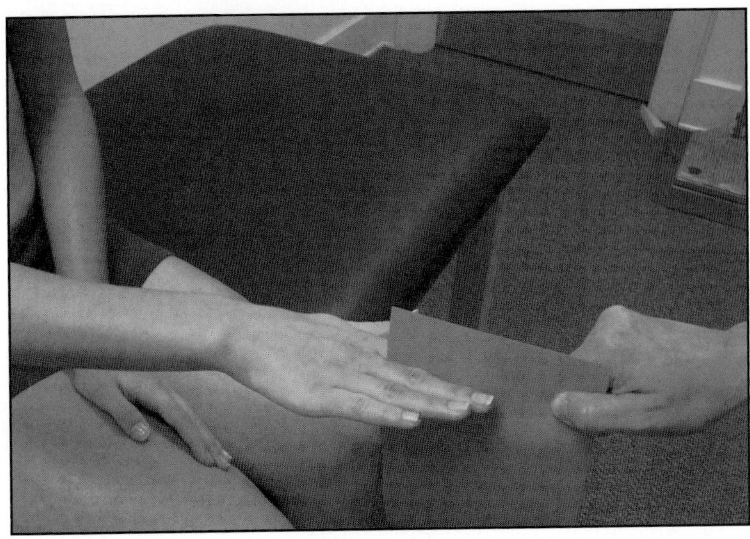

FIGURE 7-15

Chapter

8

Reflex Testing

Deep tendon reflexes are monosynaptic reflexes, meaning they are composed of an afferent (sensory) limb and an efferent (motor) limb with a synapse between the two at the level of the spinal cord. The afferent (sensory) portion of the reflex is stimulated when a quick stretch is applied to the muscle, which occurs when striking an already partially elongated muscle with a reflex hammer. This stimulation results in an efferent (motor) response, resulting in contraction of the muscle being tested.

There are multiple grading scales used when assessing deep tendon reflexes. Each scale assesses for the degree of response of the muscle being tested. Tables 8-1 and 8-2 demonstrate the two most commonly used scales for reflex testing.

Table 8-1

Reflex Grading Scale

Grade	*Clinical Finding*
0*	No reflex elicited
1	Hyporeflexive response elicited
2	Normal reflex elicited
3*	Hyperresponsive reflex elicited

*These grades are generally considered to be indicative of pathology.

Table 8-2

Alternate Reflex Grading Scale

Grade	*Clinical Finding*
0*	No reflex elicited
1+	Minimal response elicited
2+	Normal reflex elicited
3+	Brisk Response elicited
4+*	Hyperresponsive reflex elicited

*These grades are generally considered to be indicative of pathology.

The following guidelines should be followed by the clinician when performing assessment of deep tendon reflexes.

1. The patient should be encouraged to relax as much as possible prior to initiating the test.
2. The clinician should strike the tendon with the reflex hammer such that the hammer is held loosely and allowed to swing freely during testing.
3. Proper force and accuracy is crucial when striking a tendon during deep tendon reflex testing. The clinician may require practice in performing deep tendon reflex testing in order to consistently perform assessments accurately.

Muscle facilitation or reinforcement may be necessary to elicit a deep tendon reflex in some patients. Facilitation or reinforcement involves having the patient perform a strong muscular contraction in a muscle group not being tested. It is important that this facilitation not involve active contraction of a muscle in extremity being tested. Commonly used facilitation techniques for upper extremity deep tendon reflex testing include having the patient press the medial aspects of the feet together (Figure 8-1), pressing the medial aspects of the knees together (Figure 8-2), or having the patient perform isomeric knee extension against the resistance of the contralateral lower extremity (Figure 8-3). The most commonly used facilitation technique for lower extremity reflex testing is to have the patient perform the Jenrassik maneuver—clasp the fingers together and attempt to isometrically pull them apart (Figure 8-4). Alternate techniques for either upper or lower extremity reflex testing include having the patient make a fist with the uninvolved hand or clenching his or her teeth. Muscle facilitation techniques should be performed while the clinician is striking the tendon.

References

Hoppenfeld S. *Orthopaedic Neurology*, Baltimore, MD: Lippincott-Raven; 1997.

Hoppenfeld S. *Physical Examination of the Spine and Extremities*. East Norwalk, CT: Appleton-Century-Crofts; 1976.

Magee DJ. *Orthopedic Physical Assessment*. 4th ed. Philadelphia, PA: W.B. Saunders; 2002.

Meadows JTS. *Orthopedic Differential Diagnosis in Physical Therapy*. New York: McGraw-Hill; 1999.

Reese NB. *Muscle and Sensory Testing*. 2nd ed. Philadelphia, PA: W.B. Saunders; 2005.

Starkey C, Ryan JL. *Evaluation of Orthopedic and Athletic Injuries*. 2nd ed. Philadelphia, PA: F.A. Davis; 2002.

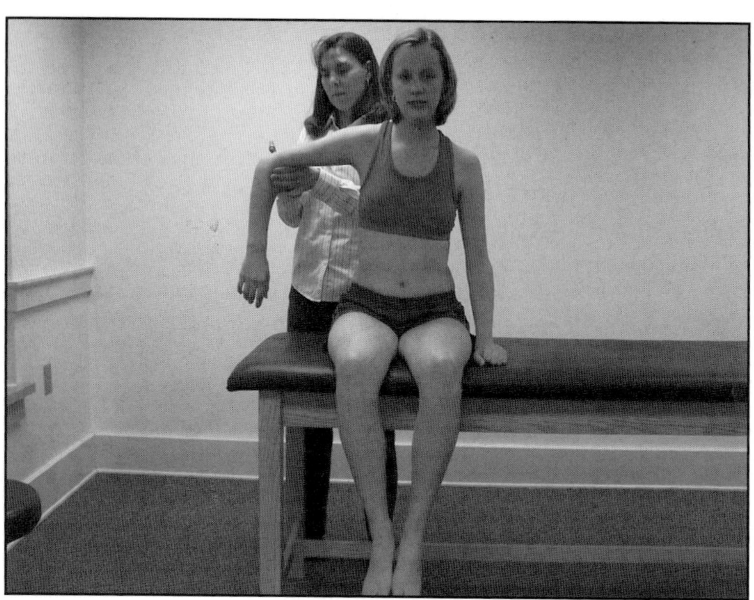

Figure 8-1

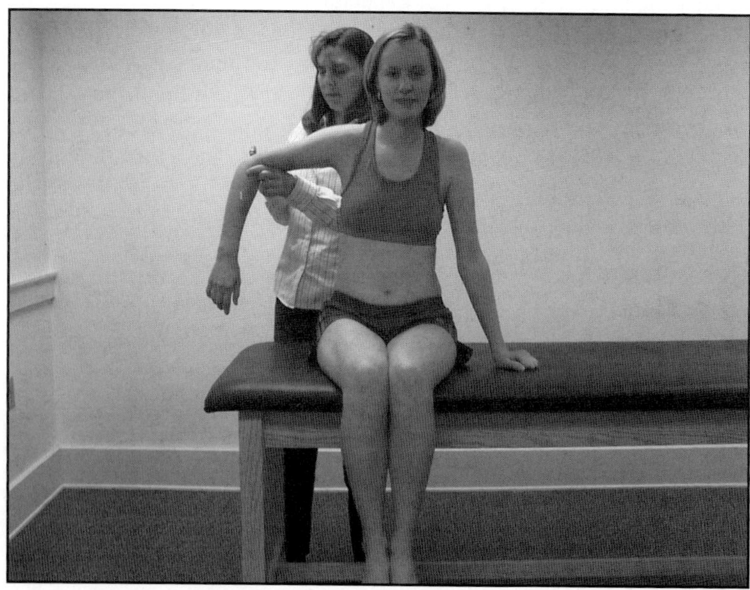

Figure 8-2

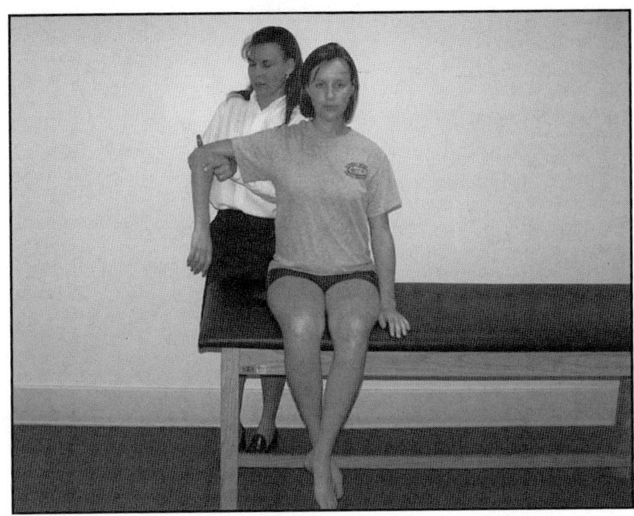

FIGURE 8-3

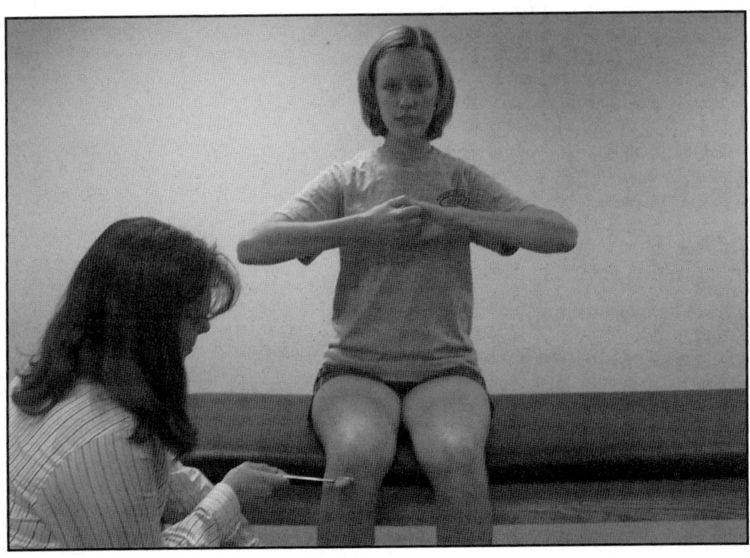

FIGURE 8-4

Biceps Brachii Reflex (C5 Nerve Root) Testing

Test Position

The patient is positioned in sitting or standing with the elbow positioned in flexion and the forearm supinated. The upper extremity on the test side should be supported by the clinician.

Action

The clinician places his thumb over the patient's distal biceps tendon. The clinician strikes the thumb overlying the biceps tendon to elicit a reflex (Figure 8-5).

Positive Finding

A normal response to this test is elbow flexion. The reflex is graded based on the tendon's response (see Tables 8-1 and 8-2).

Special Considerations

Some authors consider this reflex as testing both the C5 and C6 spinal segments. Reflexes should be compared bilaterally, assessing for variations in response that will assist the clinician in differentiating a peripheral nerve injury (unilateral deficits) from a central nervous system injury (bilateral deficits).

Specificity

.95 - .99

Sensitivity

.10 - .24

Positive Likelihood Ratio

.80 - 10

Negative Likelihood Ratio

.91 – 4.9

References

Lauder TD, Dillingham TR, Andary M. Predicting electrodiagnostic outcome in patients with upper limb symptoms: are the history and physical examination helpful? *Arch Phys Med Rehab*. 2000;81:436-441.

Reese NB. *Muscle and Sensory Testing*. 2nd ed. Philadelphia, PA: W.B. Saunders; 2005.

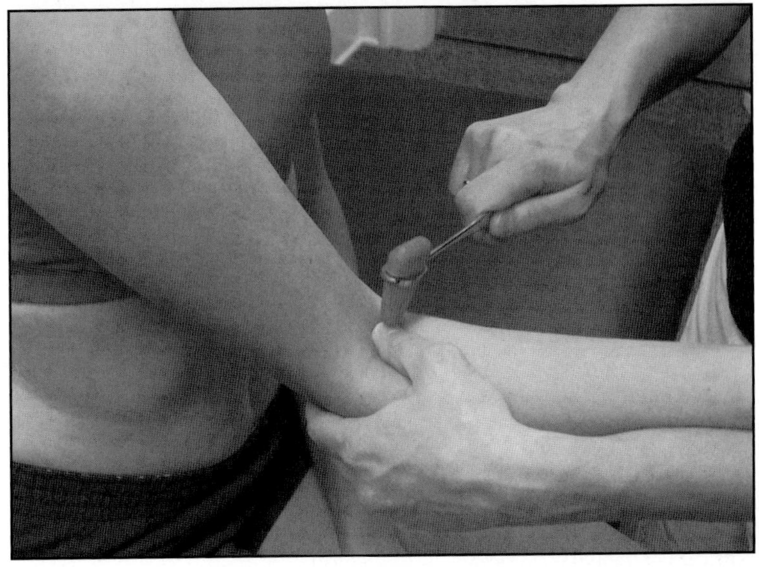

FIGURE 8-5

Starkey C, Ryan JL. *Evaluation of Orthopedic and Athletic Injuries*. 2nd ed. Philadelphia, PA: F.A. Davis; 2002.

Wainner R, Fritz J, Irrgang J, Boninger M, Delito A, Allison S. Reliability and diagnostic accuracy of the clinical examination and patient self-report measures for cervical radiculopathy. *Spine*. 2003;28:52-62.

Brachioradialis Reflex (C6 Nerve Root) Testing

Test Position

The patient is positioned in sitting or standing with the elbow positioned in flexion and the forearm in neutral. The upper extremity on the test side should be supported by the clinician.

Action

The clinician strikes the radial side of the patient's forearm, over the brachioradialis tendon, to elicit a reflex. The clinician may strike the medial side of the forearm just proximal to the radial styloid process (Figure 8-6) or over the proximal third of the medial side of the forearm (Figure 8-7).

Positive Finding

A normal response to this test is elbow flexion. The reflex is graded based on the tendon's response (see Tables 8-1 and 8-2).

Special Considerations

Some authors consider this reflex as testing both the C5 and C6 spinal segments. Reflexes should be compared bilaterally, assessing for variations in response that will assist the clinician in differentiating a peripheral nerve injury (unilateral deficits) from a central nervous system injury (bilateral deficits).

Specificity

.95 – .99

Sensitivity

.06 – .08

Positive Likelihood Ratio

.99 – 8.0

Negative Likelihood Ratio

.93 – 1.2

References

Lauder TD, Dillingham TR, Andary M. Predicting electrodiagnostic outcome in patients with upper limb symptoms: Are the history and physical examination helpful? *Arch Phys Med Rehab*. 2000;81:436-441.

Reese NB. *Muscle and Sensory Testing*. 2nd ed. Philadelphia, PA: W.B. Saunders; 2005.

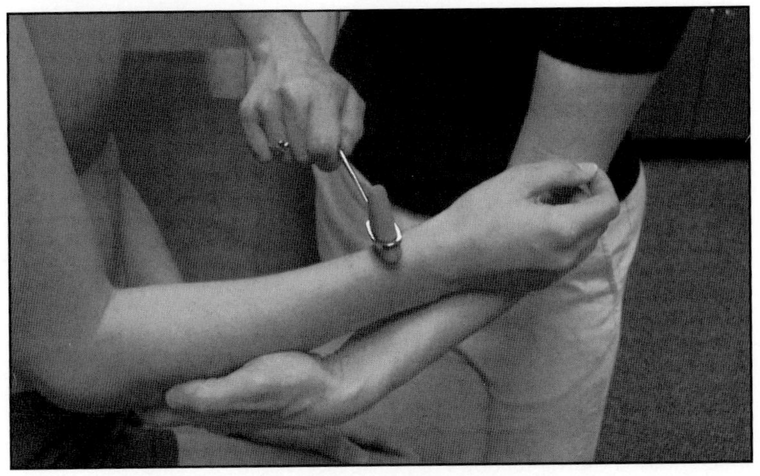

FIGURE 8-6

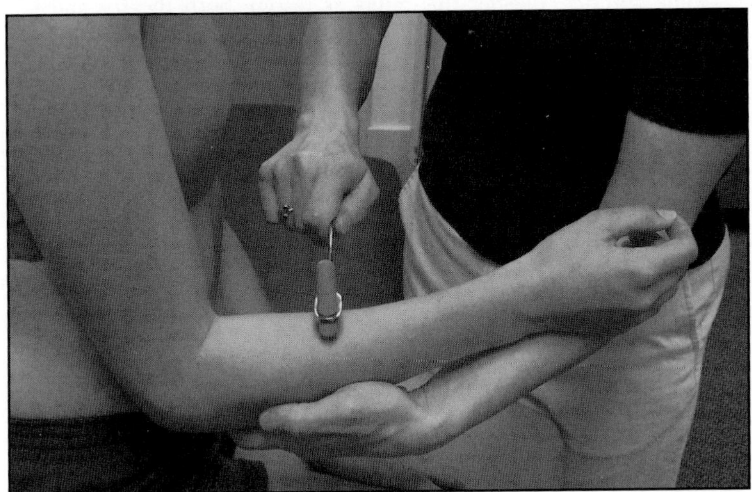

FIGURE 8-7

Starkey C, Ryan JL. *Evaluation of Orthopedic and Athletic Injuries*. 2nd ed. Philadelphia, PA: F.A. Davis; 2002.

Wainner R, Fritz J, Irrgang J, Boninger M, Delito A, Allison S. Reliability and diagnostic accuracy of the clinical examination and patient self-report measures for cervical radiculopathy. *Spine*. 2003;28:52-62.

Triceps Reflex (C7 Nerve Root) Testing

Test Position

The patient is positioned in sitting or standing with the shoulder abducted to 90 degrees with internal rotation and the elbow flexed to approximately 90 degrees. The upper extremity on the test side should be supported by the clinician.

Action

The clinician strikes the triceps tendon just proximal to the olecranon process (Figure 8-8).

Positive Finding

A normal response to this test is elbow extension. The reflex is graded based on the tendon's response (see Tables 8-1 and 8-2).

Special Considerations

Some authors consider this reflex as testing both the C6 and C7 spinal segments. Reflexes should be compared bilaterally, assessing for variations in response that will assist the clinician in differentiating a peripheral nerve injury (unilateral deficits) from a central nervous system injury (bilateral deficits).

Specificity

.93 - .95

Sensitivity

.03 - .10

Positive Likelihood Ratio

1.05 - 2.0

Negative Likelihood Ratio

.95 - 40

References

Lauder TD, Dillingham TR, Andary M. Predicting electrodiagnostic outcome in patients with upper limb symptoms: are the history and physical examination helpful? *Arch Phys Med Rehab*. 2000;81:436-441.

Reese NB. *Muscle and Sensory Testing*. 2nd ed. Philadelphia, PA: W.B. Saunders; 2005.

Starkey C, Ryan JL. *Evaluation of Orthopedic and Athletic Injuries*. 2nd ed. Philadelphia, PA: F.A. Davis; 2002.

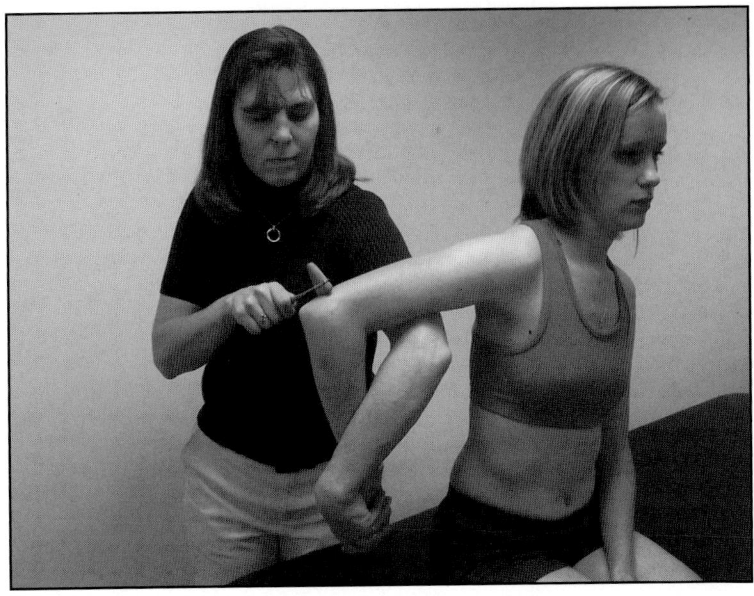

FIGURE 8-8

Tarkka IM, Hayes KC. Characteristics of the triceps brachii tendon reflex in man. *American Journal of Physical Medicine*; 1983;62(1):1-11.

Wainner R, Fritz J, Irrgang J, Boninger M, Delito A, Allison S. Reliability and diagnostic accuracy of the clinical examination and patient self-report measures for cervical radiculopathy. *Spine*. 2003;28:52-62

Chapter

9

Special Tests for the Cervical Spine

Brachial Plexus Traction Test

Test Position

The patient is positioned in sitting.

Action

The clinician places one hand on the side of the patient's head and the other hand on the superior aspect of the patient's shoulder. The clinician passively laterally flexes the cervical spine away from the test side while simultaneously applying downward pressure on the patient's shoulder (Figure 9-1).

Positive Finding

A positive test is radiating pain and symptoms into the patient's upper extremity on the side opposite the direction of cervical spine lateral flexion. For example, pain will be noted in the left upper extremity with passive cervical spine flexion to the right. A positive test opposite the direction of cervical spine lateral flexion is indicative of a traction injury to the brachial plexus.

Special Considerations

Cervical spine pain may also be found on the same side as the cervical spine lateral flexion. A positive test for pain on the side of cervical spine lateral flexion is indicative of a compression injury such as a facet dysfunction or nerve root compression. This test should be performed bilaterally.

Alternate Names

This test is also known as the *Brachial Plexus Stretch Test*.

Specificity

No data available.

Sensitivity

No data available.

References

Konin JG, Wiksten DL, Isear JA, Brader H. *Special Tests for Orthopedic Examination.* 3rd ed. Thorofare, NJ: SLACK Incorporated; 2005.

Magee DJ. *Orthopedic Physical Assessment.* 4th ed. Philadelphia, PA: W.B. Saunders; 2002.

Starkey C, Ryan JL. *Evaluation of Orthopedic and Athletic Injuries.* 2nd ed. Philadelphia, PA: F.A. Davis; 2002.

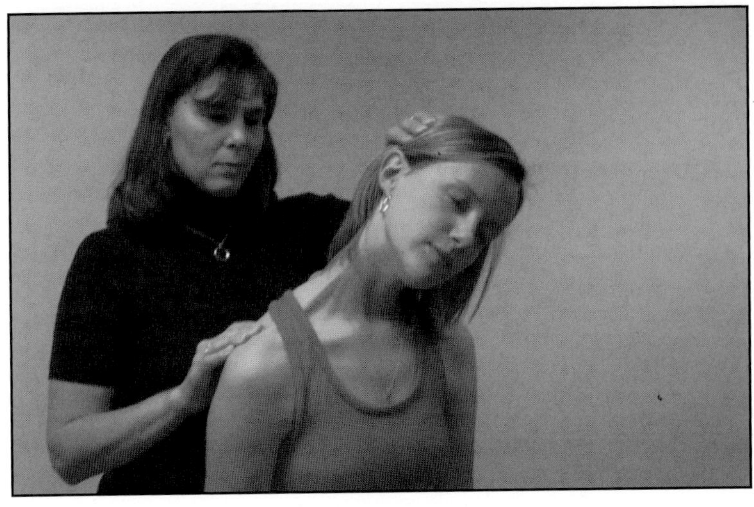

FIGURE 9-1

Upper Limb Tension Test (ULTT) 1: Median Nerve Bias

Test Position

The patient is positioned in supine.

Action

The clinician passively positions the shoulder in depression and abduction to 110 degrees, then positions the forearm in full supination, positions the wrist in full extension, positions the fingers and thumb in full extension, and lastly positions the elbow in full extension. The clinician continues to add components one at a time to the test position until all motions for the shoulder, forearm, wrist, fingers, and elbow have been completed or until the patient reports a positive test. If the test is negative, the clinician may add lateral flexion of the cervical spine to the contralateral side of testing in order to attempt to exacerbate the patient's symptoms (Figures 9-2 and 9-3).

Positive Finding

A positive test is reproduction of the patient's symptoms into the upper extremity. A positive test is indicative of brachial plexus or cervical plexus dysfunction on the side of testing. This particular test is designed to place greater stress on the median nerve.

Special Considerations

The shoulder should remain in a position of depression throughout the performance of this test. This test creates numerous false-positive findings that are related to placing tension on contractile and inert tissues of the upper extremity. Among these false-positive findings are deep aching or stretching sensations in the anterior shoulder; the cubital fossa; the anterior, radial portion of the forearm; and the radial aspect of the hand. These symptoms are often exacerbated by contralateral side-bending of the cervical spine and relieved by ipsilateral side-bending of the cervical spine.

Historical Notes

This test was initially described by Elvey as a single test in 1994. Since its inception, the test has been divided into four separate procedures to assess specific nerves of the upper extremity.

Alternate Names

This test is also known as the *Brachial Plexus Tension Test, the Brachial Plexus Tension Test of Elvey,* and the *Elvey Test.*

Reliability

Kappa values at the 95% confidence interval = .76

Specificity

.22

Sensitivity

.44

Positive Likelihood Ratio

.12

Negative Likelihood Ratio

.85

References

Burns R. Neural tension in a female varsity volleyball player. *Athletic Therapy Today*. 2004;9(5):49-51.

Coppieters MW, Stappaerts KH, Everaert DG, Staes FF. A qualitative assessment of shoulder girdle elevation during upper limb tension test I. *Manual Therapy*. 1999;4(1):33-38.

Kleinrensink GJ, Stoeckart R, Mulder PG, et al. Upper limb tension tests as tools in the diagnosis of nerve and plexus lesions: anatomical and biomechanical aspects. *Clinical Biomechanics*. 2000;15(1):9-14.

Magee DJ. *Orthopedic Physical Assessment*. 4th ed. Philadelphia, PA: W.B. Saunders; 2002.

Rubinstein SM, Pool JJ, van Tulder MW, Riphagen II, de Vet HC. A systematic review of the diagnostic accuracy of provocative tests of the neck for diagnosing cervical radiculopathy. *European Spine Journal*. 2007;16(3):307-319.

Wainner R, Fritz J, Irrgang J, Boninger M, Delitto A, Allison S. Reliability and diagnostic accuracy of the clinical examination and patient self-report measures for cervical radiculopathy. *Spine*. 2003;28(1):52-62.

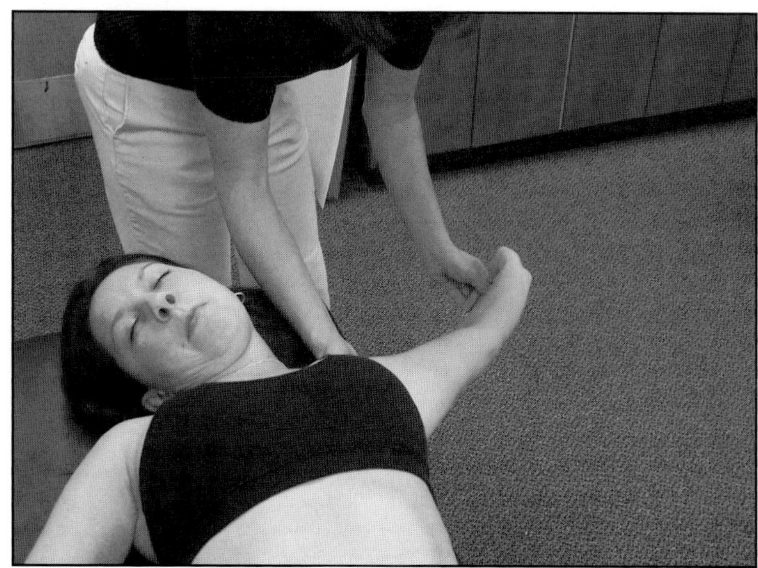

FIGURE 9-2

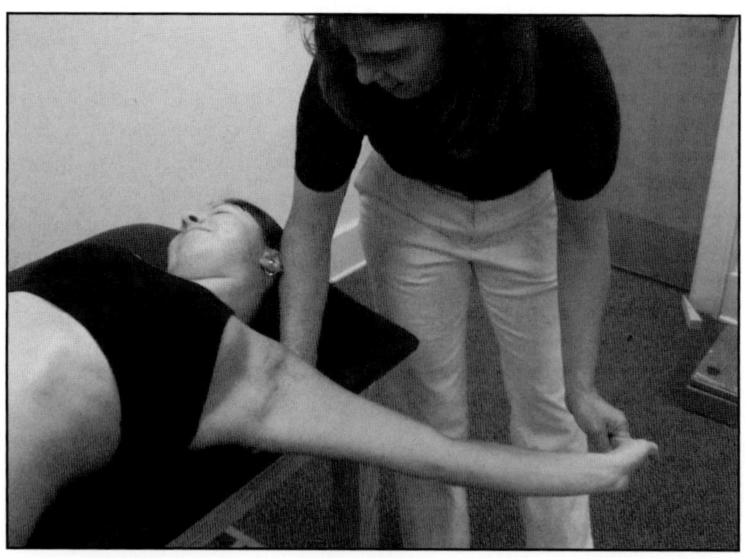

FIGURE 9-3

ULTT 2: Median, Musculocutaneous, and Axillary Nerve Bias

Test Position

The patient is positioned in supine.

Action

The clinician passively positions the shoulder in depression and abduction to 10 degrees, then positions the forearm in full supination, then positions the wrist in full extension, positions the fingers and thumb in full extension, positions the shoulder in external rotation, and lastly positions the elbow in full extension. The clinician continues to add components one at a time to the test position until all motions for the shoulder, forearm, wrist, fingers, and elbow have been completed or until the patient reports a positive test. If the test is negative, the clinician may add lateral flexion of the cervical spine to the contralateral side of testing in order to attempt to exacerbate the patient's symptoms (Figure 9-4).

Positive Finding

A positive test is reproduction of the patient's symptoms into the upper extremity. A positive test is indicative of brachial plexus or cervical plexus dysfunction on the side of testing. This particular test is designed to place greater stress on the median, musculocutaneous, and axillary nerves.

Special Considerations

The shoulder should remain in a position of depression throughout the performance of this test. This test creates numerous false-positive findings that are related to placing tension on contractile and inert tissues of the upper extremity. Among these false-positive findings are deep aching or stretching sensations in the anterior shoulder; the cubital fossa; the anterior, radial portion of the forearm; and the radial aspect of the hand. These symptoms are often exacerbated by contralateral side-bending of the cervical spine and relieved by ipsilateral side-bending of the cervical spine.

Historical Notes

This test was initially described by Elvey as a single test in 1994. Since its inception, the test has been divided into four separate procedures to assess specific nerves of the upper extremity.

Alternate Names

This test is also known as the *Brachial Plexus Tension Test*, the *Brachial Plexus Tension Test of Elvey*, and the *Elvey Test*.

Reliability

Kappa values at the 95% confidence interval = .83

Specificity

No data available.

Sensitivity

No data available.

References

Burns R. Neural tension in a female varsity volleyball player. *Athletic Therapy Today*. 2004;9(5):49-51.

Kleinrensink GJ, Stoeckart R, Mulder PG, et al. Upper limb tension tests as tools in the diagnosis of nerve and plexus lesions: anatomical and biomechanical aspects. *Clinical Biomechanics*. 2000;15(1):9-14.

Magee DJ. *Orthopedic Physical Assessment*. 4th ed. Philadelphia, PA: W.B. Saunders; 2002.

Rubinstein SM, Pool JJ, van Tulder MW, Riphagen II, de Vet HC. A systematic review of the diagnostic accuracy of provocative tests of the neck for diagnosing cervical radiculopathy. *European Spine Journal*. 2007;16(3):307-319.

Wainner R, Fritz J, Irrgang J, Boninger M, Delitto A, Allison S. Reliability and diagnostic accuracy of the clinical examination and patient self-report measures for cervical radiculopathy. *Spine*. 2003;28(1):52-62.

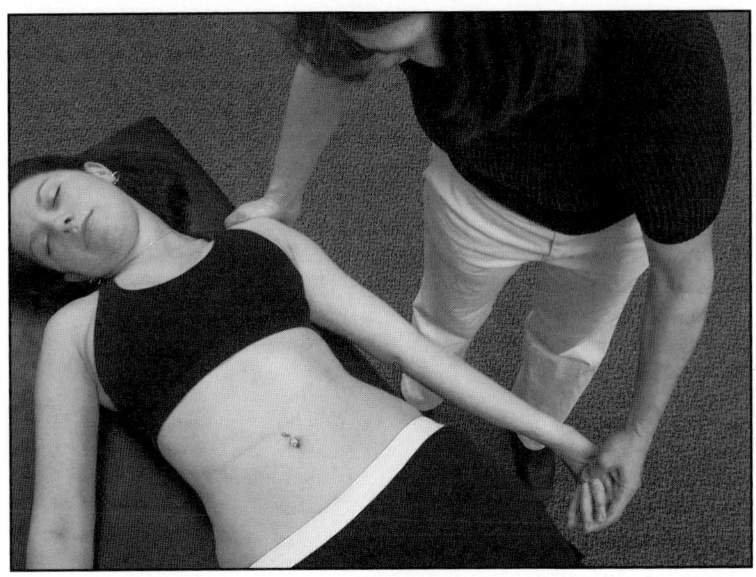

FIGURE 9-4

ULTT 3: Radial Nerve Bias

Test Position

The patient is positioned in supine.

Action

The clinician passively positions the shoulder in depression and abduction to 10 degrees, positions the forearm in full pronation, positions the wrist in full flexion and ulnar deviation, positions the fingers and thumb in full flexion, positions the shoulder in internal rotation, and lastly positions the elbow in full extension. The clinician continues to add components one at a time to the test position until all motions for the shoulder, forearm, wrist, fingers, and elbow have been completed or until the patient reports a positive test. If the test is negative, the clinician may add lateral flexion of the cervical spine to the contralateral side of testing in order to attempt to exacerbate the patient's symptoms (Figure 9-5).

Positive Finding

A positive test is reproduction of the patient's symptoms into the upper extremity. A positive test is indicative of brachial plexus or cervical plexus dysfunction on the side of testing. This particular test is designed to place greater stress on the radial nerve.

Special Considerations

The shoulder should remain in a position of depression throughout the performance of this test. This test creates numerous false-positive findings that are related to placing tension on contractile and inert tissues of the upper extremity. Among these false-positive findings are deep aching or stretching sensations in the anterior shoulder; the cubital fossa; the anterior, radial portion of the forearm; and the radial aspect of the hand. These symptoms are often exacerbated by contralateral side-bending of the cervical spine and relieved by ipsilateral side-bending of the cervical spine.

Historical Notes

This test was initially described by Elvey as a single test in 1994. Since its inception, the test has been divided into four separate procedures to assess specific nerves of the upper extremity.

Alternate Names

This test is also known as the *Brachial Plexus Tension Test*, the *Brachial Plexus Tension Test of Elvey*, and the *Elvey Test*.

Specificity

.33

Sensitivity

.97

Positive Likelihood Ratio

.85

Negative Likelihood Ratio

1.1

References

Burns R. Neural tension in a female varsity volleyball player. *Athletic Therapy Today*. 2004;9(5):49-51.

Kleinrensink GJ, Stoeckart R, Mulder PG, et al. Upper limb tension tests as tools in the diagnosis of nerve and plexus lesions: Anatomical and biomechanical aspects. *Clinical Biomechanics*. 2000;15(1):9-14.

Magee DJ. *Orthopedic Physical Assessment*. 4th ed. Philadelphia, PA: W.B. Saunders; 2002.

Rubinstein SM, Pool JJ, van Tulder MW, Riphagen II, de Vet HC. A systematic review of the diagnostic accuracy of provocative tests of the neck for diagnosing cervical radiculopathy. *European Spine Journal*. 2007;16(3):307-319.

Wainner R, Fritz J, Irrgang J, Boninger M, Delitto A, Allison S. Reliability and diagnostic accuracy of the clinical examination and patient self-report measures for cervical radiculopathy. *Spine*. 2003;28(1):52-62.

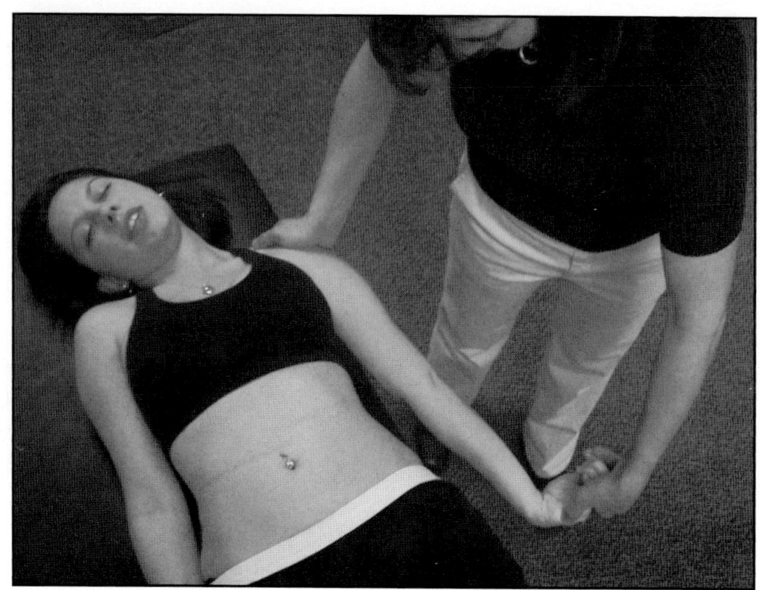

Figure 9-5

ULTT 4: Ulnar Nerve Bias

Test Position

The patient is positioned in supine.

Action

The clinician passively positions the shoulder in depression and abduction to 90 degrees, positions the forearm in full supination, positions the wrist in full extension with radial deviation, positions the fingers and thumb in full extension, positions the shoulder in external rotation, and lastly positions the elbow in full flexion. The clinician continues to add components one at a time to the test position until all motions for the shoulder, forearm, wrist, fingers, and elbow have been completed or until the patient reports a positive test. If the test is negative, the clinician may add lateral flexion of the cervical spine to the contralateral side of testing in order to attempt to exacerbate the patient's symptoms (Figures 9-6 and 9-7).

Positive Finding

A positive test is reproduction of the patient's symptoms into the upper extremity. A positive test is indicative of brachial plexus or cervical plexus dysfunction on the side of testing. This particular test is designed to place greater stress on the ulnar nerve.

Special Considerations

The shoulder should remain in a position of depression throughout the performance of this test. This test creates numerous false-positive findings that are related to placing tension on contractile and inert tissues of the upper extremity. Among these false-positive findings are deep aching or stretching sensations in the anterior shoulder; the cubital fossa; the anterior, radial portion of the forearm; and the radial aspect of the hand. These symptoms are often exacerbated by contralateral side-bending of the cervical spine and relieved by ipsilateral side-bending of the cervical spine.

Historical Notes

This test was initially described by Elvey as a single test in 1994. Since its inception, the test has been divided into four separate procedures to assess specific nerves of the upper extremity.

Alternate Names

This test is also known as the *Brachial Plexus Tension Test*, the *Brachial Plexus Tension Test of Elvey*, and the *Elvey Test*.

Specificity

No data available.

Sensitivity

No data available.

References

Burns R. Neural tension in a female varsity volleyball player. *Athletic Therapy Today*. 2004;9(5):49-51.

Kleinrensink GJ, Stoeckart R, Mulder PG, et al. Upper limb tension tests as tools in the diagnosis of nerve and plexus lesions: Anatomical and biomechanical aspects. *Clinical Biomechanics*. 2000;15(1):9-14.

Magee DJ. *Orthopedic Physical Assessment*. 4th ed. Philadelphia, PA: W.B. Saunders; 2002.

Rubinstein SM, Pool JJ, van Tulder MW, Riphagen II, de Vet HC. A systematic review of the diagnostic accuracy of provocative tests of the neck for diagnosing cervical radiculopathy. *European Spine Journal*. 2007;16(3):307-319.

Wainner R, Fritz J, Irrgang J, Boninger M, Delitto A, Allison S. Reliability and diagnostic accuracy of the clinical examination and patient self-report measures for cervical radiculopathy. *Spine*. 2003;28(1):52-62.

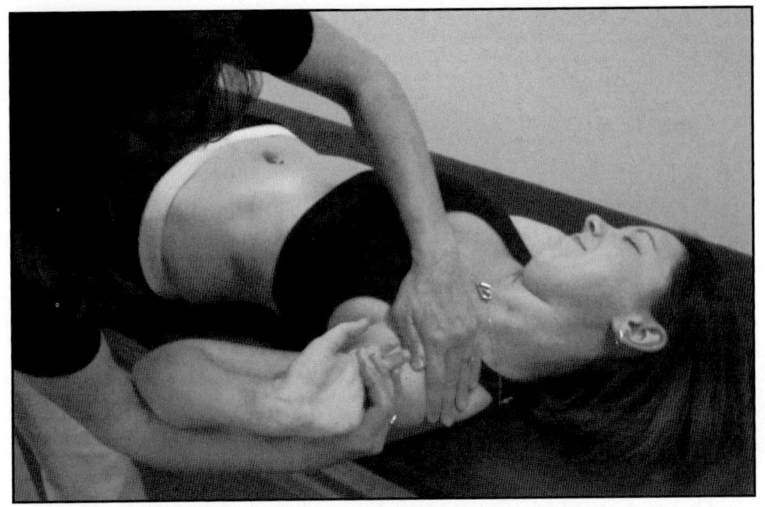

FIGURE 9-6

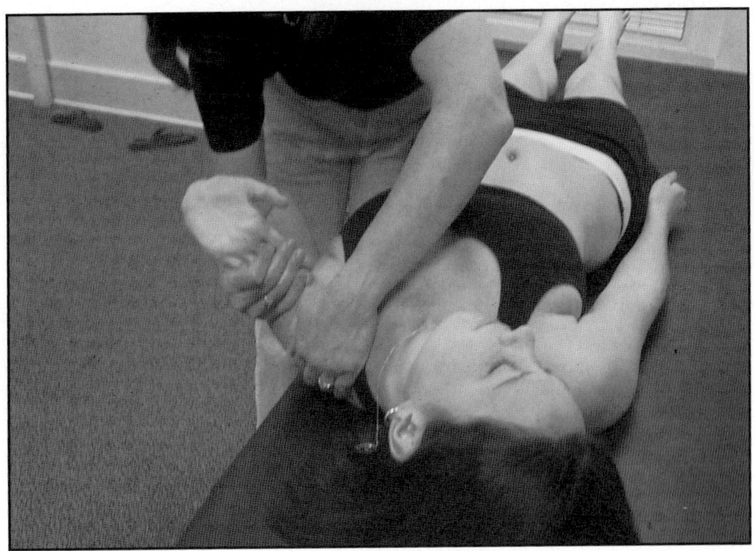

FIGURE 9-7

Shoulder Abduction Test

Test Position

The patient is positioned in sitting.

Action

The clinician instructs the patient to actively abduct the shoulder so that his or her hand rests on top of his or her head (Figure 9-8).

Positive Finding

A positive test is a decrease in the patient's cervical spine pain or upper extremity symptoms, indicating a disc herniation or nerve root compression. A decrease in the patient's pain is hypothesized to be secondary to decreased tension on the involved nerve root.

Special Considerations

This test should be performed bilaterally. The patient may voluntarily demonstrate this posture in order to relieve pain.

Alternate Names

This test is also known as the *Relief Test*.

Reliability

Kappa values at the 95% confidence interval for this range from .20 to .40.

References

Davidson RI, Dunn EJ, Metzmaker JN. The shoulder abduction test in the diagnosis of radicular pain in cervical extradural compressive monoradiculopathies. *Spine*. 1981;6(5):441-446.

Magee DJ. *Orthopedic Physical Assessment*. 4th ed. Philadelphia, PA: W.B. Saunders; 2002.

Malanga GA, Landes P, Nadler SF. Provocative tests in cervical spine examination: historical basis and scientific analyses. *Pain Physician*. 2003;6(2):199-205.

Rubinstein SM, Pool JJ, van Tulder MW, Riphagen II, de Vet HC. A systematic review of the diagnostic accuracy of provocative tests of the neck for diagnosing cervical radiculopathy. *European Spine Journal*. 2007;16(3):307-319.

Viikari-Juntura E. Interexaminer reliability of observations in physical examinations of the neck. *Physical Therapy*. 1987;67:1526-1532.

Viikari-Juntura E, Porras M, Laasonen EM. Validity of clinical tests in the diagnosis of root compression in cervical disc disease. *Spine*. 1989;14(3):253-257.

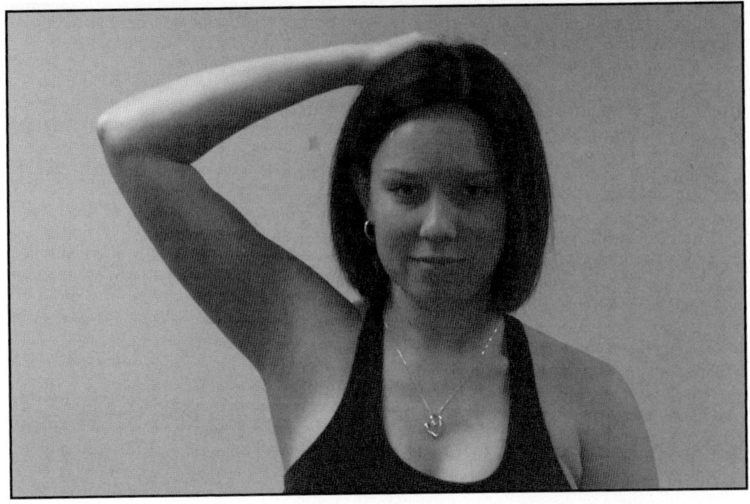

FIGURE 9-8

Wainner R, Fritz J, Irrgang J, Boninger M, Delitto A, Allison, S. Reliability and diagnostic accuracy of the clinical examination and patient self-report measures for cervical radiculopathy. *Spine*. 2003;28:52-62.

Cervical Compression Test

Test Position

The patient is positioned in sitting with the cervical spine in neutral.

Action

The clinician places the volar aspect of both hands on the superior aspect of the patient's head. The clinician applies a compressive force downward on the patient's head (Figure 9-9).

Positive Finding

A positive finding is an increase in pain in the cervical spine, indicative of facet dysfunction or fracture, or increased pain in the upper extremity, indicative of disc herniation, spinal stenosis, or nerve root compression.

Special Considerations

The vertebral artery test should be performed prior to performing a cervical compression test. Caution should be taken when performing this test on a patient with suspected or known spinal stenosis, osteoporosis, osteoarthritis, or rheumatoid arthritis.

Reliability

Kappa values at the 95% confidence interval for this range from .34 to .44, depending on the clinician's knowledge of the patient's history.

References

Bertilson B, Grunnesjo M, Strender L. Reliability of clinical tests in the assessment of patients with neck and shoulder problems. *Spine*; 2003;28:2222-2231.

Konin JG, Wiksten DL, Isear JA, Brader, H. *Special Tests for Orthopedic Examination*. 3rd ed. Thorofare, NJ: SLACK Incorporated; 2006.

Magee DJ. *Orthopedic Physical Assessment*. 4th ed. Philadelphia, PA: W.B. Saunders; 2002.

Starkey C, Ryan JL. *Evaluation of Orthopedic and Athletic Injuries*. 2nd ed. Philadelphia, PA: F.A. Davis; 2002.

Viikari-Juntura E, Porras M, Laasonen EM. Validity of clinical tests in the diagnosis of root compression in cervical disc disease. *Spine*. 1989;14(3):253-257.

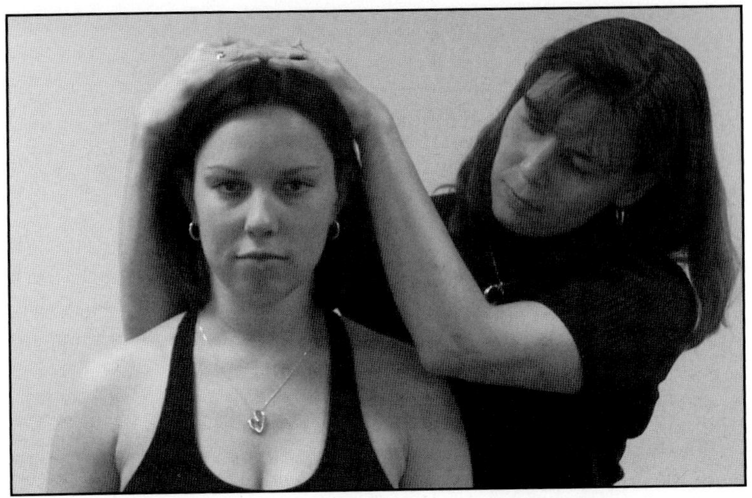

FIGURE 9-9

Spurling's Test

Test Position

The patient is positioned in sitting with the cervical spine in neutral.

Action

The clinician places the volar aspect of both hands on the superior aspect of the patient's head. The clinician applies a compressive force downward on the patient's head while the patient actively laterally flexes his or her cervical spine. The test is repeated with the patient laterally flexing to the opposite side (Figure 9-10).

Test Variations

The clinician may alter the performance of this test by passively laterally flexing the patient's cervical spine while simultaneously applying a compressive force. Additional variations of this test include positioning the patient in slight cervical spine extension and lateral flexion when applying a compressive force (Figure 9-11).

Positive Finding

A positive finding is pain in the upper extremity on the side of lateral flexion. A positive test is indicative of foraminal stenosis and/or nerve root compression on the side of lateral flexion. A finding of cervical spine pain without upper extremity symptoms may indicate the presence of facet dysfunction or fracture.

Special Considerations

This test should be performed bilaterally. The vertebral artery test should be performed prior to performing a cervical compression test. Caution should be taken when performing this test on a patient with suspected or known spinal stenosis, osteoporosis, osteoarthritis, or rheumatoid arthritis.

Historical Notes

This test is named for neurosurgeon Roy Glenwood Spurling, who first described the test in the 1930s.

Alternate Names

This test is also known as *Spurling's Maneuver* and *Spurling's Sign*.

Reliability

Kappa values at the 95% confidence interval for this range from .28 to .62.

References

Bertilson B, Grunnesjo M, Strender L. Reliability of clinical tests in the assessment of patients with neck and shoulder problems. *Spine*. 2003;28:2222-2231.

Konin JG, Wiksten DL, Isear JA, Brader, H. *Special Tests for Orthopedic Examination*. 3rd ed. Thorofare, NJ: SLACK Incorporated; 2006.

Magee DJ. *Orthopedic Physical Assessment*. 4th ed. Philadelphia, PA: W.B. Saunders; 2002.

Malanga GA, Landes P, Nadler SF. Provocative tests in cervical spine examination: historical basis and scientific analyses. *Pain Physician*. 2003;6(2): 199-205.

Rubinstein SM, Pool JJ, van Tulder MW, Riphagen II, de Vet HC. A systematic review of the diagnostic accuracy of provocative tests of the neck for diagnosing cervical radiculopathy. *European Spine Journal*. 2007;16(3):307-319.

Shah KC, Rajshekhar V. Reliability of diagnosis of soft cervical disc prolapse using Spurling's Test. *British Journal of Neurosurgery*. 2004;18(5):480-483.

Starkey C, Ryan JL. *Evaluation of Orthopedic and Athletic Injuries*. 2nd ed. Philadelphia, PA: F.A. Davis; 2002.

Tong HC, Haig AJ, Yamakawa K. The Spurling test and cervical radiculopathy. *Spine*. 2002;27(2):156-159.

Wainner R, Fritz J, Irrgang J, Boninger M, Delitto A, Allison S. Reliability and diagnostic accuracy of the clinical examination and patient self-report measures for cervical radiculopathy. *Spine*. 2003;28:52-62.

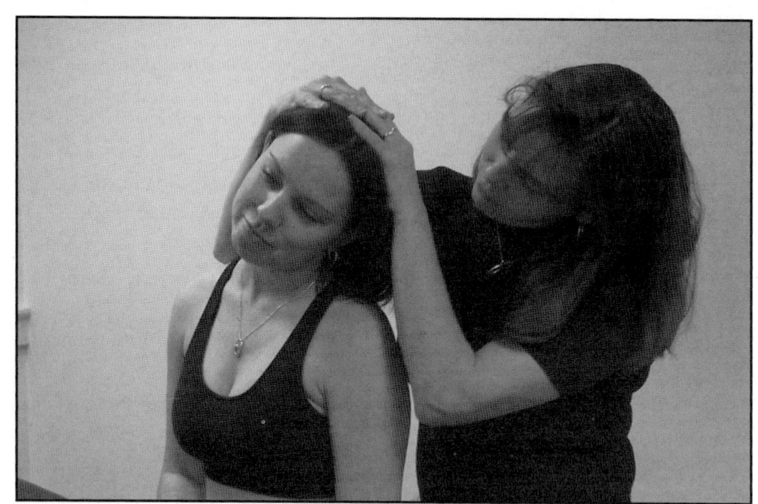

FIGURE 9-10

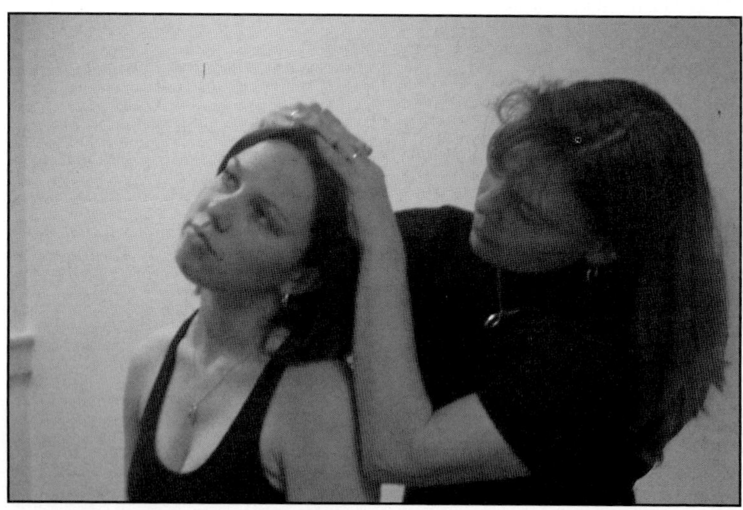

FIGURE 9-11

Cervical Distraction Test

Test Position

The patient is positioned in sitting or supine with the cervical spine in neutral.

Action

The clinician instructs the patient to relax and then applies a traction force to the head, causing distraction of the cervical spine (Figures 9-12 and 9-13).

Positive Finding

A positive finding is a decrease in pain and is indicative of nerve root compression or facet dysfunction.

Special Considerations

This test should not be performed in the presence of known cervical spine instability. A second finding when performing this test is an increase in cervical spine pain and is indicative of a spinous process fracture or ligamentous sprain of the cervical spine.

Alternate Names

This test is also known as the *Foraminal Distraction Test*.

Reliability

Kappa values at the 95% confidence interval for this range from .41 to .88.

References

Bertilson B, Grunnesjo M, Strender L. Reliability of clinical tests in the assessment of patients with neck and shoulder problems. *Spine*. 2003;28:2222-2231.

Konin JG, Wiksten DL, Isear JA, Brader, H. *Special Tests for Orthopedic Examination*. 3rd ed. Thorofare, NJ: SLACK Incorporated; 2006.

Magee DJ. *Orthopedic Physical Assessment*. 4th ed. Philadelphia, PA: W.B. Saunders; 2002.

Malanga GA, Landes P, Nadler SF. Provocative tests in cervical spine examination: historical basis and scientific analyses. *Pain Physician*. 2003;6(2):199-205.

Rubinstein SM, Pool JJ, van Tulder MW, Riphagen II, de Vet HC. A systematic review of the diagnostic accuracy of provocative tests of the neck for diagnosing cervical radiculopathy. *European Spine Journal*. 2007;16(3):307-319.

Starkey C, Ryan JL. *Evaluation of Orthopedic and Athletic Injuries*. 2nd ed. Philadelphia, PA: F.A. Davis; 2002.

Viikari-Juntura E. Interexaminer reliability of observations in physical examinations of the neck. *Physical Therapy*. 1987;67:1526-1532.

Viikari-Juntura E, Porras M, Laasonen EM. Validity of clinical tests in the diagnosis of root compression in cervical disc disease. *Spine*. 1989;14(3): 253-257.

Wainner R, Fritz J, Irrgang J, Boninger M, Delitto A, Allison S. Reliability and diagnostic accuracy of the clinical examination and patient self-report measures for cervical radiculopathy. *Spine*. 2003;28:52-62.

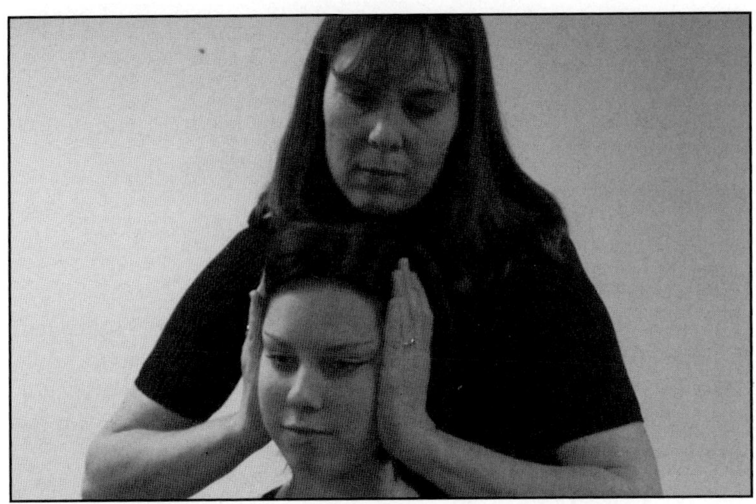

FIGURE 9-12

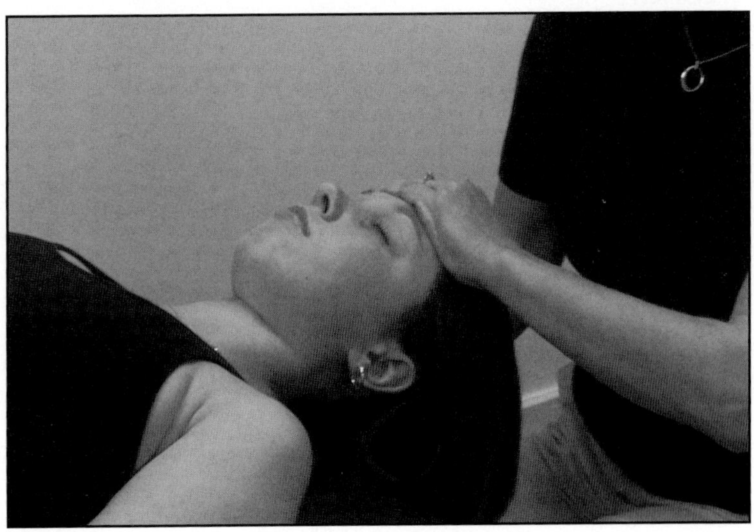

FIGURE 9-13

Swallowing Test

Test Position

The patient is positioned in sitting with the cervical spine in neutral.

Action

The clinician instructs the patient to swallow.

Positive Finding

A positive test is a finding of increased pain or difficulty swallowing. Increased pain as a positive test is indicative of disc herniation, while difficulty swallowing is indicative of anterior cervical spine dysfunction such as tumor, vertebral subluxation, osteophyte formation, or soft tissue swelling.

Special Considerations

A false-positive may occur if the patient is positioned with the cervical spine in extension.

Specificity

No data available.

Sensitivity

No data available.

References

Magee DJ. *Orthopedic Physical Assessment.* 4th ed. Philadelphia, PA: W.B. Saunders; 2002.

Tinel's Sign

Test Position

The patient is positioned in sitting.

Action

The clinician gently taps the cervical spine just anterior to the transverse process of C6, approximately 2 centimeters superior to the clavicle (Figure 9-14).

Positive Finding

A positive finding is the report of increased pain or altered sensation into the ipsilateral upper extremity. A positive test is indicative of a brachial plexus lesion.

Special Considerations

This test should be performed bilaterally. The anatomical region where this test is performed is known as Erb's Point and is believed to be the area where the proximal portion of the brachial plexus is most superficial. The procedure can also be performed in the upper and lower extremities to assess for neurologic dysfunction. These tests are discussed elsewhere in this text.

Historical Notes

This test is named for Jules Tinel, who, in 1915, described the process of nerve regeneration after injury and described a test that involved pressing on the nerve area. In reality, however, it was Paul Hoffmann who, also in 1915, originally described the tapping test to assess for median nerve injury in cases of carpal tunnel syndrome.

Alternate Names

This test is also known as the *Hoffmann-Tinel Sign*, the *Tinel-Hoffmann Sign*, and *Tinel's Symptom*.

Specificity

.83

Sensitivity

.69

Positive Likelihood Ratio

4.06

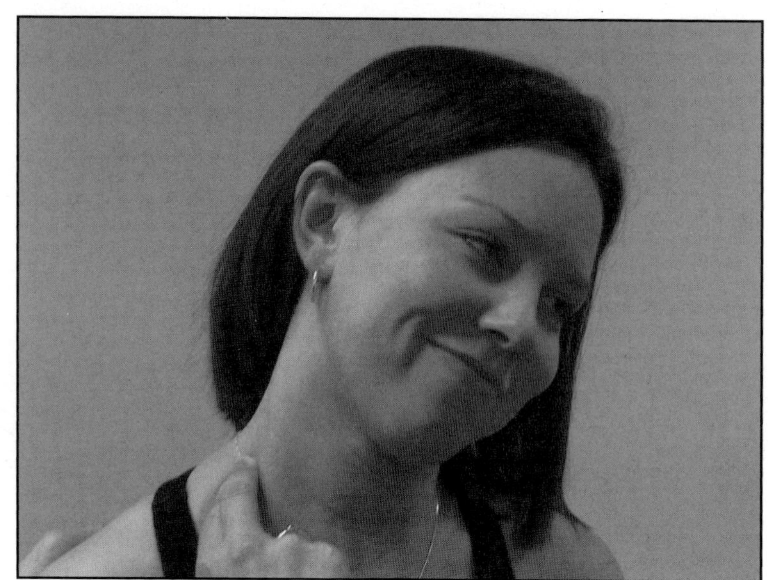

Figure 9-14

Negative Likelihood Ratio

.37

References

Konin JG, Wiksten DL, Isear JA, Brader, H. *Special Tests for Orthopedic Examination.* 3rd ed. Thorofare, NJ: SLACK Incorporated; 2006.

Magee DJ. *Orthopedic Physical Assessment.* 4th ed. Philadelphia, PA: W.B. Saunders; 2002.

Starkey C, Ryan JL. *Evaluation of Orthopedic and Athletic Injuries.* 2nd ed. Philadelphia, PA: F.A. Davis; 2002.

Uchihara T, Furukawa T, Tsukagoshi H. Compression of brachial plexus as a diagnostic test of cervical cord lesion. *Spine.* 1994;19:2170-2173.

Valsalva's Maneuver

Test Position

The patient is positioned in sitting.

Action

The clinician instructs the patient to take a deep breath. The clinician next instructs the patient exhale forcefully into a closed fist (Figure 9-15). An alternate test is to instruct the patient to take a deep breath and hold while bearing down, as if having a bowel movement.

Positive Finding

A positive finding is an increase in spinal pain or peripheral symptoms (pain, numbness or tingling) indicating a space-occupying lesion, such as a disc herniation, tumor, or osteophyte.

Special Considerations

A positive Valsalva's Maneuver results in increased intrathecal pressure which may alter venous return, resulting in dizziness or loss of consciousness. Therefore, the clinician should always be in close proximity to the patient, ready to intervene as needed when performing this test.

Historical Notes

This procedure is named for Antonio Maria Valsalva, a physician who first described the test in the 17th century. The test was first used to assess the patency of Eustachian tubes.

Alternate Names

This test is also known as *Valsalva's Test*.

Specificity

No data available.

Sensitivity

No data available.

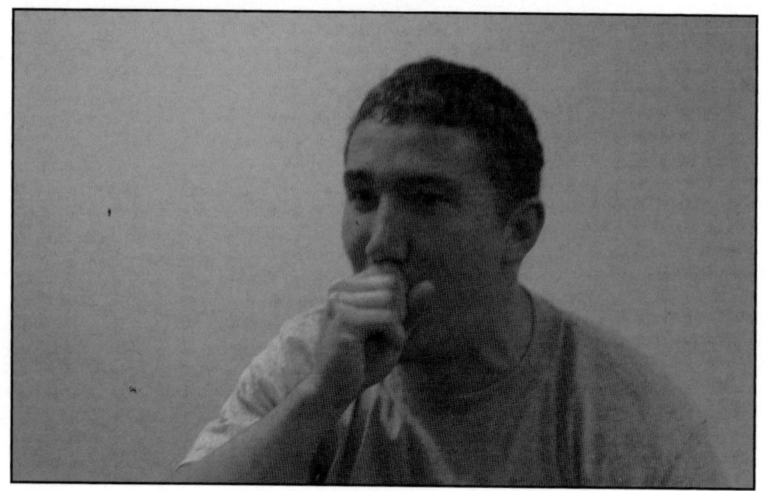

FIGURE 9-15

REFERENCES

Konin JG, Wiksten DL, Isear JA, Brader, H. *Special Tests for Orthopedic Examination*. 3rd ed. Thorofare, NJ: SLACK Incorporated; 2006.

Rubinstein SM, Pool JJ, van Tulder MW, Riphagen II, de Vet HC. A systematic review of the diagnostic accuracy of provocative tests of the neck for diagnosing cervical radiculopathy. *European Spine Journal*. 2007;16(3):307-319.

Starkey C, Ryan JL. *Evaluation of Orthopedic and Athletic Injuries*. 2nd ed. Philadelphia, PA: F.A. Davis; 2002.

Section

THREE

Thoracic Spine

Chapter 10

Dermatome Testing

The following chart presents an overview of selected dermatome testing locations for thoracic spine dermatomes (Figure 10-1). Dermatome testing is most commonly assessed by testing light touch sensation over the desired region. Testing is always performed bilaterally for comparative purposes. Additional tests that may be employed include sharp-dull sensation, two-point discrimination, and temperature sensation. Each of these test procedures is described in greater detail in Chapter 6.

The most common positive test finding during dermatome testing is a loss or a decrease in sensation, indicating injury to a spinal nerve root. However, increased sensitivity during sensory testing, known as hyperesthesia, can also be a positive finding. Hyperesthesia can present in several forms. Extreme sensitivity to pain is known as hyperpathia. Neuralgia is described as "shock-like" sensations throughout a dermatome distribution, while paresthesia (also known as dysesthesia) is described as burning, numbness, and tingling in a dermatome or peripheral nerve distribution in the absence of external stimulus application.

REFERENCES

Hoppenfeld S. *Orthopaedic Neurology*. Baltimore, MD: Lippincott-Raven; 1997.

Hoppenfeld S. *Physical Examination of the Spine and Extremities*. East Norwalk, CT: Appleton-Century-Crofts; 1976.

Magee DJ. *Orthopedic Physical Assessment*. 4th ed. Philadelphia, PA: W.B. Saunders; 2002.

Meadows JTS. *Orthopedic Differential Diagnosis in Physical Therapy*. New York: McGraw-Hill; 1999.

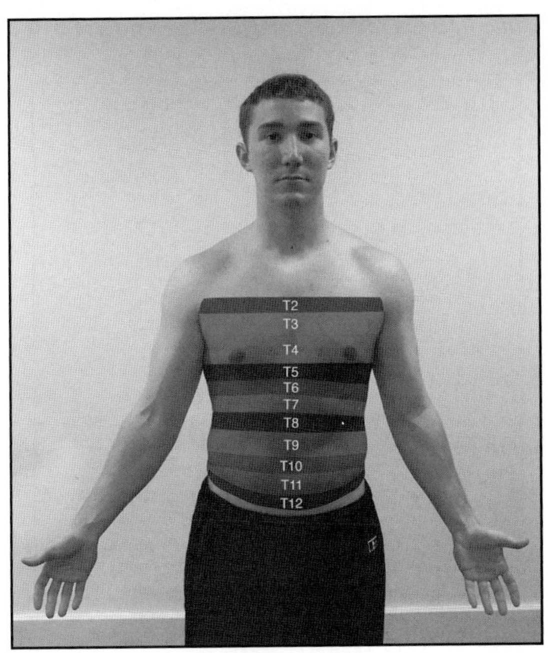

FIGURE 10-1

Table 10-1

THORACIC SPINE DERMATOME TESTING

Nerve Root	*Dermatome*
T1	Medial aspect of upper arm to the axilla
T2	Axilla
T4	Nipple line
T7	Xiphoid process, costal margin
T10	Umbilicus
T12	Anterior superior iliac spine (ASIS)

Individual dermatome locations (Figures 10-2 through 10-6).

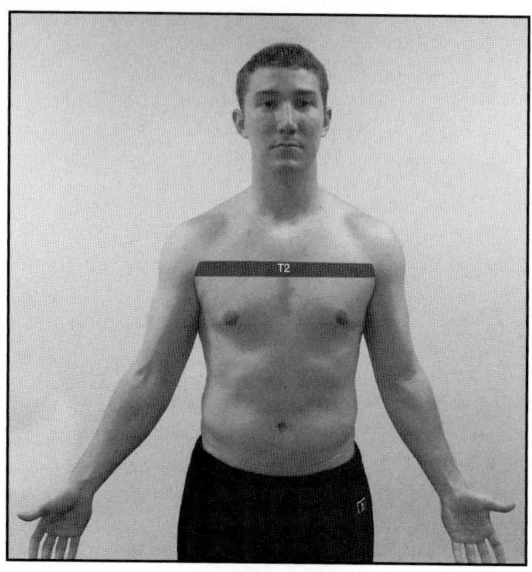

FIGURE 10-2

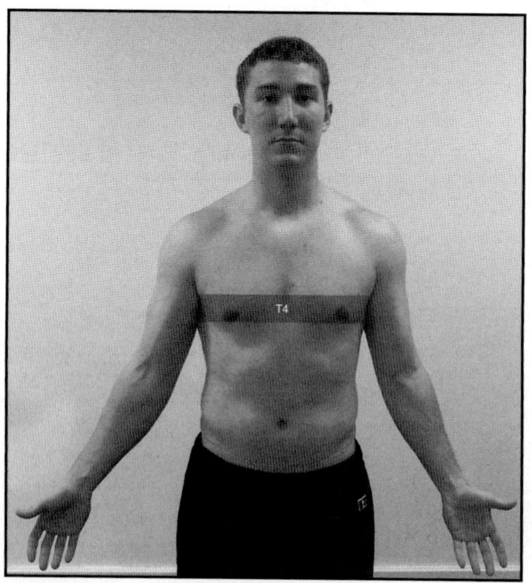

FIGURE 10-3

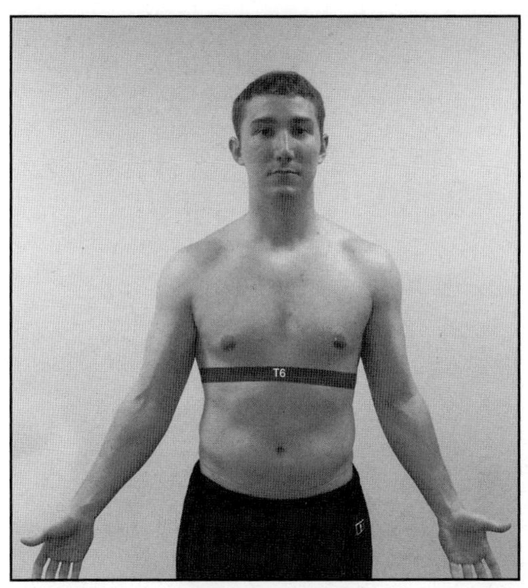

FIGURE 10-4

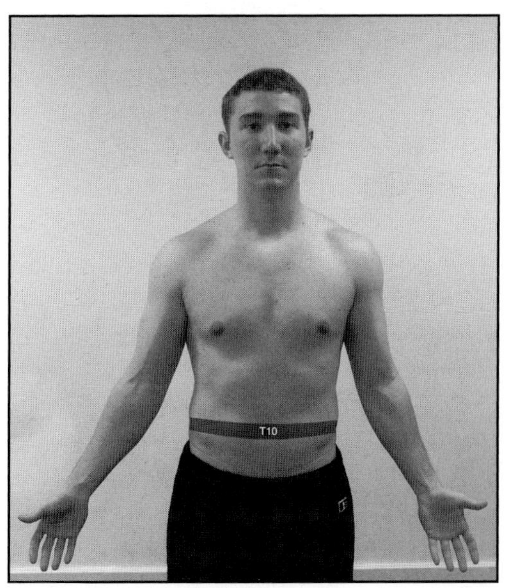

FIGURE 10-5

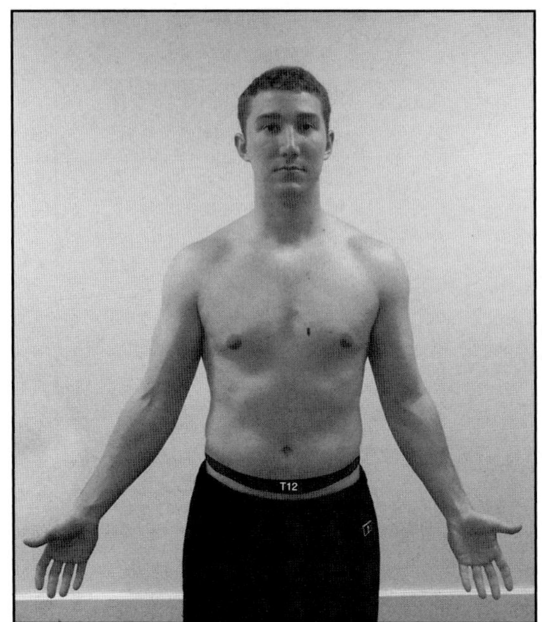

FIGURE 10-6

Chapter

11

Myotome Testing

The following chart presents an overview of myotome testing for spinal nerve roots T2 – T12. Myotome testing involves the performance of "functional tests" to assess muscle strength of the thoracic spine. When testing for myotome function of the thoracic spine, the clinician is assessing multiple spinal levels simultaneously. Myotome testing is not intended to be diagnostic for individual muscle weakness—this is accomplished through the application of specific manual muscle testing—but rather to identify weakness of a group of muscles corresponding to an activity.

Table 11-1

THORACIC SPINE MYOTOMES

Action	*Muscles Active (Nerve Root)*
Trunk Flexion (Thoracic Spine Flexion)	Rectus Abdominus (T5-T12) External Oblique (T7-T12) Internal Oblique (T7-T12)
Trunk Extension (Thoracic Spine Extension)	Spinalis Thoracis (T1-T12) Iliocostalis Thoracis (T1-T12) Longissimus Thoracis (T1-T12) Semispinalis Thoracis (T1-T12) Multifidus (T1-T12) Rotatores (T1-T12)
Trunk Lateral Flexion & Rotation (to the same side)	Iliocostalis Thoracis (T1-T12) Longissimus Thoracis (T1-T12 Internal Oblique (T7-T12
Trunk Lateral Flexion & Rotation (to the opposite side)	Semispinalis Thoracis (T1-T12) External Oblique (T7-T12) Multifidus (T1-T12 Rotatores (T1-T12)
Abdominal Compression	Transverse Abdominus (T7-T12)

Table 11-2

Thoracic Spine Myotome Testing

Muscle (Nerve Root)	*Test Procedure*
Rectus Abdominus (T5–T12)	Supine Trunk Flexion (sit-up) (Figure 11-1)
Internal Obliques (T8–T12) External Obliques (T7–T12)	Trunk Rotation (sit-up with rotation) (Figure 11-2)
Transverse Abdominus (T7–T12)	Assess for anterior abdominal wall bulging during trunk flexion (sit-up) (Figure 11-3)
Spinalis Thoracis (T1–T12) Iliocostalis Thoracis (T1–T12) Longissimus Thoracis (T1–T12) Semispinalis Thoracis (T1–T12) Multifidus (T1–T12) Rotatores (T1–T12)	Prone Trunk Extension (Figure 11-4)

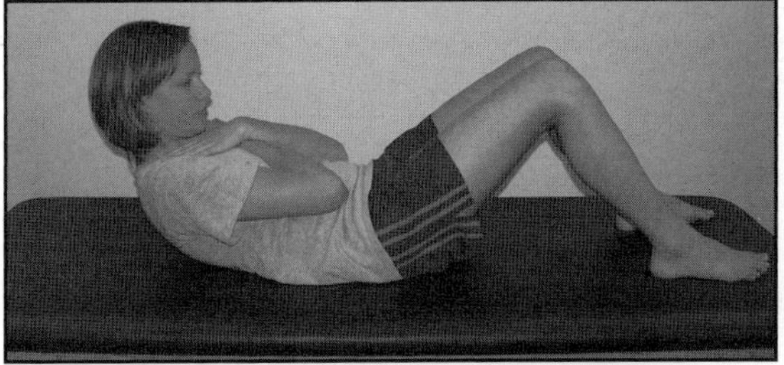

Figure 11-1

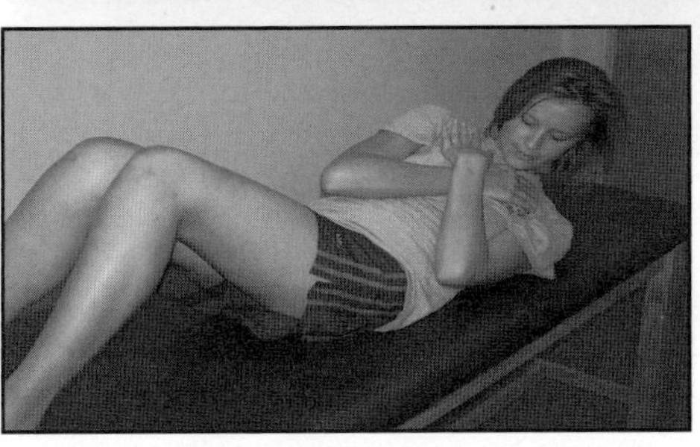

Figure 11-2

References

Hislop H, Montgomery J. *Daniels & Worthingham's Muscle Testing.* 8th ed. Philadelphia, PA: W.B. Saunders.

Kendall FP, Rodgers MM, McCreary EK, Provance PG, Romani WA. *Muscles: Testing and Function with Posture and Pain.* 5th ed. Baltimore, MD: Lippincott, Williams & Wilkins; 2006.

Magee DJ. *Orthopedic Physical Assessment.* 4th ed. Philadelphia, PA: W.B. Saunders; 2002.

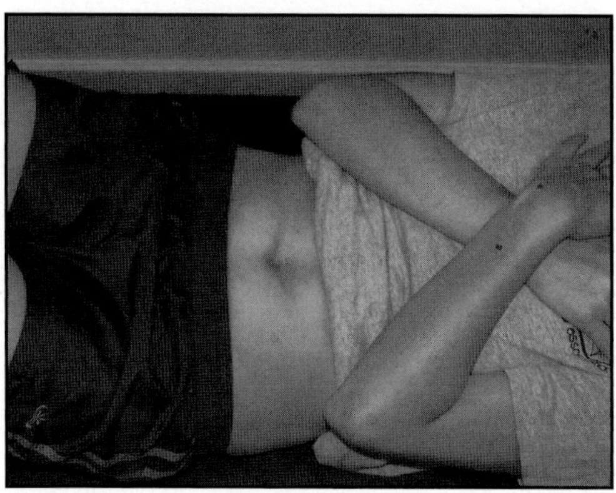

Figure 11-3

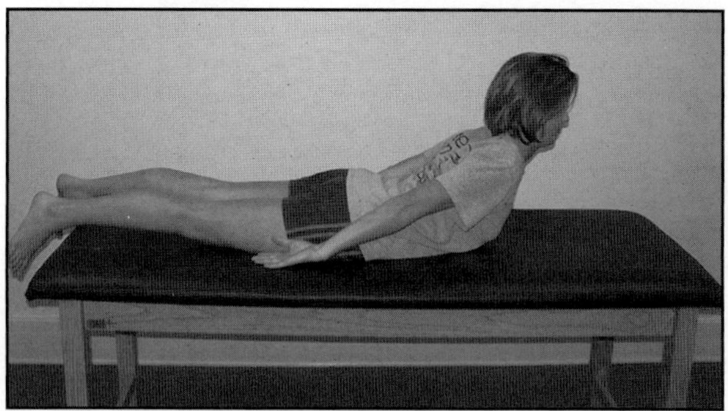

Figure 11-4

Section FOUR

Lumbar Spine

Chapter 12

Dermatome Testing

The following chart presents an overview of dermatome testing location for dermatomes L1 – S2 (Figures 12-1 and 12-2). Dermatome testing is most commonly assessed by testing light touch sensation over the desired region. Testing is always performed bilaterally for comparative purposes. Additional tests that may be employed include sharp-dull sensation, two-point discrimination, and temperature sensation. Each of these test procedures is described in greater detail in Chapter 6.

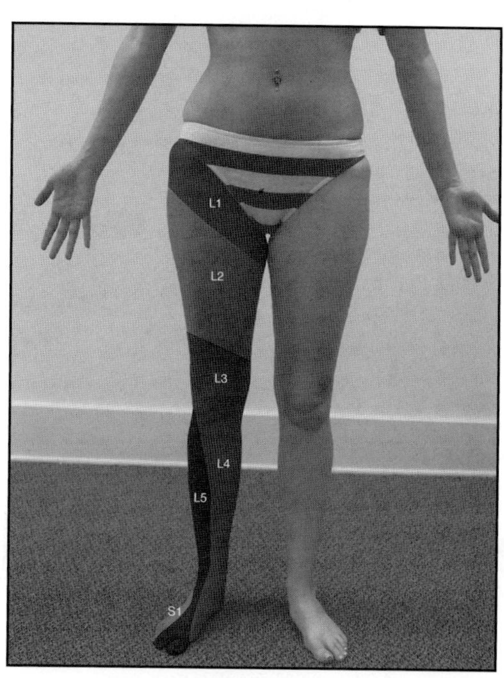

FIGURE 12-1

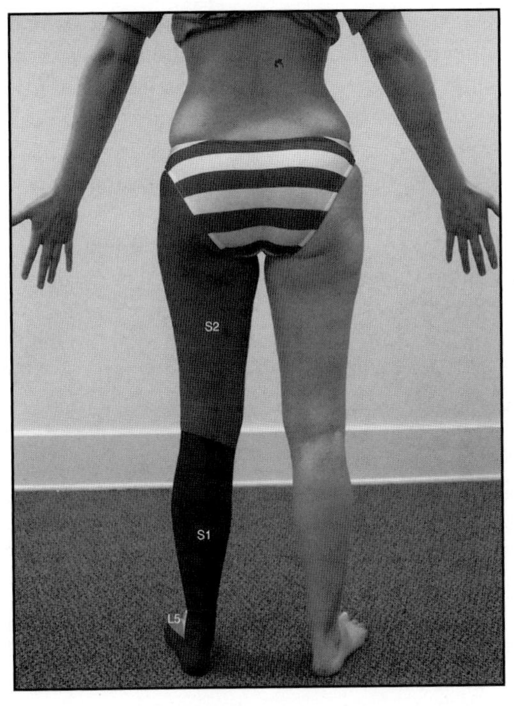

FIGURE 12-2

Table 12-1

LUMBAR SPINE DERMATOMES

Nerve Root	*Dermatome*
L1	Superior lateral hip and groin
L2	Anterior thigh
L3	Patellar region
L4	Inferior knee, medial lower leg, and medial arch
L5	Dorsum of foot and lateral lower leg
S1	Lateral foot and posterior lower leg
S2	Popliteal space and posterior thigh

The most common positive test finding during dermatome testing is a loss or a decrease in sensation, indicating injury to a spinal nerve root or a peripheral nerve. However, increased sensitivity during sensory testing, known as hyperesthesia, can also be a positive finding. Hyperesthesia can present in several forms. Extreme sensitivity to pain is known as hyperpathia. Neuralgia is described as "shock-like" sensations throughout a dermatome or peripheral nerve distribution, while paresthesia (also known as dysesthesia) is described as burning, numbness, and tingling in a dermatome or peripheral nerve distribution in the absence of external stimulus application. Sensory testing of the lumbar dermatomes L3–S1 using pin-prick has been found to demonstrate sensitivity values of .50, specificity values of .62, a positive likelihood ratio of 1.32, and a negative likelihood ratio of .81.

References

Hoppenfeld S. *Orthopaedic Neurology*. Baltimore, MD: Lippincott-Raven; 1997.

Hoppenfeld S. *Physical Examination of the Spine and Extremities*. East Norwalk, CT: Appleton-Century-Crofts; 1976.

Lauder TD, Dillingham TR, Andary M. Effect of history and exam in predicting electrodiagnostic outcome among patients with suspected lumbosacral radicukopathy. *Am J Phys Med Rehab*. 2000;79:60-68.

Magee DJ. *Orthopedic Physical Assessment*. 4th ed. Philadelphia, PA: W.B. Saunders; 2002.

Meadows JTS. *Orthopedic Differential Diagnosis in Physical Therapy*. New York: McGraw-Hill; 1999.

Individual dermatome locations (Figures 12-3 through 12-9):

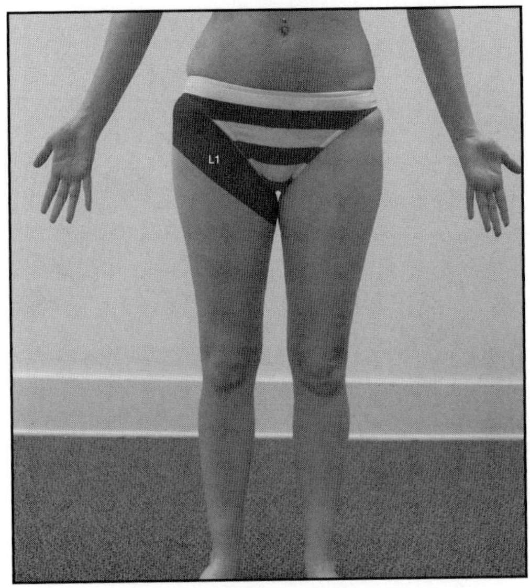

FIGURE 12-3

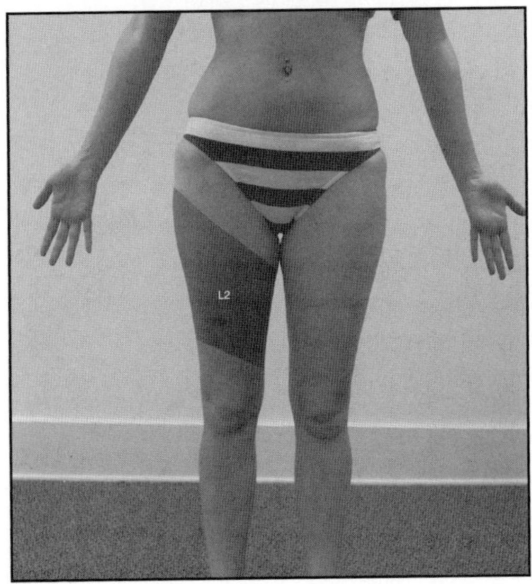

FIGURE 12-4

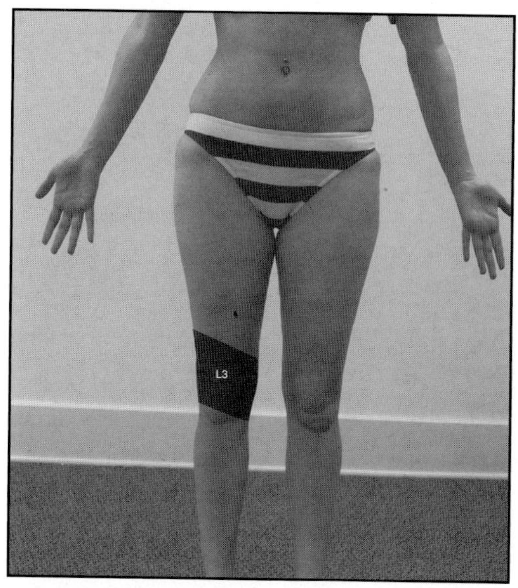

FIGURE 12-5

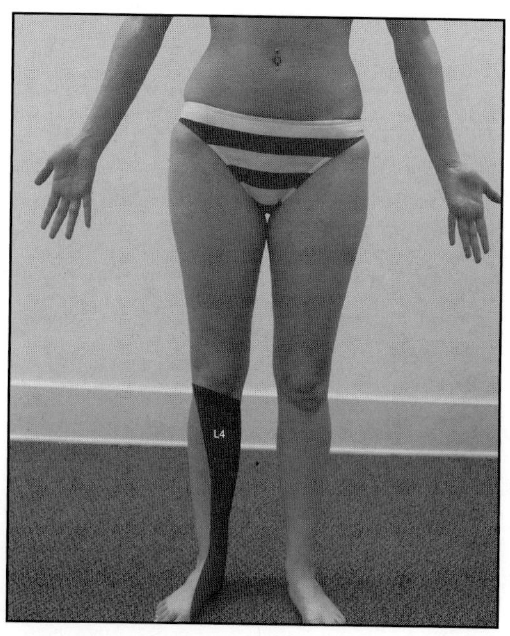

FIGURE 12-6

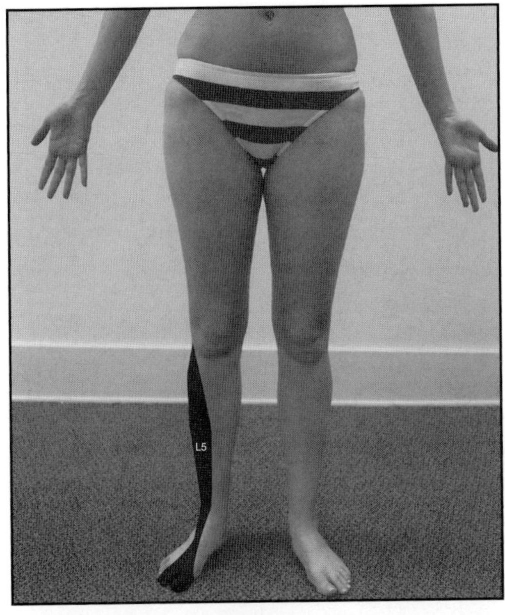

FIGURE 12-7

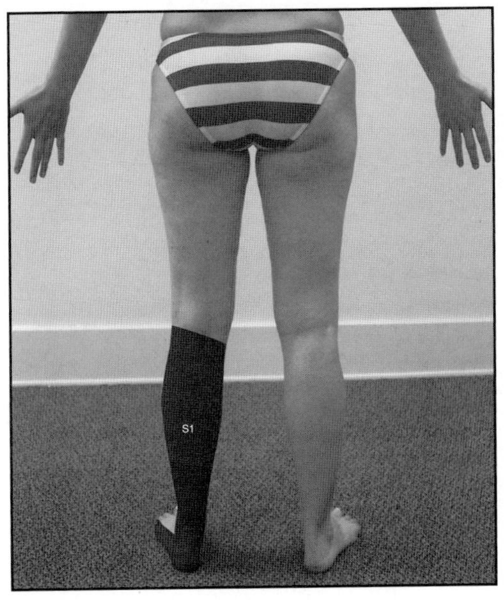

FIGURE 12-8

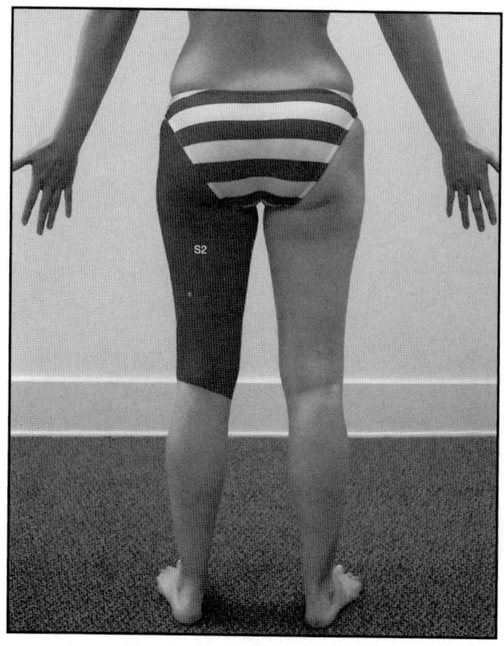

FIGURE 12-9

Chapter

13

Myotome Testing

The following chart presents an overview of myotome testing for spinal nerve roots L1 – S2. Myotome testing involves the performance of "break tests" to assess muscle strength for a given motion. Myotome testing is not intended to be diagnostic for individual muscle weakness—this is accomplished through the application of specific manual muscle testing—but rather to identify weakness of a group of muscles corresponding to a single joint motion. Patterns of muscle weakness can then be related to a single spinal nerve root level. Each of these test procedures will be described in greater detail in this chapter.

Table 13-1

LUMBAR SPINE MYOTOME TESTING

Nerve Root	*Myotome*
L1	Hip flexion
L2	Hip flexion
L3	Knee extension
L4	Ankle dorsiflexion
	Ankle inversion
L5	Great toe extension
S1	Ankle plantarflexion
	Ankle eversion
S2	Knee flexion

REFERENCES

Hoppenfeld S. *Orthopaedic Neurology*. Baltimore, MD: Lippincott-Raven; 1997.

Hoppenfeld S. *Physical Examination of the Spine and Extremities*. East Norwalk, CT: Appleton-Century-Crofts; 1976.

Magee DJ. *Orthopedic Physical Assessment*. 4th ed. Philadelphia, PA: W.B. Saunders; 2002.

Meadows JTS. *Orthopedic Differential Diagnosis in Physical Therapy*. New York: McGraw-Hill; 1999.

L1 and L2 Myotome Test

Test Position

The patient is positioned in sitting with the hip and knee flexed to 90 degrees.

Action

The clinician instructs the patient to flex his or her hip, as if marching in place. The clinician then instructs the patient to hold his or her hip in this position while the clinician applies resistance. The clinician places the stabilization hand on the anterior aspect of the hip and places the resistance hand on the anterior aspect of the thigh, just proximal to the knee. The clinician applies a force in the direction of hip extension while instructing the patient to hold against the resistance (Figure 13-1).

Positive Finding

A positive finding is weakness; the patient is unable to withstand the clinician's resistance, indicating possible involvement of the L1 or L2 spinal nerve root. Bilateral strength deficits could be indicative of a central nervous system lesion or simply of weakness of the iliacus, psoas major, or rectus femoris musculature.

Special Considerations

An alternate test is to have the patient perform a supine straight leg raise with the clinician stabilizing at the anterior hip and providing resistance just proximal to the patella in the direction of hip extension. Perform the test bilaterally to allow for strength comparisons. The clinician should apply the resistance in a slow, controlled manner, progressing in intensity as tolerated by the patient. A finding of pain or pain and weakness is more indicative of contractile tissue involvement (muscle, tendon, or bony insertion of tendon) and is not indicative of spinal nerve root involvement.

Specificity

.84

Sensitivity

.7

Positive Likelihood Ratio

4.38

Negative Likelihood Ratio

.36

References

Hoppenfeld S. *Orthopaedic Neurology*. Baltimore, MD: Lippincott-Raven; 1997.

Hoppenfeld S. *Physical Examination of the Spine and Extremities*. East Norwalk, CT: Appleton-Century-Crofts; 1976.

Lauder TD, Dillingham TR, Andary M. Effect of history and exam in predicting electrodiagnostic outcome among patients with suspected lumbosacral radiculopathy. *Am J Phys Med Rehab*. 2000;79:60-68.

Magee DJ. *Orthopedic Physical Assessment*. 4th ed. Philadelphia, PA: W.B. Saunders; 2002.

Meadows JTS. *Orthopedic Differential Diagnosis in Physical Therapy*. New York: McGraw-Hill; 1999.

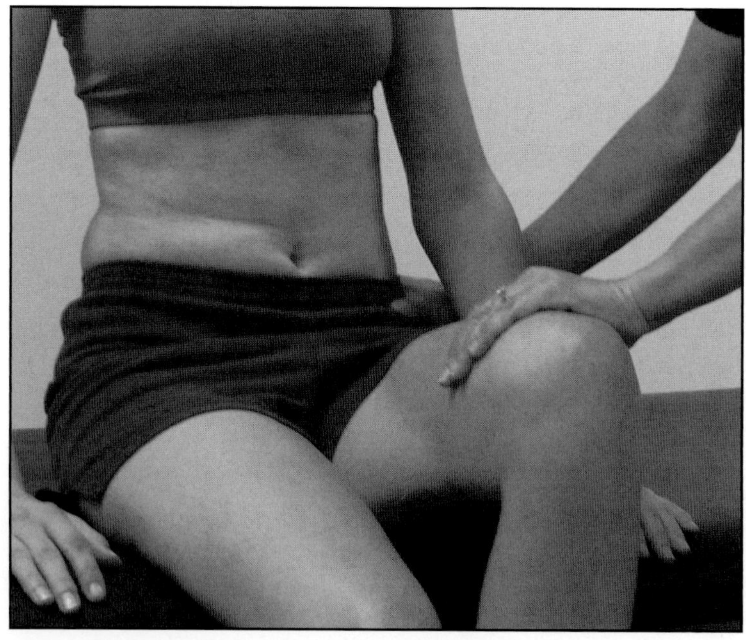

Figure 13-1

L3 Myotome Test

Test Position

The patient is positioned in sitting with the hip and knee flexed to 90 degrees.

Action

The clinician instructs the patient to extend his or her knee to between 30 to 45 degrees from full extension. The clinician then instructs the patient to hold his or her knee in this position while the clinician applies resistance. The clinician places the stabilization hand on the anterior aspect of the thigh just superior to the patella and places the resistance hand on the anterior aspect of the lower leg, just proximal to the ankle. The clinician applies a force in the direction of knee flexion while instructing the patient to hold against the resistance (Figure 13-2).

Positive Finding

A positive finding is weakness; the patient is unable to withstand the clinician's resistance, indicating possible involvement of the L3 spinal nerve root. Bilateral strength deficits could be indicative of a central nervous system lesion or simply of weakness of the quadriceps muscle group.

Special Considerations

Perform the test bilaterally to allow for strength comparisons. The clinician should apply the resistance in a slow, controlled manner, progressing in intensity as tolerated by the patient. A finding of pain or pain and weakness is more indicative of contractile tissue involvement (muscle, tendon, or bony insertion of tendon) and is not indicative of spinal nerve root involvement. The clinician should avoid the terminal ranges of knee extension while performing this test due to an increased risk of patellofemoral joint compression, resulting in patient discomfort.

Specificity

.89

Sensitivity

.40

Positive Likelihood Ratio

3.64

Negative Likelihood Ratio

.67

References

Hoppenfeld S. *Orthopaedic Neurology*. Baltimore, MD: Lippincott-Raven; 1997.

Hoppenfeld S. *Physical Examination of the Spine and Extremities*. East Norwalk, CT: Appleton-Century-Crofts; 1976.

Lauder TD, Dillingham TR, Andary M. Effect of history and exam in predicting electrodiagnostic outcome among patients with suspected lumbosacral radiculopathy. *Am J Phys Med Rehab*. 2000;79:60-68.

Magee DJ. *Orthopedic Physical Assessment*. 4th ed. Philadelphia, PA: W.B. Saunders; 2002.

Meadows JTS. *Orthopedic Differential Diagnosis in Physical Therapy*. New York: McGraw-Hill; 1999.

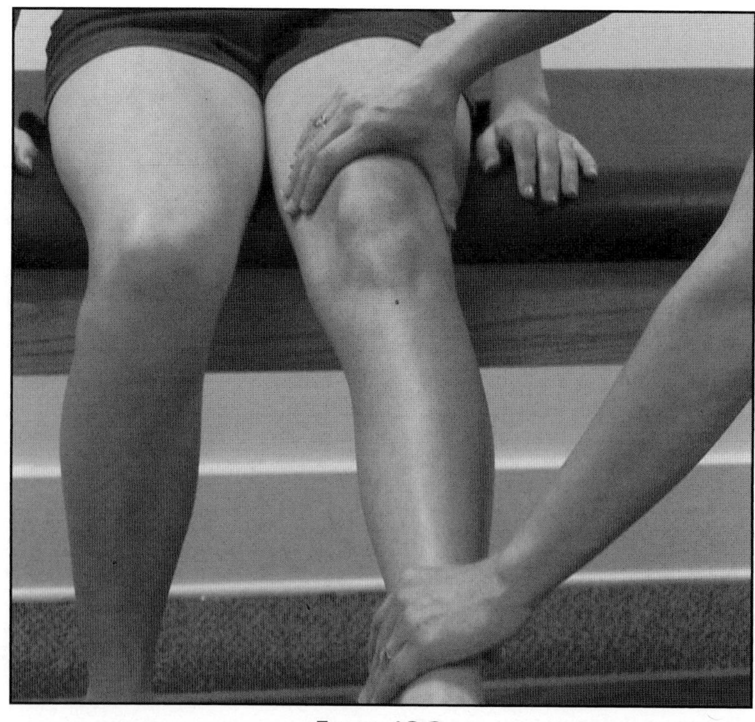

Figure 13-2

L4 Myotome Test: Ankle Dorsiflexion

Test Position

The patient is positioned in sitting with the hip and knee flexed to 90 degrees or in long sitting with the foot and ankle off the end of the table.

Action

The clinician instructs the patient to dorsiflex his or her ankle to end-range. The clinician then instructs the patient to hold his or her ankle in this position while the clinician applies resistance. The clinician places the stabilization hand on the anterior aspect of the lower leg just proximal to the ankle and places the resistance hand on the dorsum of the foot, just proximal to the MTP joints. The clinician applies a force in the direction of ankle plantarflexion while instructing the patient to hold against the resistance (Figure 13-3).

Positive Finding

A positive finding is weakness; the patient is unable to withstand the clinician's resistance, indicating possible involvement of the L4 spinal nerve root. A complementary finding of weakness in ankle inversion increases the likelihood of L4 nerve root involvement. Bilateral strength deficits could be indicative of a central nervous system lesion or simply of weakness of the tibialis anterior and fibularis tertius muscles.

Special Considerations

Perform the test bilaterally to allow for strength comparisons. The clinician should apply the resistance in a slow, controlled manner, progressing in intensity as tolerated by the patient. A finding of pain or pain and weakness is more indicative of contractile tissue involvement (muscle, tendon, or bony insertion of tendon) and is not indicative of spinal nerve root involvement. The clinician may opt to instruct the patient to dorsiflex and invert his or her ankle in combination and resist both motions simultaneously when assessing the L4 myotome.

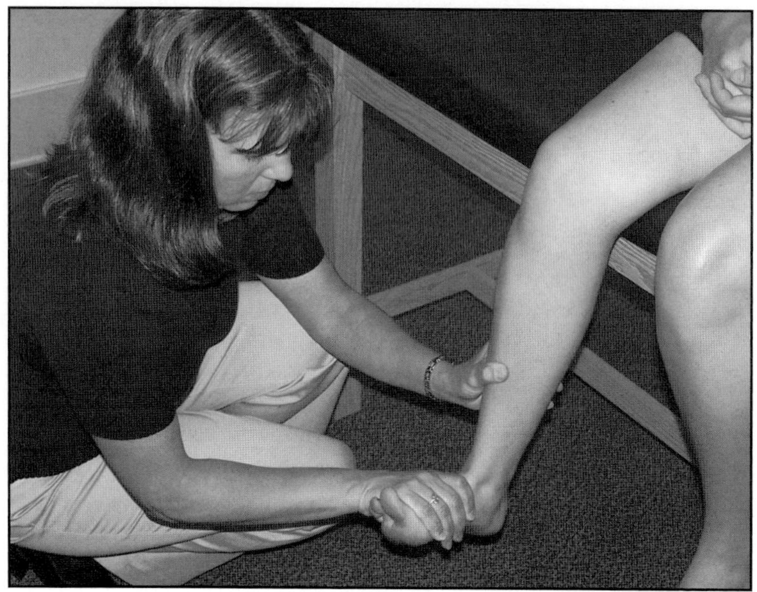

FIGURE 13-3

REFERENCES

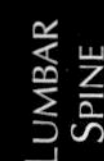

Hoppenfeld S. *Orthopaedic Neurology*. Baltimore, MD: Lippincott-Raven; 1997.

Hoppenfeld S. *Physical Examination of the Spine and Extremities*. East Norwalk, CT: Appleton-Century-Crofts; 1976.

Magee DJ. *Orthopedic Physical Assessment*. 4th ed. Philadelphia, PA: W.B. Saunders; 2002.

Meadows JTS. *Orthopedic Differential Diagnosis in Physical Therapy*. New York: McGraw-Hill; 1999.

L4 Myotome Test: Ankle Inversion

Test Position

The patient is positioned in sitting with the hip and knee flexed to 90 degrees or in long sitting with the foot and ankle off the end of the table.

Action

The clinician instructs the patient to invert his or her ankle to end-range. The clinician then instructs the patient to hold his or her ankle in this position while the clinician applies resistance. The clinician places the stabilization hand on the anterior aspect of the lower leg just proximal to the ankle and places the resistance hand on the medial aspect of the foot, just proximal to the MTP joints. The clinician applies a force in the direction of ankle eversion while instructing the patient to hold against the resistance (Figure 13-4).

Positive Finding

A positive finding is weakness; the patient is unable to withstand the clinician's resistance, indicating possible involvement of the L4 spinal nerve root. A complementary finding of weakness in ankle dorsiflexion increases the likelihood of L4 nerve root involvement. Bilateral strength deficits could be indicative of a central nervous system lesion or simply of weakness of the tibialis anterior and tibialis posterior muscles.

Special Considerations

Perform the test bilaterally to allow for strength comparisons. The clinician should apply the resistance in a slow, controlled manner, progressing in intensity as tolerated by the patient. A finding of pain or pain and weakness is more indicative of contractile tissue involvement (muscle, tendon, or bony insertion of tendon) and is not indicative of spinal nerve root involvement. The clinician may opt to instruct the patient to dorsiflex and invert his ankle in combination and resist both motions simultaneously when assessing the L4 myotome.

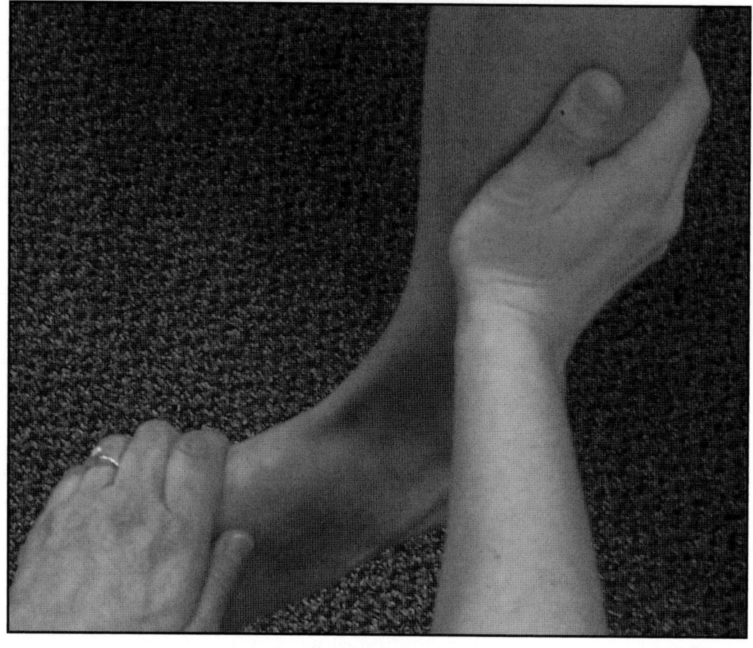

FIGURE 13-4

REFERENCES

Hoppenfeld S. *Orthopaedic Neurology*. Baltimore, MD: Lippincott-Raven; 1997.

Hoppenfeld S. *Physical Examination of the Spine and Extremities*. East Norwalk, CT: Appleton-Century-Crofts; 1976.

Magee DJ. *Orthopedic Physical Assessment*. 4th ed. Philadelphia, PA: W.B. Saunders; 2002.

Meadows JTS. *Orthopedic Differential Diagnosis in Physical Therapy*. New York: McGraw-Hill; 1999.

L5 Myotome Test

Test Position

The patient is positioned in sitting with the hip and knee flexed to 90 degrees or in long sitting with the foot and ankle off the end of the table.

Action

The clinician instructs the patient to extend his or her great toe to end-range. The clinician then instructs the patient to hold his or her great toe in this position while the clinician applies resistance. The clinician places the stabilization hand on the dorsum of the foot just proximal to the first MTP joint and places the resistance finger on the proximal phalanx of the great toe. The clinician applies a force in the direction of great toe flexion while instructing the patient to hold against the resistance (Figure 13-5).

Positive Finding

A positive finding is weakness; the patient is unable to withstand the clinician's resistance, indicating possible involvement of the L5 spinal nerve root. Bilateral strength deficits could be indicative of a central nervous system lesion or simply of weakness of the extensor hallicus muscles.

Special Considerations

The clinician should apply resistance to the great toe using only one finger. Perform the test bilaterally to allow for strength comparisons. The clinician should apply the resistance in a slow, controlled manner, progressing in intensity as tolerated by the patient. A finding of pain or pain and weakness is more indicative of contractile tissue involvement (muscle, tendon, or bony insertion of tendon) or a first MTP joint pathology and is not indicative of spinal nerve root involvement.

Specificity

.55

Sensitivity

.61

Positive Likelihood Ratio

1.36

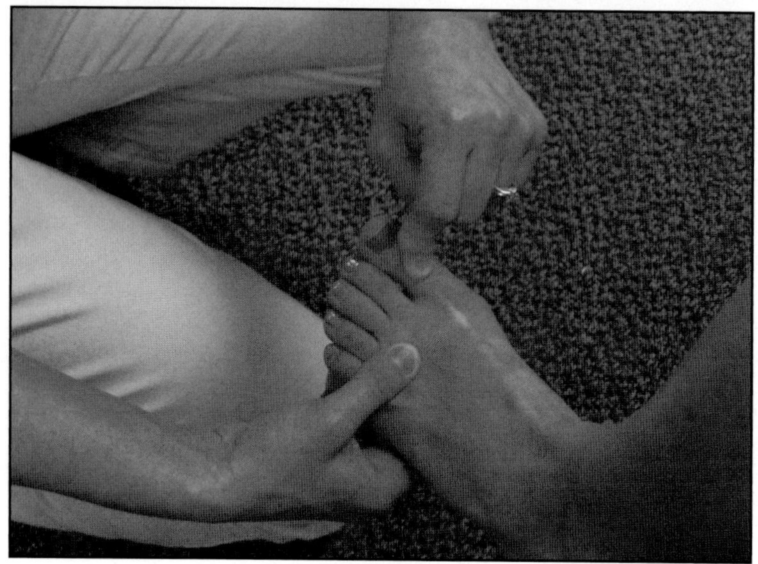

FIGURE 13-5

NEGATIVE LIKELIHOOD RATIO

.71

REFERENCES

Hoppenfeld S. *Orthopaedic Neurology*. Baltimore, MD: Lippincott-Raven; 1997.

Hoppenfeld S. *Physical Examination of the Spine and Extremities*. East Norwalk, CT: Appleton-Century-Crofts; 1976.

Lauder TD, Dillingham TR, Andary M. Effect of history and exam in predicting electrodiagnostic outcome among patients with suspected lumbosacral radicukopathy. *Am J Phys Med Rehab*. 2000;79:60-68.

Magee DJ. *Orthopedic Physical Assessment*. 4th ed. Philadelphia, PA: W.B. Saunders; 2002.

Meadows JTS. *Orthopedic Differential Diagnosis in Physical Therapy*. New York: McGraw-Hill; 1999.

S1 Myotome Test: Ankle Plantarflexion

Test Position

The patient is positioned in sitting with the hip and knee flexed to 90 degrees or in long sitting with the foot and ankle off the end of the table.

Action

The clinician instructs the patient to plantarflex his or her ankle to end-range. The clinician then instructs the patient to hold his or her ankle in this position while the clinician applies resistance. The clinician places the stabilization hand on the anterior aspect of the lower leg just proximal to the ankle and places the resistance hand on the plantar aspect of the foot, just proximal to the MTP joints. The clinician applies a force in the direction of ankle dorsiflexion while instructing the patient to hold against the resistance (Figure 13-6).

Positive Finding

A positive finding is weakness; the patient is unable to withstand the clinician's resistance, indicating possible involvement of the S1 spinal nerve root. A complementary finding of weakness in ankle eversion increases the likelihood of S1 nerve root involvement. Bilateral strength deficits could be indicative of a central nervous system lesion or simply of weakness of the gastrocnemius and soleus muscles.

Special Considerations

Perform the test bilaterally to allow for strength comparisons. The clinician should apply the resistance in a slow, controlled manner, progressing in intensity as tolerated by the patient. A finding of pain or pain and weakness is more indicative of contractile tissue involvement (muscle, tendon, or bony insertion of tendon) and is not indicative of spinal nerve root involvement. The clinician may opt to instruct the patient to plantarflex and evert his or her ankle in combination and resist both motions simultaneously when assessing the S1 myotome.

Specificity

.76

Sensitivity

.47

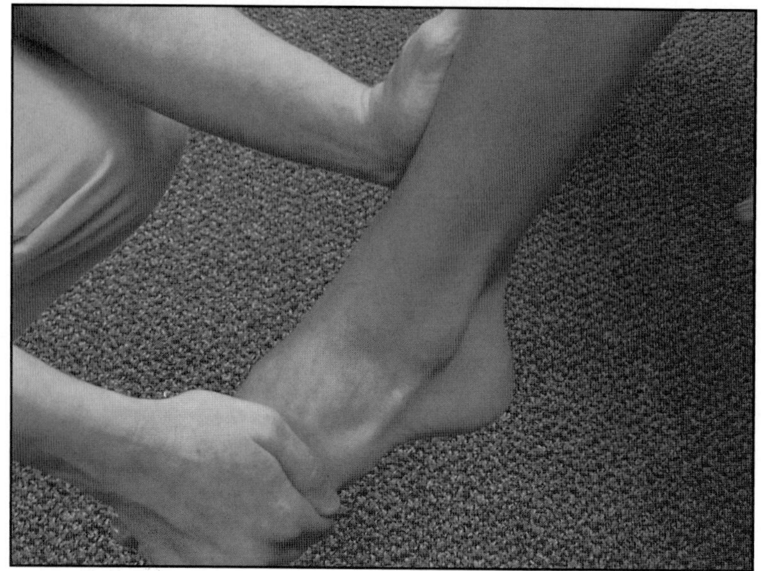

FIGURE 13-6

POSITIVE LIKELIHOOD RATIO

1.96

NEGATIVE LIKELIHOOD RATIO

.70

REFERENCES

Hoppenfeld S. *Orthopaedic Neurology*. Baltimore, MD: Lippincott-Raven; 1997.

Hoppenfeld S. *Physical Examination of the Spine and Extremities*. East Norwalk, CT: Appleton-Century-Crofts; 1976.

Lauder TD, Dillingham TR, Andary M. Effect of history and exam in predicting electrodiagnostic outcome among patients with suspected lumbosacral radiculopathy. *Am J Phys Med Rehab*. 2000;79:60-68.

Magee DJ. *Orthopedic Physical Assessment*. 4th ed. Philadelphia, PA: W.B. Saunders; 2002.

Meadows JTS. *Orthopedic Differential Diagnosis in Physical Therapy*. New York: McGraw-Hill; 1999.

S1 Myotome Test: Ankle Eversion

Test Position

The patient is positioned in sitting with the hip and knee flexed to 90 degrees or in long sitting with the foot and ankle off the end of the table.

Action

The clinician instructs the patient to evert his or her ankle to end-range. The clinician then instructs the patient to hold his or her ankle in this position while the clinician applies resistance. The clinician places the stabilization hand on the anterior aspect of the lower leg just proximal to the ankle and places the resistance hand on the lateral aspect of the foot, just proximal to the MTP joints. The clinician applies a force in the direction of ankle inversion while instructing the patient to hold against the resistance (Figure 13-7).

Positive Finding

A positive finding is weakness; the patient is unable to withstand the clinician's resistance, indicating possible involvement of the S1 spinal nerve root. A complementary finding of weakness in ankle plantarflexion increases the likelihood of S1 nerve root involvement. Bilateral strength deficits could be indicative of a central nervous system lesion or simply of weakness of the fibularis muscles (tertius, brevis, and longus).

Special Considerations

Perform the test bilaterally to allow for strength comparisons. The clinician should apply the resistance in a slow, controlled manner, progressing in intensity as tolerated by the patient. A finding of pain or pain and weakness is more indicative of contractile tissue involvement (muscle, tendon, or bony insertion of tendon) and is not indicative of spinal nerve root involvement. The clinician may opt to instruct the patient to plantarflex and evert his ankle in combination and resist both motions simultaneously when assessing the S1 myotome.

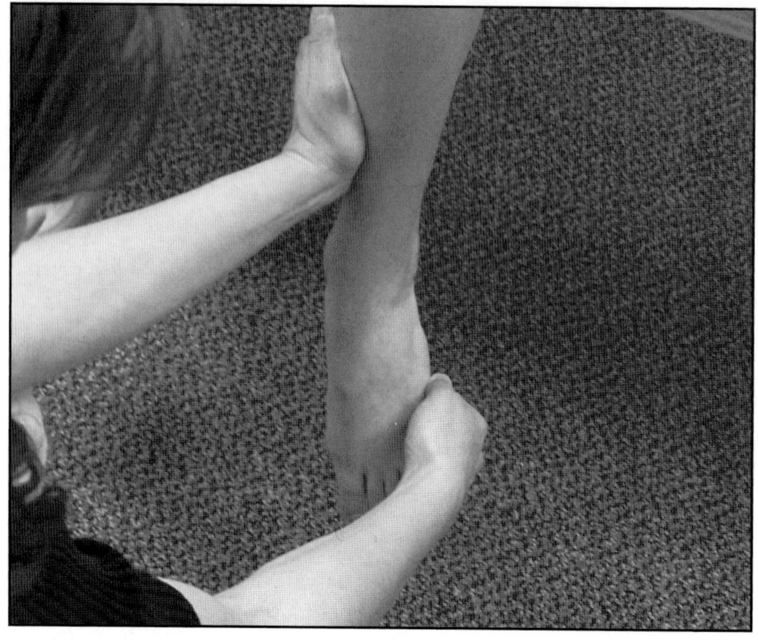

FIGURE 13-7

REFERENCES

Hoppenfeld S. *Orthopaedic Neurology*. Baltimore, MD: Lippincott-Raven; 1997.

Hoppenfeld S. *Physical Examination of the Spine and Extremities*. East Norwalk, CT: Appleton-Century-Crofts; 1976.

Magee DJ. *Orthopedic Physical Assessment*. 4th ed. Philadelphia, PA: W.B. Saunders; 2002.

Meadows JTS. *Orthopedic Differential Diagnosis in Physical Therapy*. New York: McGraw-Hill; 1999.

S2 Myotome Test

Test Position

The patient is positioned in prone with the hip in neutral.

Action

The clinician instructs the patient to flex his or her knee to 90 degrees. The clinician then instructs the patient to hold his or her knee in this position while the clinician applies resistance. The clinician places the stabilization hand on the posterior aspect of the thigh just inferior to the gluteal fold and places the resistance hand on the posterior aspect of the lower leg, just proximal to the ankle. The clinician applies a force in the direction of knee extension while instructing the patient to hold against the resistance (Figure 13-8). This test may also be performed in sitting with stabilization provided over the distal thigh (Figure 13-9).

Positive Finding

A positive finding is weakness; the patient is unable to withstand the clinician's resistance, indicating possible involvement of the S2 spinal nerve root. Bilateral strength deficits could be indicative of a central nervous system lesion or simply of weakness of the hamstring muscle group.

Special Considerations

Perform the test bilaterally to allow for strength comparisons. The clinician should apply the resistance in a slow, controlled manner, progressing in intensity as tolerated by the patient. A finding of pain or pain and weakness is more indicative of contractile tissue involvement (muscle, tendon, or bony insertion of tendon) and is not indicative of spinal nerve root involvement.

References

Hoppenfeld S. *Orthopaedic Neurology*. Baltimore, MD: Lippincott-Raven; 1997.

Hoppenfeld S. *Physical Examination of the Spine and Extremities*. East Norwalk, CT: Appleton-Century-Crofts; 1976.

Magee DJ. *Orthopedic Physical Assessment*. 4th ed. Philadelphia, PA: W.B. Saunders; 2002.

Meadows JTS. *Orthopedic Differential Diagnosis in Physical Therapy*. New York: McGraw-Hill; 1999.

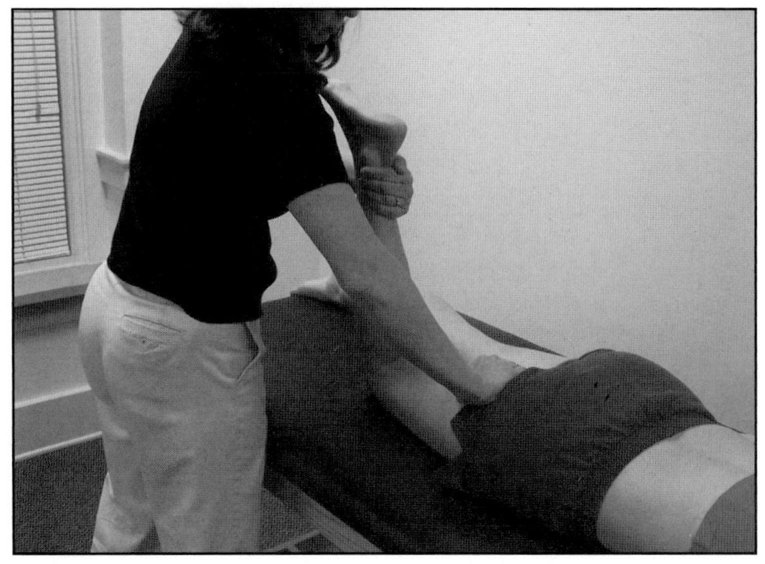

Figure 13-8

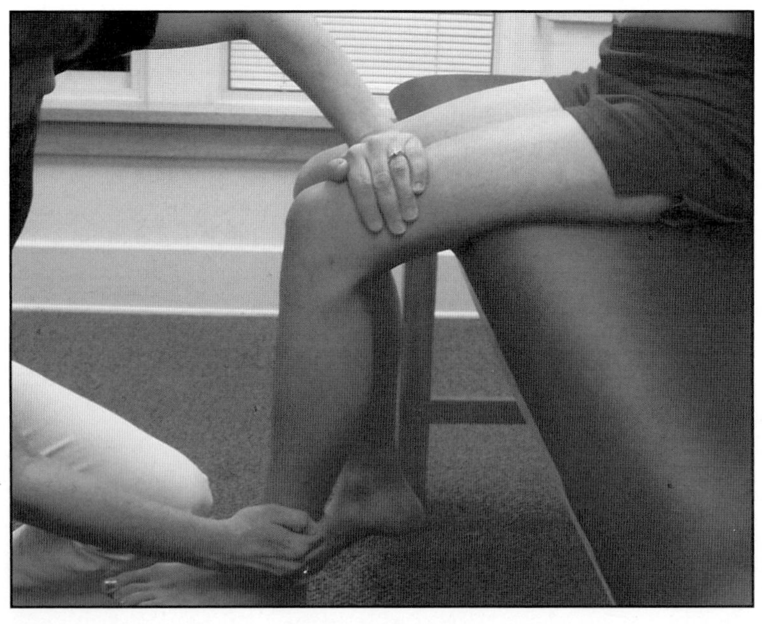

Figure 13-9

Chapter

14

Reflex Testing

Patellar Tendon Reflex (L4 Nerve Root) Testing

Test Position

The patient is positioned in sitting with the knee flexed to 90 degrees off the end of the table.

Action

The clinician strikes the patellar tendon to elicit a reflex (Figure 14-1).

Positive Finding

A normal response to this test is knee extension. The reflex is graded based on the tendon's response (see Tables 8-1 and 8-2).

Special Considerations

Some authors consider this reflex as testing the L2, L3, and L4 spinal segments.

Specificity

.93

Sensitivity

.50

Positive Likelihood Ratio

7.14

Negative Likelihood Ratio

.54

References

Lauder TD, Dillingham TR, Andary M. Effect of history and exam in predicting electrodiagnostic outcome among patients with suspected lumbosacral radiculopathy. *Am J Phys Med Rehab*. 2000;79:60-68.

Reese NB. *Muscle and Sensory Testing*. 2nd ed. Philadelphia, PA: W.B. Saunders; 2005.

Starkey C, Ryan JL. *Evaluation of Orthopedic and Athletic Injuries*. 2nd ed. Philadelphia, PA: F.A. Davis; 2002.

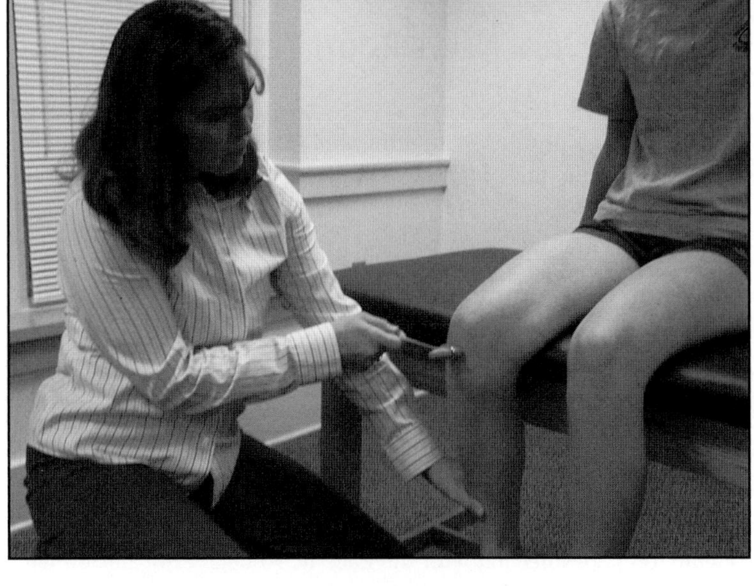

FIGURE 14-1

Achilles Tendon Reflex (S1 Nerve Root) Testing

Test Position

The patient is positioned in sitting with the knee flexed to 90 degrees off the end of the table and the ankle placed passively in slight dorsiflexion (Figure 14-2).

Action

The clinician strikes the Achilles tendon to elicit a reflex.

Positive Finding

A normal response to this test is ankle plantarflexion. The reflex is graded based on the tendon's response (see Tables 8-1 and 8-2).

Special Considerations

Alternate test positions include the patient in supine with the knee extended off the end of the table with the ankle in slight dorsiflexion (Figure 14-3) or kneeling with the knee in 90 degrees of flexion with the ankle in slight dorsiflexion (Figure 14-4). Some authors consider this reflex as testing both the S1 and S2 spinal segments.

Specificity

.90

Sensitivity

.47

Positive Likelihood Ratio

4.7

Negative Likelihood Ratio

.59

References

Lauder TD, Dillingham TR, Andary M. Effect of history and exam in predicting electrodiagnostic outcome among patients with suspected lumbosacral radiculopathy. *Am J Phys Med Rehab*. 2000;79:60-68.

Reese NB. *Muscle and Sensory Testing*. 2nd ed. Philadelphia, PA: W.B. Saunders; 2005.

Starkey C, Ryan JL. *Evaluation of Orthopedic and Athletic Injuries*. 2nd ed. Philadelphia, PA: F.A. Davis; 2002.

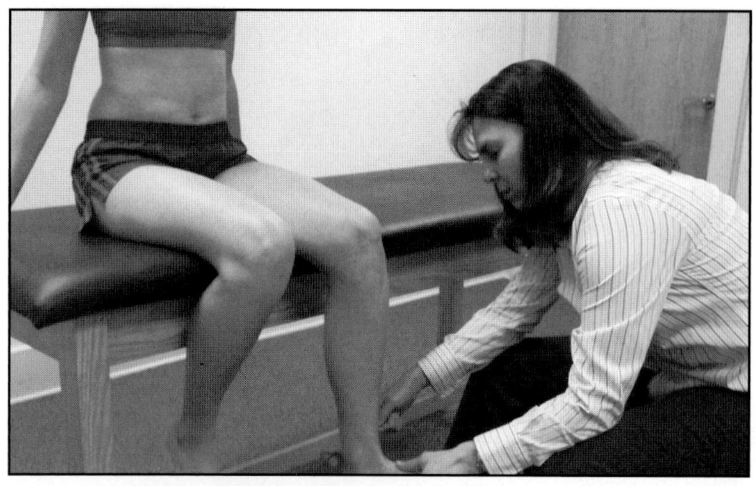

FIGURE 14-2

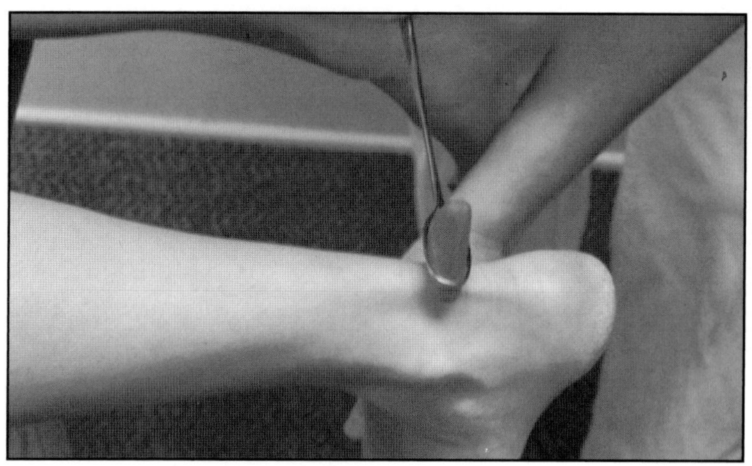

FIGURE 14-3

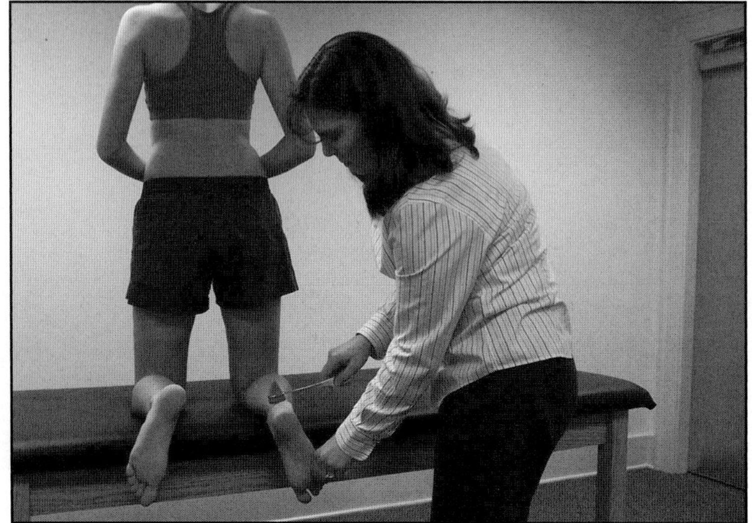

FIGURE 14-4

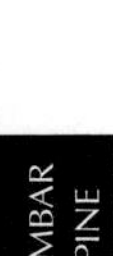

Chapter 15

Special Tests for the Thoracic and Lumbar Spine

Beevor's Sign

Test Position

The patient is positioned in a hook-lying position.

Action

The clinician instructs the patient to perform a partial sit-up while observing for movement of the umbilicus (Figure 15-1).

Positive Finding

A positive finding is superior, inferior, or lateral movement of the umbilicus as the patient performs or attempts to perform a partial sit-up. A positive test is indicative of inhibition of the rectus abdominus, possibly due to compromise of the T5–T12 nerve roots.

Special Considerations

The umbilicus will always move toward the stronger muscle group in the presence of pathology.

Historical Notes

This test is named for its originator, neurologist Charles Edward Beevor.

Specificity

No data available.

Sensitivity

No data available.

References

Awerbuch GI, Nigro MA, Wishnow R. Beevor's sign and facioscapulohumeral dystrophy. *Arch Neurol*. 1990;47(11):1208-9.

Pearce JM. Beevor's sign. *Eur Neurol*. 2005;53(4):208-9.

Starkey C, Ryan JL. *Evaluation of Orthopedic and Athletic Injuries*. 2nd ed. Philadelphia, PA: F.A. Davis; 2002.

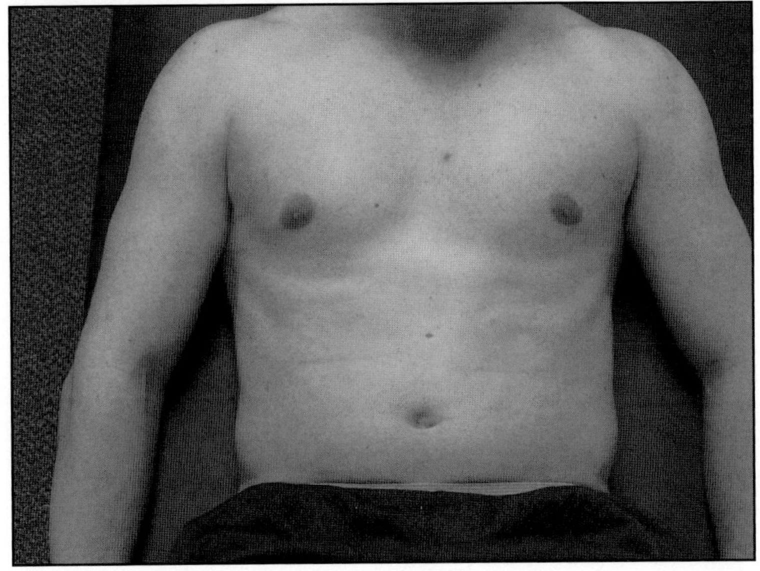

FIGURE 15-1

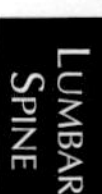

Milgram's Test

Test Position

The patient is positioned in supine with the knees fully extended.

Action

The clinician instructs the patient to perform a bilateral straight leg raise to a height of approximately 2 to 6 inches above the table. The clinician instructs the patient to hold this position for 30 seconds (Figure 15-2).

Positive Finding

A positive test is the patient's inability to maintain the test position for a full 30 seconds, inability to initiate or complete the bilateral straight leg raise, or reproduction of symptoms into the lower extremity during performance of the test. A positive test is indicative of a space-occupying lesion, such as a disc herniation, tumor, or osteophyte.

Special Considerations

This test results in an increase in intrathecal pressure, which may alter venous return, resulting in dizziness or loss of consciousness. This test is difficult to complete for a full 30 seconds, leading to the potential for numerous false-positive findings.

Historical Notes

The test is named for Joseph Elias Milgram, an orthopedist who developed the test in the late 1950s.

Specificity

No data available.

Sensitivity

No data available.

References

Magee DJ. *Orthopedic Physical Assessment.* 4th ed. Philadelphia, PA: W.B. Saunders; 2002.

Starkey C, Ryan JL. *Evaluation of Orthopedic and Athletic Injuries.* 2nd ed. Philadelphia, PA: F.A. Davis; 2002.

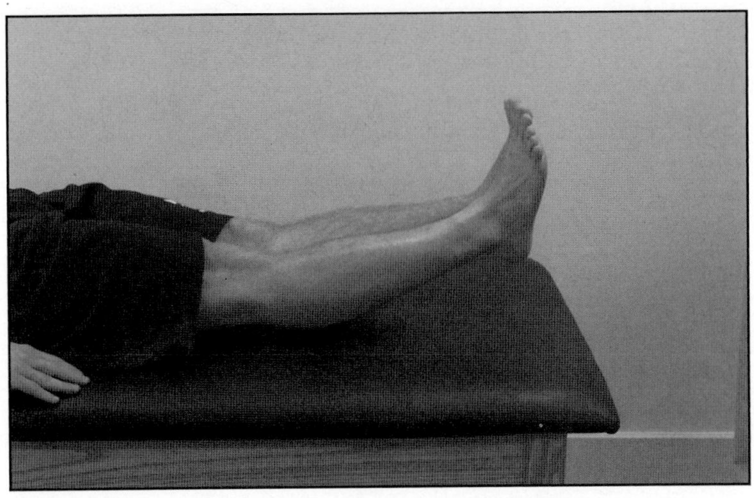

FIGURE 15-2

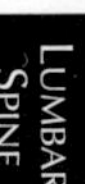

Brudzinski's Sign

Test Position

The patient is positioned in supine with his or her hands cupped behind his or her head.

Action

The clinician instructs the patient to passively flex his cervical spine by placing his or her hands behind his or her head and passively lifting his or her head off the table. The patient is then instructed to actively flex his or her hip (with the knee in full extension) on the test side to end-range or to the point of pain. The clinician next instructs the patient to actively flex his or her knee to 90 degrees, while maintaining the hip in flexion on the test side. The opposite lower extremity should remain flat on the table during testing (Figures 15-3 and 15-4).

Positive Finding

A positive test is spine pain or lower extremity symptoms that are increased with neck and hip flexion, but relieved with knee flexion. A positive test is indicative of nerve root impingement, irritation of the dura, and meningeal irritation.

Special Considerations

Performance of Brudzinski's Sign is recommended if the clinician suspects bacterial or viral meningitis.

Historical Notes

This test is named for Josef Brudzinski, who initially presented the addition of cervical spine flexion to Kernig's Test in order to increase tension on the neurologic structures of the spine.

Alternate Names

This test is also known as *Brudzinki's Test, Brudzinski's Symptom, Brudzinski-Kernig Test, Kernig-Brudzinski Test, Brudzinski-Kernig Sign,* and *Kernig-Brudzinski Sign*.

Sensitivity

.05 for detecting meningitis in adults

Positive Likelihood Ratio

.97 for detecting meningitis in adults

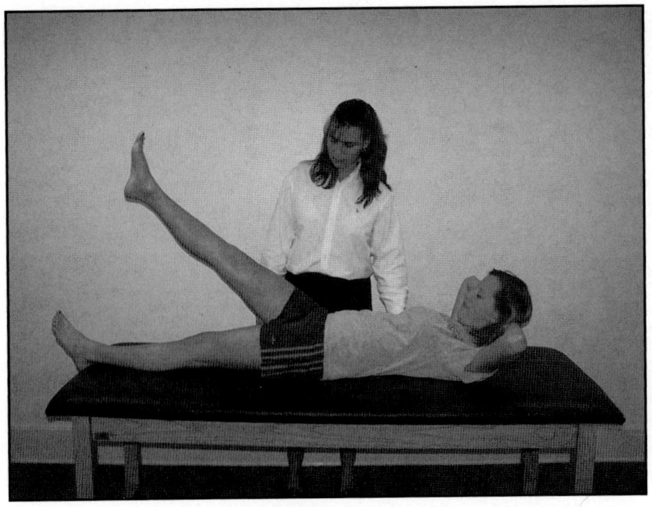

FIGURE 15-3

REFERENCES

Konin JG, Wiksten DL, Isear JA, Brader H. *Special Tests for Orthopedic Examination*. 3rd ed. Thorofare, NJ: SLACK Incorporated; 2006.

Magee DJ. *Orthopedic Physical Assessment*. 4th ed. Philadelphia, PA: W.B. Saunders; 2002.

Starkey C, Ryan JL. *Evaluation of Orthopedic and Athletic Injuries*. 2nd ed. Philadelphia, PA: FA Davis; 2002.

Thomas KE, Hasbun R, Jekel J, Quagliarello VJ. The diagnostic accuracy of Kernig's sign, Brudzinski's sign and nuchal rigidity in adults with suspected meningitis. *Clinical Infection Discussion*. 2002;35(1):46-52.

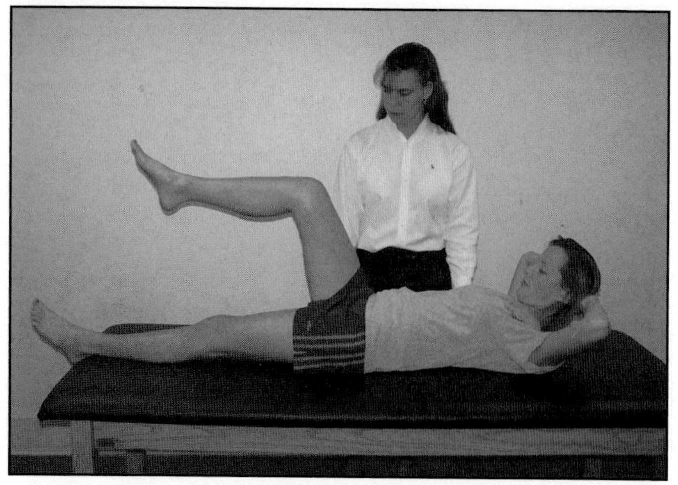

FIGURE 15-4

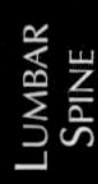

Kernig's Test

Test Position

The patient is positioned in supine.

Action

The clinician instructs the patient to actively flex his or her hip (with the knee in full extension) on the test side to end-range or to the point of pain. The clinician next instructs the patient to actively flex his or her knee to 90 degrees, while maintaining the hip in flexion on the test side. The opposite lower extremity should remain flat on the table during testing (Figures 15-5 and 15-6).

Positive Finding

A positive test is spine pain or lower extremity symptoms that are increased with hip flexion, but relieved with knee flexion. A positive test is indicative of nerve root impingement, irritation of the dura, and meningeal irritation.

Special Considerations

Performance of Kernig's Test is recommended if the clinician suspects bacterial or viral meningitis.

Historical Notes

This test is named for Vladimir Mikhailovich Kernig, who initially described the test in 1882 as a method to increase tension on the neurologic structures of the spine as a primary test for meningitis. The test was later adapted by Brudzinski to include cervical spine flexion.

Alternate Names

This test is also known as *Kernig's Sign*, *Kernig's Phenomenon*, *Kernig's Symptom*, *Brudzinski-Kernig Test*, *Kernig-Brudzinski Test*, *Brudzinski-Kernig Sign*, and *Kernig-Brudzinski Sign*.

Sensitivity

.05 for detecting meningitis in adults

Positive Likelihood Ratio

.97 for detecting meningitis in adults

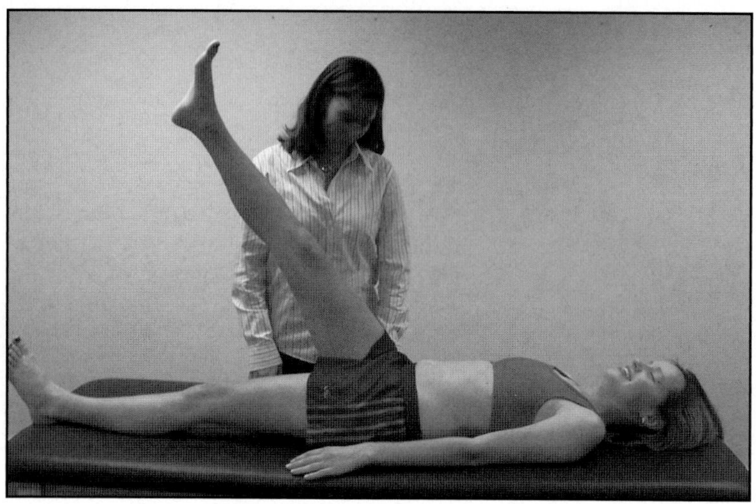

FIGURE 15-5

REFERENCES

Konin JG, Wiksten DL, Isear JA, Brader H. *Special Tests for Orthopedic Examination*. 3rd ed. Thorofare, NJ: SLACK Incorporated; 2006.

Magee DJ. *Orthopedic Physical Assessment*. 4th ed. Philadelphia, PA: W.B. Saunders; 2002.

Starkey C, Ryan JL. *Evaluation of Orthopedic and Athletic Injuries*. 2nd ed. Philadelphia, PA: FA Davis; 2002.

Thomas KE, Hasbun R, Jekel J, Quagliarello VJ. The diagnostic accuracy of Kernig's sign, Brudzinski's sign and nuchal rigidity in adults with suspected meningitis. *Clinical Infection Discussion*. 2002;35(1):46-52.

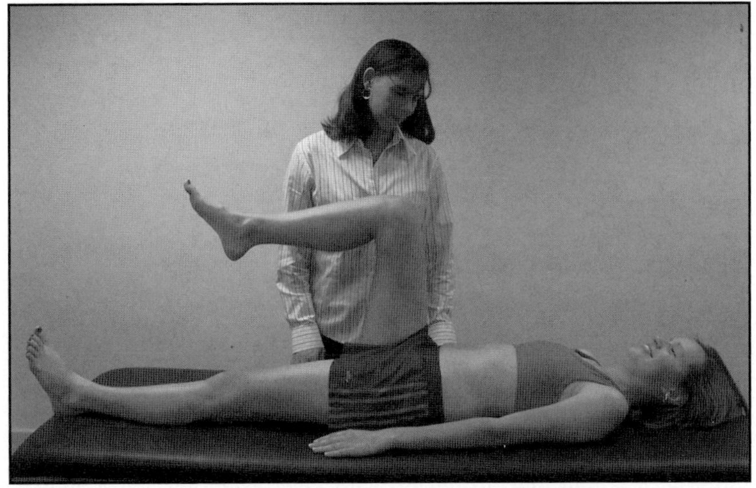

FIGURE 15-6

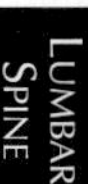

Straight Leg Raise Test

Test Position

The patient is positioned in supine with the hips and knees in full extension.

Action

The clinician passively flexes the involved hip, while maintaining full knee extension. Hip flexion is continued until end-range is reached (typically between 70 and 90 degrees) or the patient reports discomfort in the spine or lower extremity. The opposite lower extremity should remain flat on the table during testing (Figure 15-7).

Positive Finding

A positive test is indicated by the presence of pain or discomfort prior to reaching full hip flexion with knee extension and is indicative of disc herniation, sciatic nerve irritation, or hamstring tightness. Typically, the presence of spine pain (with or without lower extremity pain) indicates disc herniation or sciatic nerve involvement, while lower extremity discomfort alone is more indicative of hamstring tightness.

Special Considerations

In order to differentiate the cause of the patient's discomfort between neurologic involvement and hamstring tightness, the clinician may perform a modified Straight Leg Raise Test as follows. If the patient reports discomfort prior to reaching the end-range of motion, the hip is lowered until the discomfort subsides. The clinician then passively dorsiflexes the ankle on the test side and/or instructs the patient to actively or passively flex his or her cervical spine. In the presence of irritation of the dura mater, the patient will again complain of discomfort. If the patient's original discomfort was the result of hamstring tightness, ankle dorsiflexion and cervical spine flexion will not exacerbate the patient's discomfort.

Historical Notes

The test was originally developed by Ernest-Charles Lasegue in the 1870s as he searched for a test to identify malingerers simulating sciatica. The test remained unpublished until 1880, when Laza K. Lazarevic published the test.

Alternate Names

This test is also known as *Lasegue's Test* and *Lasegue's Sign*. The addition of cervical spine flexion to the straight leg raise test has been described

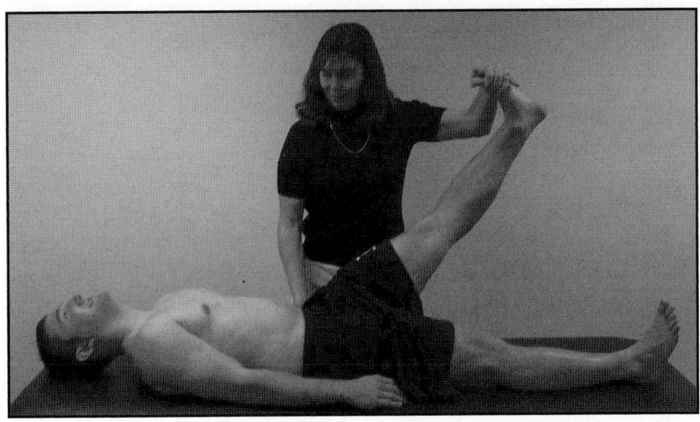

FIGURE 15-7

as *Hyndman's Sign, Brudzinski's Sign, Lidner's Sign,* and the *Soto-Hall Test*. The addition of the ankle dorsiflexion movement is also known as *Bragard's Test*.

SPECIFICITY

.10 – .57 for detecting disc herniation

SENSITIVITY

.78 – .97 for detecting disc herniation

POSITIVE LIKELIHOOD RATIO

1.0 – 1.98 for detecting disc herniation

NEGATIVE LIKELIHOOD RATIO

.05 – 3.5 for detecting disc herniation

RELIABILITY

Kappa values at the 95% confidence interval for this range from .32 to .68.

REFERENCES

Cleland J. *Orthopaedic Clinical Examination: An Evidence-Based Approach for Physical Therapists*. Carlstadt, NJ: Icon Learning Systems; 2005.

Magee DJ. *Orthopedic Physical Assessment.* 4th ed. Philadelphia, PA: W.B. Saunders; 2002.

Starkey C, Ryan JL. *Evaluation of Orthopedic and Athletic Injuries.* 2nd ed. Philadelphia, PA: F.A. Davis; 2002.

Well Straight Leg Raise Test

Test Position

The patient is positioned in supine with the hips and knees in full extension.

Action

The clinician passively flexes the uninvolved hip, while maintaining full knee extension. Hip flexion is continued until end-range is reached (typically between 70 and 90 degrees) or the patient reports discomfort in the spine or opposite lower extremity. The opposite lower extremity should remain flat on the table during testing (Figure 15-8).

Positive Finding

A positive test is a report of pain in the opposite (involved) lower extremity during passive straight leg raising of the uninvolved lower extremity. A positive test is indicative of a large space-occupying lesion such as a central disc herniation or tumor.

Special Considerations

A positive well straight leg raise test is typically indicative of a poor prognosis without surgical intervention.

Historical Notes

This test was first described by Fajersztajn.

Alternate Names

This test is also known as the *Well Leg Raising Test of Fajersztajn*, *Lhermitt's Test*, the *Prostrate Leg Raising Test*, the *Cross-over Sign*, and the *Sciatic Phenomenon*.

Specificity

.88 – 1.0 for detecting disc herniation

Sensitivity

.15 – .57 for detecting disc herniation

Positive Likelihood Ratio

1.92 – 6.14 for detecting disc herniation

Negative Likelihood Ratio

.43 – .88 for detecting disc herniation

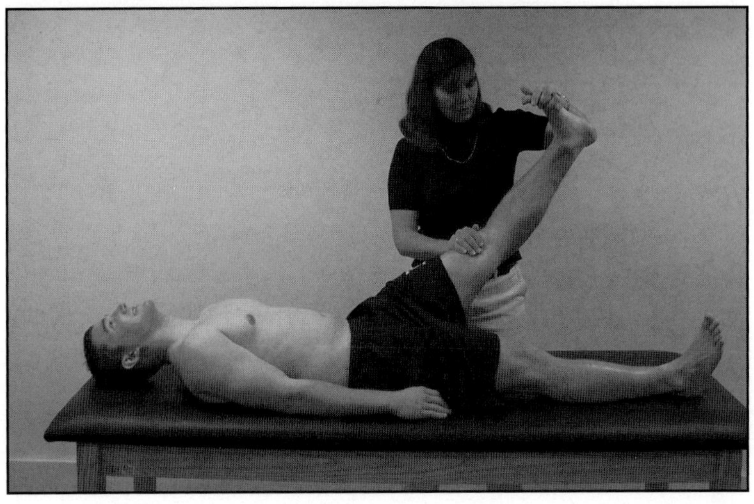

FIGURE 15-8

REFERENCES

Cleland J. *Orthopaedic Clinical Examination: An Evidence-Based Approach for Physical Therapists*. Carlstadt, NJ: Icon Learning Systems; 2005.

Konin JG, Wiksten DL, Isear JA, Brader H. *Special Tests for Orthopedic Examination*. 3rd ed. Thorofare, NJ: SLACK Incorporated; 2006.

Magee DJ. *Orthopedic Physical Assessment*. 4th ed. Philadelphia, PA: W.B. Saunders; 2002.

Starkey C, Ryan JL. *Evaluation of Orthopedic and Athletic Injuries*. 2nd ed. Philadelphia, PA: F.A. Davis; 2002.

Quadrant Test

Test Position

The patient is positioned in standing with his or her feet shoulder-width apart and hands on hips.

Action

The clinician instructs the patient to perform spine extension, lateral flexion, and rotation to the affected side. The clinician places his or her hands on the superior aspect of the patient's shoulders and applies overpressure (Figure 15-9).

Positive Finding

A positive finding is spine pain, indicating involvement of the facets or reproduction of the patient's lower extremity symptoms, indicating disc herniation, nerve root entrapment, or other space-occupying lesion.

Special Considerations

Symptoms isolated to the sacroiliac joint during testing indicate SI dysfunction.

Specificity

No data available.

Sensitivity

No data available.

References

Lyle MA, Manes S, McGuinness M, Ziaei S, Iversen MD. Relationship of physical examination findings and self-reported symptoms severity and physical function in patients with degenerative lumbar conditions. *Phys Ther.* 2005;85(2):120-133.

Magee DJ. *Orthopedic Physical Assessment.* 4th ed. Philadelphia, PA: W.B. Saunders; 2002.

Starkey C, Ryan JL. *Evaluation of Orthopedic and Athletic Injuries.* 2nd ed. Philadelphia, PA: F.A. Davis; 2002.

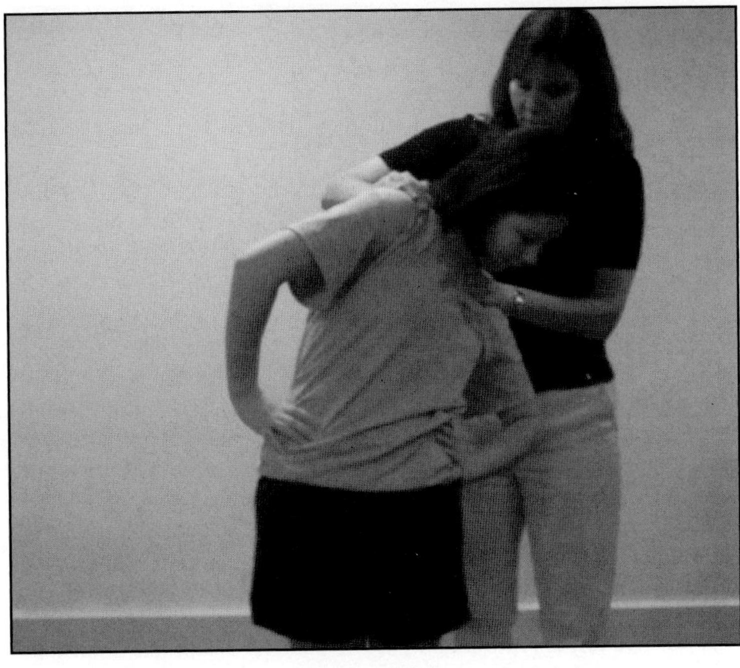

FIGURE 15-9

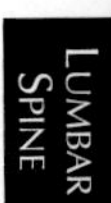

Slump Test

Test Position

The patient is positioned in sitting with both the knees and hips flexed to 90 degrees (Figure 15-10).

Action

The patient is instructed to slump forward and round his or her shoulders while maintaining the cervical spine in neutral (Figure 15-11). The patient is instructed to maintain this position and the clinician assesses for reproduction of symptoms. Next, the clinician flexes the patient's cervical spine and holds this position assessing for reproduction of symptoms (Figure 15-12). If no changes are noted, the clinician passively extends the patient's knee and, again, observes for reproduction of symptoms (Figure 15-13). If no symptoms are noted, the clinician passively dorsiflexes the patient's ankle while maintaining knee extension, and assesses for reproduction of symptoms (Figure 15-14). The test should then be repeated on the opposite side.

Positive Finding

A positive test is reproduction of the patient's symptoms, indicating involvement of the dura, the spinal cord, or the spinal nerve roots.

Special Considerations

The motions of cervical spine flexion, knee extension, and ankle dorsiflexion can be performed either passively or actively when completing this exam. If the patient reports a reproduction of symptoms, further provocation is not required and the test is discontinued.

Alternate Names

This test is also known as the *Slouch Test*.

Specificity

No data available.

Sensitivity

No data available.

References

Cleland JA, Childs JD, Palmer JA, Eberhart S. Slump stretching in the management of non-radicular low back pain: a pilot clinical trial. *Manual Therapy*. 2006;11(4):279-286.

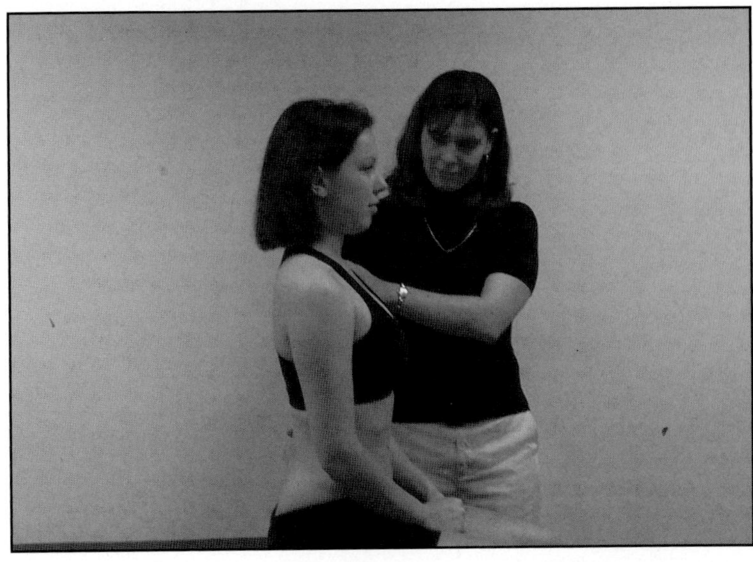

FIGURE 15-10

George SZ. Characteristics of patients with lower extremity symptoms treated with slump stretching: a case series. *J Orthop Sports Phys Ther*. 2002;32(8):391-398.

Johnson EK, Chiarello CM. The slump test: the effects of head and lower extremity position on knee extension. *J Orthop Sports Phys Ther*. 1997;26(6): 310-317.

Konin JG, Wiksten DL, Isear JA, Brader H. *Special Tests for Orthopedic Examination*. 3rd ed. Thorofare, NJ: SLACK Incorporated; 2006.

Magee DJ. *Orthopedic Physical Assessment*. 4th ed. Philadelphia, PA: W.B. Saunders; 2002.

Stankovic R, Johnell O, Maly P, Wilner S. Use of lumbar extension, slump test, physical and neurological examination in the evaluation of patients with suspected herniated nucleus pulposus: a prospective clinical study. *Manual Therapy*. 1999;4(1):25-32.

Starkey C, Ryan JL. *Evaluation of Orthopedic and Athletic Injuries*. 2nd ed. Philadelphia, PA: F.A. Davis; 2002.

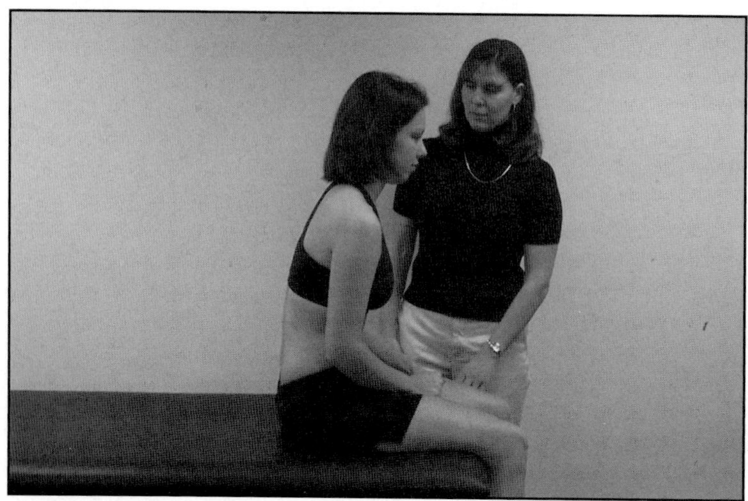

Figure 15-11

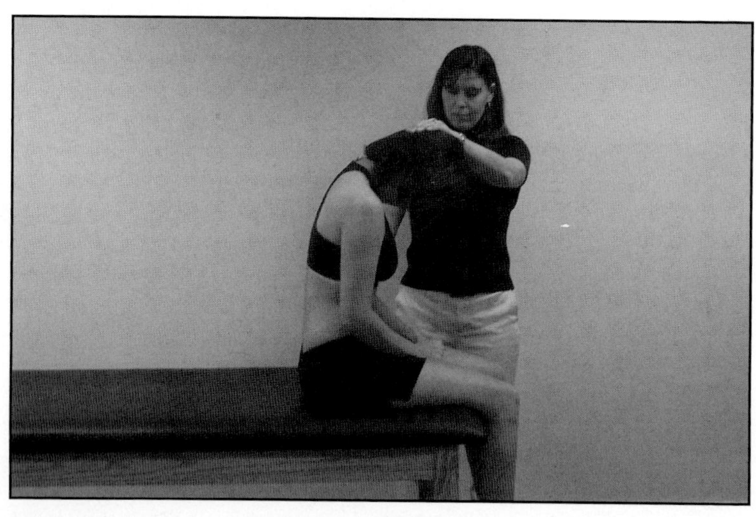

Figure 15-12

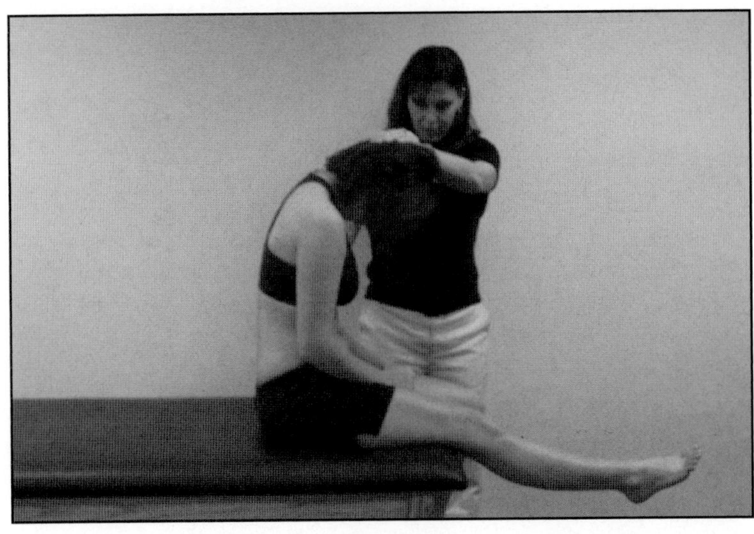

FIGURE 15-13

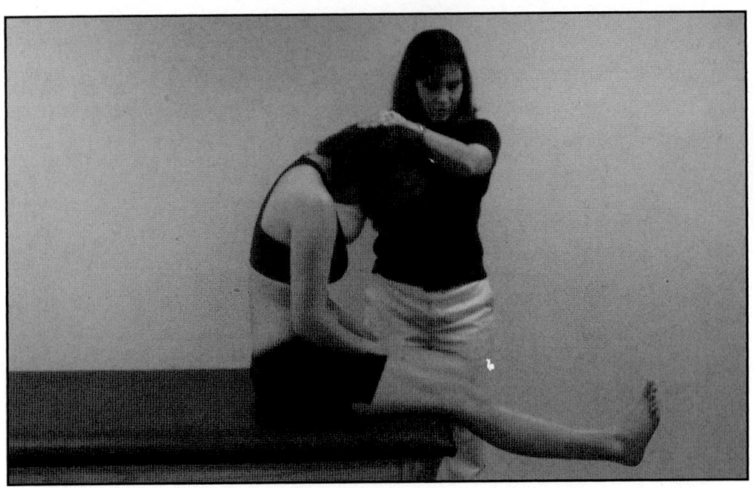

FIGURE 15-14

Bowstring Test

Test Position

The patient is positioned in supine.

Action

The clinician performs a passive Straight Leg Raise on the involved side (Figure 15-15). If the patient reports radiating pain during the straight leg raise, the clinician passively flexes the involved knee approximately 20 degrees in order to relieve the patient's radicular symptoms. The clinician then palpates the sciatic nerve in the popliteal space in an attempt to reproduce the patient's symptoms (Figure 15-16).

Positive Finding

A positive finding is radicular symptoms during straight leg raising that are relieved with knee flexion and exacerbated with palpation of the popliteal space. A positive test indicates sciatic nerve pathology.

Special Considerations

The patient should be maintained in the same degree of hip flexion throughout the performance of this test.

Alternate Names

This test is also known as the *Cram Test* and the *Popliteal Pressure Sign*. The test can be modified to be performed in sitting and is referred to as the *Sciatic Tension Test* or *Deyerle's Sign*.

Specificity

No data available.

Sensitivity

No data available.

References

Konin JG, Wiksten DL, Isear JA, Brader H. *Special Tests for Orthopedic Examination*. 3rd ed. Thorofare, NJ: SLACK Incorporated; 2006.

Magee DJ. *Orthopedic Physical Assessment*. 4th ed. Philadelphia, PA: W.B. Saunders; 2002.

Starkey C, Ryan JL. *Evaluation of Orthopedic and Athletic Injuries*. 2nd ed. Philadelphia, PA: F.A. Davis; 2002.

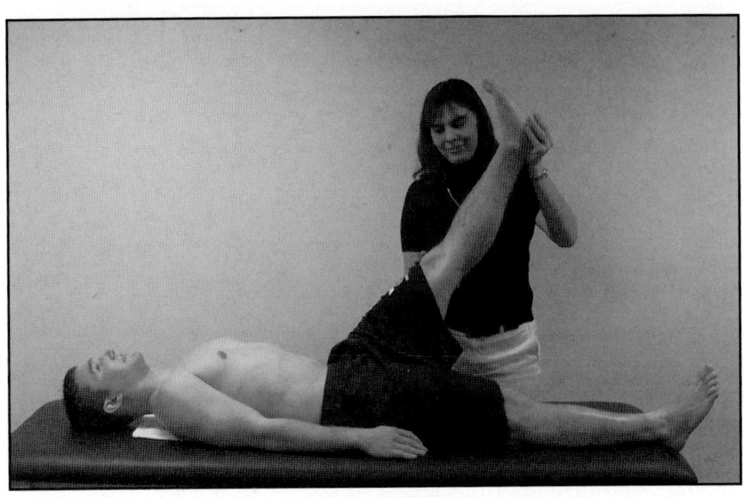

FIGURE 15-15

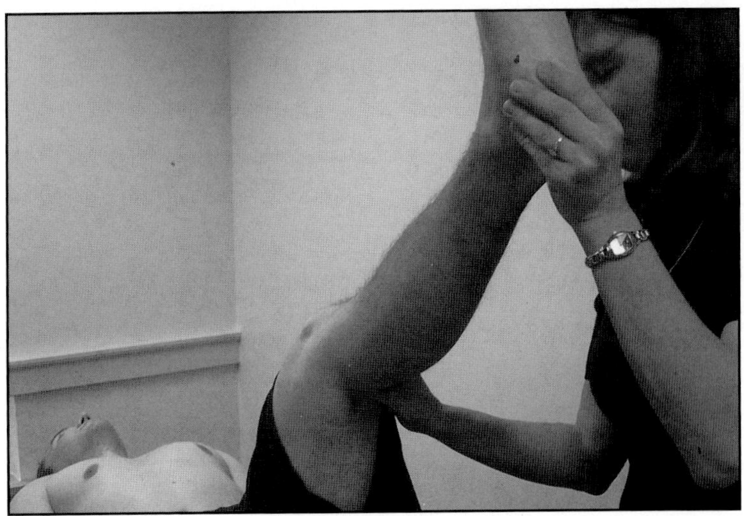

FIGURE 15-16

Tension Sign

Test Position

The patient is positioned in supine.

Action

The clinician performs passive hip flexion to 90 degrees while allowing knee flexion to 90 degrees (Figure 15-17). The clinician then extends the knee to end-range while palpating the sciatic nerve in the popliteal space (Figure 15-18).

Positive Finding

A positive finding is tenderness in the popliteal space that is exacerbated during palpation with the knee in full extension and relieved with knee flexion. Reproduction of sciatic symptoms is also a positive finding. A positive tests indicates sciatic nerve pathology.

Special Considerations

This test is a modified version of the Bowstring Test.

Alternate Names

This test is also known as the *Tension Test*.

Specificity

No data available.

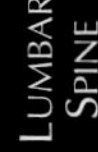

Sensitivity

No data available.

References

Magee DJ. *Orthopedic Physical Assessment.* 4th ed. Philadelphia, PA: W.B. Saunders; 2002.

Sugiura K, Yoshida T, Katoh S, Mimatsu M. A study of tension signs in lumbar disc hernia. *Int Orthop*. 1979;3(3):225-228.

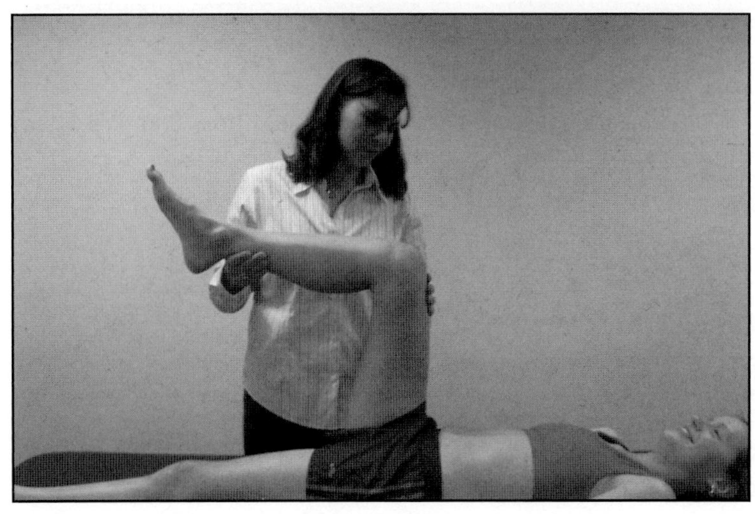

FIGURE 15-17

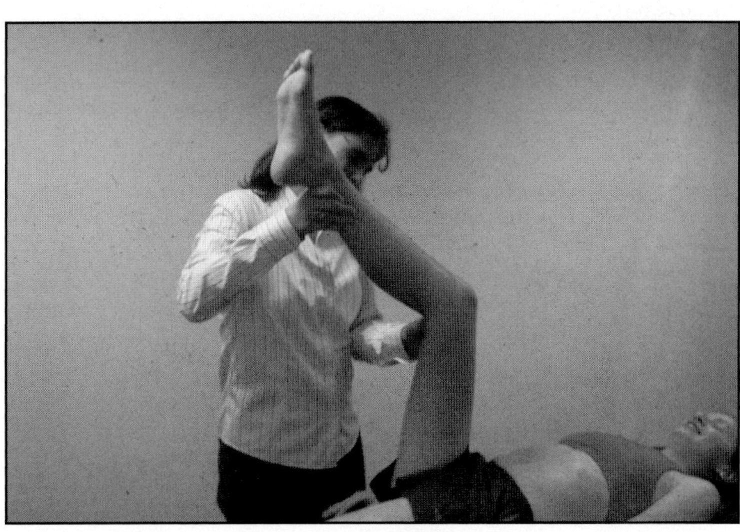

FIGURE 15-18

Sitting Root Test

Test Position

The patient is positioned in sitting with the knees and hips flexed to 90 degrees and the cervical spine in slight flexion.

Action

The clinician instructs the patient to actively extend his or her knee (Figure 15-19).

Positive Finding

A positive finding is a complaint of pain in the buttock, posterior thigh, or posterior lower leg, indicating involvement of the sciatic nerve. The clinician may also observe the patient arching or leaning backward in an attempt to decrease tension on the sciatic nerve. This finding is also considered to be a positive test.

Special Considerations

The test can also be performed by having the clinician perform passive knee extension.

Historical Notes

This test is a modification of the *Slump Test*.

Specificity

No data available.

Sensitivity

No data available.

References

Konin JG, Wiksten DL, Isear JA, Brader H. *Special Tests for Orthopedic Examination*. 3rd ed. Thorofare, NJ: SLACK Incorporated; 2006.

Magee DJ. *Orthopedic Physical Assessment*. 4th ed. Philadelphia, PA: W.B. Saunders; 2002.

Starkey C, Ryan JL. *Evaluation of Orthopedic and Athletic Injuries*. 2nd ed. Philadelphia, PA: F.A. Davis; 2002.

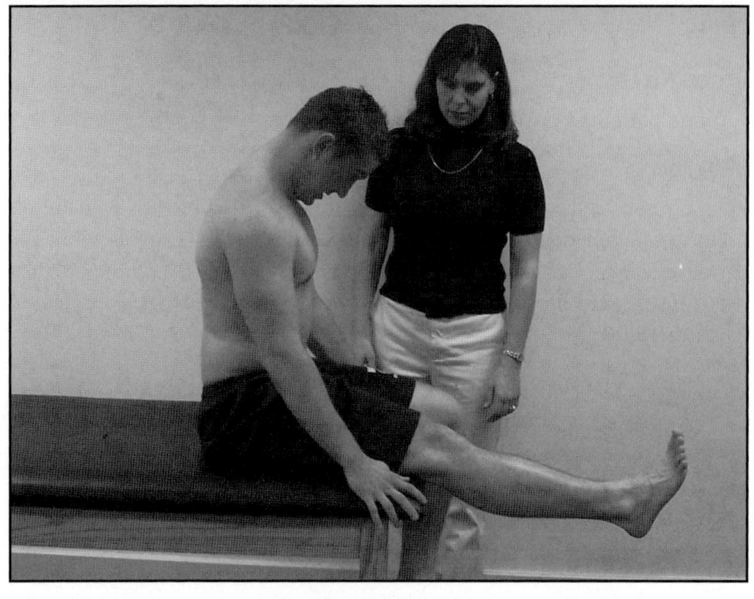

FIGURE 15-19

Prone Knee Bending Test

Test Position

The patient is positioned in prone.

Action

The clinician passively flexes the patient's knee until the patient's heel rests against his or her buttocks. If full knee flexion, allowing the heel to contact the buttock, cannot be achieved, the clinician may perform passive hip extension while maintaining maximal knee flexion (Figure 15-20).

Positive Finding

A positive test is unilateral neurologic pain in the lumbar spine, the buttock or the posterior thigh and is indicative of L2–L3 nerve root pathology. This test may also result in anterior thigh pain due to tension on the femoral nerve.

Special Considerations

The clinician must ensure that no hip rotation occurs during the performance of this test, especially in the presence of a tight rectus femoris muscle.

Alternate Names

This test is also known as *Nachlas Test*.

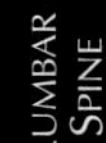

Specificity

No data available.

Sensitivity

No data available.

References

Magee DJ. *Orthopedic Physical Assessment.* 4th ed. Philadelphia, PA: W.B. Saunders; 2002.

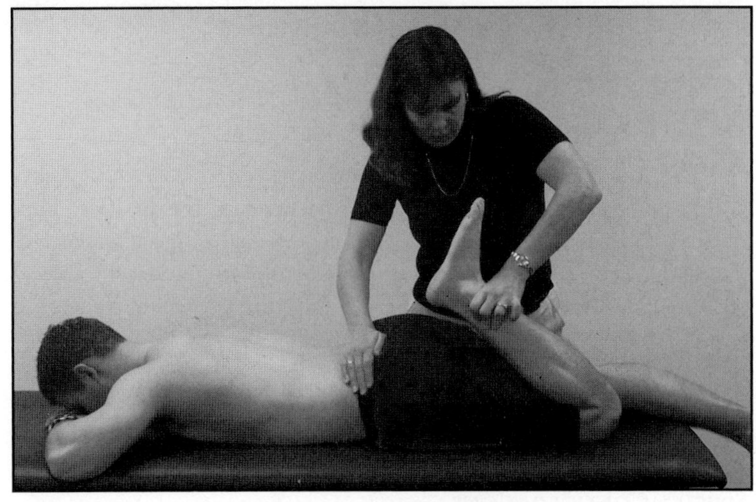

FIGURE 15-20

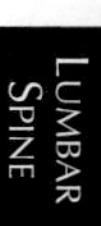

Valsalva's Maneuver

Test Position

The patient is positioned in sitting.

Action

The clinician instructs the patient to take a deep breath. The clinician next instructs the patient to exhale forcefully into a closed fist (Figure 15-21). An alternate test is to instruct the patient to take a deep breath and hold while bearing down, as if having a bowel movement.

Positive Finding

A positive finding is an increase in spinal pain or peripheral symptoms (pain, numbness, or tingling), indicating a space-occupying lesion, such as a disc herniation, tumor, or osteophyte.

Special Considerations

A positive Valsalva Maneuver results in increased intrathecal pressure, which may alter venous return, resulting in dizziness or loss of consciousness. Therefore, the clinician should always be in close proximity to the patient, ready to intervene as needed when performing this test.

Historical Notes

This procedure is named for Antonio Maria Valsalva, a physician who first described the test in the 17th century. The test was first used to assess the patency of Eustachian tubes.

Alternate Names

This test is also known as *Valsalva's Test*.

Specificity

No data available.

Sensitivity

No data available.

References

Konin JG, Wiksten DL, Isear JA, Brader H. *Special Tests for Orthopedic Examination*. 3rd ed. Thorofare, NJ: SLACK Incorporated; 2006.

Magee DJ. *Orthopedic Physical Assessment*. 4th ed. Philadelphia, PA: W.B. Saunders; 2002.

Starkey C, Ryan JL. *Evaluation of Orthopedic and Athletic Injuries*. 2nd ed. Philadelphia, PA: F.A. Davis; 2002.

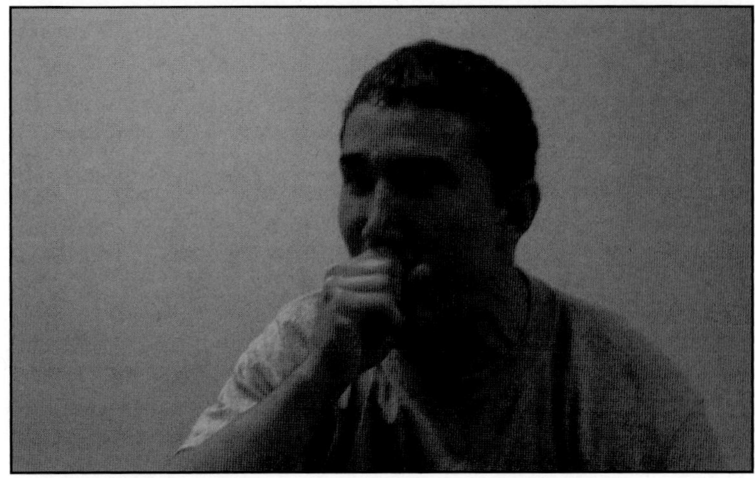

FIGURE 15-21

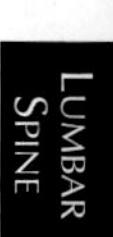

Section

FIVE

Upper Extremity

Chapter

16

Peripheral Nerve Pathology of the Upper Extremity

Axillary Nerve

Mechanism

Axillary nerve compression occurs due to trauma to the nerve, typically caused by anterior glenohumeral joint dislocation or proximal humerus fracture. A less common cause of axillary nerve impingement may occur secondary to the repeated trauma of leaning on the axillary pads while using crutches.

Clinical Findings

Common neurologic findings following axillary nerve compression include loss of sensation over the lateral aspect of the upper arm (C5 dermatome). The patient may also demonstrate flattening or atrophy of the deltoid and weakness in shoulder abduction and external rotation due to loss of the deltoids and the teres minor muscles.

Diagnostic Procedures

The clinician should carefully assess sensation of the C4 and C5 dermatomes in the presence of suspected axillary nerve injury. Additionally, the clinician should inspect for deltoid atrophy and assess active range of motion and strength of the shoulder abduction.

References

Gallaspy J, May JD. *Signs and Symptoms of Athletic Injuries*. Boston, MA: McGraw-Hill; 1996.

Magee DJ. Orthopedic Physical Assessment. 4th ed. Philadelphia, PA: W.B. Saunders; 2002.

Starkey C, Ryan JL. *Evaluation of Orthopedic and Athletic Injuries*. 2nd ed. Philadelphia, PA: F.A. Davis; 2002.

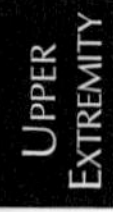

Long Thoracic Nerve Injury

Mechanism

The long thoracic nerve is injured due to indirect trauma to the shoulder or the lateral thoracic wall. The nerve may also be injured due to prolonged traction or overuse. Long thoracic nerve injury is commonly observed in swimmers, throwing athletes, and weight-lifters.

Clinical Findings

The most commonly observed finding in the presence of long thoracic nerve injury is winging of the scapula. Scapular winging is due to paralysis of the serratus anterior muscle.

Diagnostic Procedures

The clinician should observe the patient performing a wall push-up, assessing for scapular winging. The patient may also demonstrate difficulty completing active range of motion in shoulder flexion and abduction due to an alteration of scapulohumeral rhythm.

Special Considerations

Long thoracic nerve injury may be confirmed by EMG testing.

References

Brukner P, Khan K. *Clinical Sports Medicine.* 3rd ed. Auckland, NZ: McGraw-Hill Book Co; 2006.

Magee DJ. *Orthopedic Physical Assessment.* 4th ed. Philadelphia, PA: W.B. Saunders; 2002.

Peterson L, Renstrom L. *Sports Injuries: Their Prevention and Treatment.* Champaign, IL: Human Kinetics; 2001.

Starkey C, Ryan JL. *Evaluation of Orthopedic and Athletic Injuries.* 2nd ed. Philadelphia, PA: F.A. Davis; 2002.

Cubital Tunnel Syndrome

Mechanism

The cubital tunnel is defined as the area on the posterior, medial aspect of the elbow found between the medial epicondyle and the olecranon process. Cubital tunnel syndrome is identified as injury to the ulnar nerve as it passes through the tunnel. Common causes of ulnar nerve compression include direct trauma, traction in throwing athletes, and compression secondary to medial elbow edema. Injury to the nerve often accompanies ulnar collateral ligament injury in throwing athletes.

Clinical Findings

The patient will report medial elbow pain, as well as pain, numbness and tingling into the ulnar nerve distribution (the medial aspect of the forearm and hand). The ulnar nerve will be tender to palpation in the cubital tunnel.

Diagnostic Procedures

The clinician should perform sensory testing of the C8 dermatome. Additional testing should include palpation of the medial elbow and Tinel's Sign to reproduce the patient's neurologic symptoms.

Special Considerations

Cubital tunnel syndrome should be differentiated from other neurologic conditions resulting in loss of sensation to the medial hand. These include C8 nerve root injury, brachial plexus injury, and Guyon's Canal Syndrome (also known as Handlebar Palsy). Ulnar nerve compression, as the nerve enters the flexor carpi ulnaris, may also be observed in patients suffering from medial epicondylitis.

References

Magee DJ. *Orthopedic Physical Assessment.* 4th ed. Philadelphia, PA: W.B. Saunders; 2002.

Peterson L, Renstrom L. *Sports Injuries: Their Prevention and Treatment.* Champaign, IL: Human Kinetics; 2001.

Starkey C, Ryan JL. *Evaluation of Orthopedic and Athletic Injuries.* 2nd ed. Philadelphia, PA: F.A. Davis; 2002.

Cubital Fossa Syndrome

Mechanism

The cubital fossa is found between the pronator teres and brachioradialis on the anterior aspect of the elbow and contains the biceps tendon, the brachial artery, and the median nerve. Cubital fossa syndrome is identified as compression of the median nerve as it passes through the fossa. Common causes of median nerve compression include direct trauma, overuse due to repeated elbow flexion, and compression secondary to anterior elbow edema.

Clinical Findings

The patient will report cubital fossa pain and numbness and tingling into the median nerve distribution (the middle of the hand and digits 2 to 4).

Diagnostic Procedures

The clinician should perform sensory testing of the C7 dermatome. Additional testing should include palpation of the cubital fossa and performance of the Elbow Flexion Test in order to reproduce the patient's neurologic symptoms.

Special Considerations

Cubital fossa syndrome should be differentiated from other nerve compression injuries involving the median nerve distribution. These conditions include C7 nerve root compression, brachial plexus injury, pronator teres syndrome, and carpal tunnel syndrome.

References

Brukner P, Khan K. *Clinical Sports Medicine*. 3rd ed. Auckland, NZ: McGraw-Hill Book Co; 2006.

Magee DJ. *Orthopedic Physical Assessment*. 4th ed. Philadelphia, PA: W.B. Saunders; 2002.

Peterson L, Renstrom L. *Sports Injuries: Their Prevention and Treatment*. Champaign, IL: Human Kinetics; 2001.

Starkey C, Ryan JL. *Evaluation of Orthopedic and Athletic Injuries*. 2nd ed. Philadelphia, PA: F.A. Davis; 2002.

Radial Tunnel Syndrome/Supinator Syndrome

Mechanism

Radial Tunnel Syndrome, also known as Supinator Syndrome, refers to compression of the posterior interosseous branch of the radial nerve as it passes through the Arcade of Frohse in the supinator muscle.

Clinical Findings

Palpation will exhibit tenderness over the supinator muscle belly, distal to the lateral epicondyle and common extensor tendon. The patient may demonstrate pain and/or weakness with resisted forearm supination, but will demonstrate weakness only upon resisted wrist extension. The posterior interosseous branch of the radial nerve is a motor only branch, meaning the patient will not report sensory loss over the radial nerve distribution.

Diagnostic Procedures

The key diagnostic procedures to perform are palpation of the supinator muscle, as well as resistive testing in forearm supination and wrist extension. Electromyographic (EMG) and Nerve Conduction Velocity (NCV) testing may be helpful in identifying radial nerve entrapment.

Special Considerations

Symptoms of Radial Tunnel Syndrome will mimic those of lateral epicondylitis. The differentiating factor will be the assessment of resisted wrist extension. In the presence of lateral epicondylitis, the patient will demonstrate both pain and weakness during manual muscle testing of the wrist and finger extensors. Patients suffering from radial nerve entrapment will demonstrate only weakness in wrist and finger extension. The location of point tenderness may also aid the clinician in differentiating lateral epicondylitis from Supinator Syndrome.

References

Brukner P, Khan K. *Clinical Sports Medicine*. 3rd ed. Auckland, NZ: McGraw-Hill Book Co; 2006.

Magee DJ. *Orthopedic Physical Assessment*. 4th ed. Philadelphia, PA: W.B. Saunders; 2002.

Peterson L, Renstrom L. *Sports Injuries: Their Prevention and Treatment*. Champaign, IL: Human Kinetics; 2001.

Pronator Teres Syndrome

Mechanism

Pronator Teres Syndrome is a rare condition that occurs when the median nerve (anterior interosseous branch) is compressed as it passes through the pronator teres muscle.

Clinical Findings

The patient will report sensory loss over the median nerve distribution (C7 dermatome). Point tenderness may be reported over the anterior aspect of the elbow. Pain is exacerbated by resisted forearm pronation and elbow flexion. The patient may demonstrate weakness in finger flexion.

Diagnostic Procedures

The clinician should assess the pronator teres muscle by way of palpation and manual muscle testing. Additionally, the Pinch Grip Test will be positive.

Special Considerations

Pronator Teres Syndrome should be differentiated from other nerve compression injuries involving the median nerve distribution. These conditions include C7 nerve root compression, brachial plexus injury, Cubital Fossa Syndrome, and Carpal Tunnel Syndrome. The anterior interosseous branch of the median nerve is responsible for motor innervation of the pronator quadratus, the flexor pollicis longus, and the flexor digitorum profundus.

References

Brukner P, Khan K. *Clinical Sports Medicine*. 3rd ed. Auckland, NZ: McGraw-Hill Book Co; 2006.

Magee DJ. *Orthopedic Physical Assessment*. 4th ed. Philadelphia, PA: W.B. Saunders; 2002.

Peterson L, Renstrom L. *Sports Injuries: Their Prevention and Treatment*. Champaign, IL: Human Kinetics; 2001.

Carpal Tunnel Syndrome

Mechanism

Carpal Tunnel Syndrome occurs due to compression of the median nerve as it passes beneath the flexor retinaculum on the volar aspect of the wrist. The condition is most often caused by overuse of the wrist and finger flexors, resulting in swelling of the flexor tendons and compression of the median nerve in the carpal tunnel.

Clinical Findings

Classic symptoms of Carpal Tunnel Syndrome include numbness and tingling over the second, third, and fourth digits. The patient may report point tenderness to palpation of the carpal tunnel. Loss of hand dexterity and grip strength may be seen in chronic conditions, along with atrophy of the thenar eminence.

Diagnostic Procedures

Phalen's and Reverse Phalen's Tests should be performed in an attempt to reproduce the patient's neurologic symptoms. Palpation of the palmar aspect of the wrist may also prove beneficial in diagnosing this condition. EMG and NCV testing is helpful in confirming a diagnosis of Carpal Tunnel Syndrome.

Special Considerations

Carpal Tunnel Syndrome should be differentiated from other nerve compression injuries involving the median nerve distribution. These conditions include C7 nerve root compression, brachial plexus injury, Cubital Fossa Syndrome, and Pronator Teres Syndrome.

References

Brukner P, Khan K. *Clinical Sports Medicine*. 3rd ed. Auckland, NZ: McGraw-Hill Book Co; 2006.

Gallaspy J, May JD. *Signs and Symptoms of Athletic Injuries*. Boston, MA: McGraw-Hill; 1996.

Magee DJ. *Orthopedic Physical Assessment*. 4th ed. Philadelphia, PA: W.B. Saunders; 2002.

Peterson L, Renstrom L. *Sports Injuries: Their Prevention and Treatment*. Champaign, IL: Human Kinetics; 2001.

Starkey C, Ryan JL. *Evaluation of Orthopedic and Athletic Injuries*. 2nd ed. Philadelphia, PA: F.A. Davis; 2002.

Tunnel of Guyon Syndrome

Mechanism

Tunnel of Guyon Syndrome is defined as compression of the ulnar nerve as it passes between the pisiform and the hook of the hamate. The nerve is most commonly injured as a result of repeated trauma as occurs from compression in sports such as cycling. The condition is commonly referred to as Handlebar Palsy.

Clinical Findings

Symptoms of distal ulnar neuritis include pain and neurologic symptoms in the fourth and fifth digits, as well as the medial border of the hand (C8 dermatome). Finger abduction strength may be diminished upon resistive testing.

Diagnostic Procedures

Palpation of the Tunnel of Guyon and performance of a Tinel's Test are useful in diagnosing this condition.

Special Considerations

Tunnel of Guyon Syndrome is also known as *Guyon's Canal Syndrome* and *Handlebar Palsy*.

References

Brukner P, Khan K. *Clinical Sports Medicine*. 3rd ed. Auckland, NZ: McGraw-Hill Book Co; 2006.

Magee DJ. *Orthopedic Physical Assessment*. 4th ed. Philadelphia, PA: W.B. Saunders; 2002.

Peterson L, Renstrom L. *Sports Injuries: Their Prevention and Treatment*. Champaign, IL: Human Kinetics; 2001.

Drop Wrist Deformity

Mechanism

Drop Wrist results from injury to the radial nerve, causing paralysis and atrophy of the wrist extensor muscles.

Clinical Findings

The wrist will assume a position of flexion due to paralysis of the wrist extensor muscles. Additionally, the patient will be unable to complete active finger extension (Figure 16-1).

Diagnostic Procedures

Active range of motion and manual muscle testing will demonstrate wrist and finger extensor weakness caused by radial nerve injury.

Special Considerations

Drop wrist deformity can also be observed in the presence of supinator syndrome or radial tunnel syndrome.

References

Magee DJ. *Orthopedic Physical Assessment.* 4th ed. Philadelphia, PA: W.B. Saunders; 2002.

FIGURE 16-1

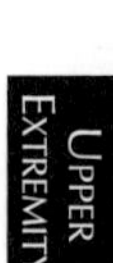

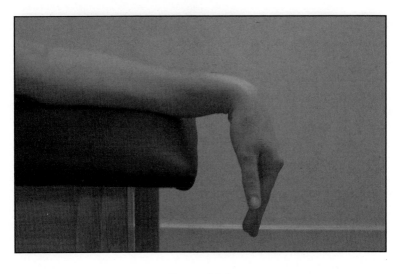

Ape Hand Deformity

Mechanism

Ape Hand Deformity is the result of median nerve palsy.

Clinical Findings

The classic sign of Ape Hand Deformity is atrophy of the thenar eminence. The thumb will also fall back in line with the fingers due to the pull of the extensor muscles. The patient will be unable to flex or oppose the thumb (Figures 16-2 and 16-3).

Diagnostic Procedures

This condition is best diagnosed upon visual inspection.

References

Magee DJ. *Orthopedic Physical Assessment.* 4th ed. Philadelphia, PA: W.B. Saunders; 2002.

Starkey C, Ryan JL. *Evaluation of Orthopedic and Athletic Injuries.* 2nd ed. Philadelphia, PA: F.A. Davis; 2002.

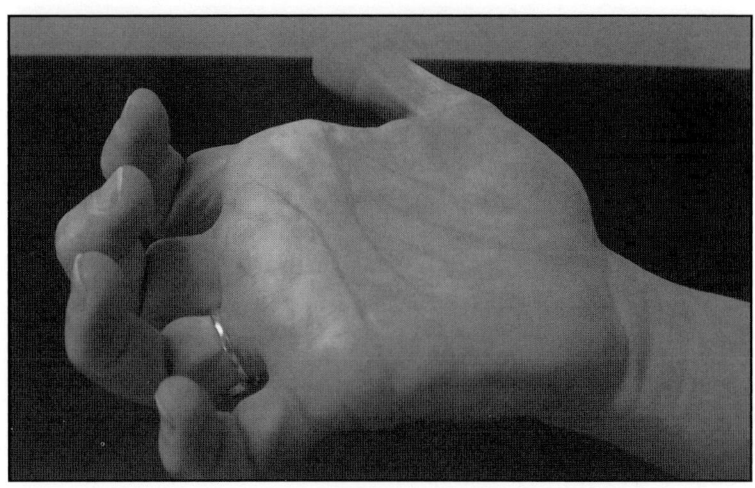

FIGURE 16-2

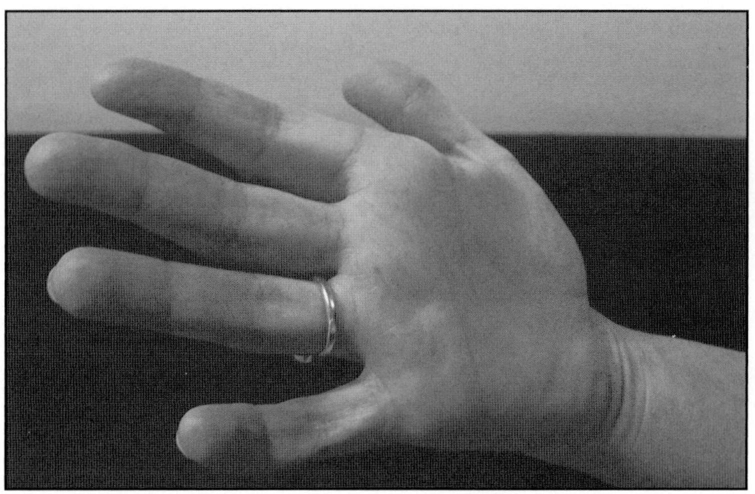

FIGURE 16-3

Bishop's Hand Deformity

Mechanism

Bishop's Hand Deformity results from atrophy of the hypothenar eminence, interossei, and medial lumbrical muscles due to ulnar nerve pathology.

Clinical Findings

The fingers will assume a posture of PIP and DIP flexion that is most pronounced in the fourth and fifth digits (Figure 16-4). Atrophy of the hypothenar eminence will be observed.

Diagnostic Procedures

This condition is best diagnosed upon visual inspection.

Special Considerations

This condition is also known as *Benediction Hand Deformity*.

References

Magee DJ. *Orthopedic Physical Assessment.* 4th ed. Philadelphia, PA: W.B. Saunders; 2002.

Starkey C, Ryan JL. *Evaluation of Orthopedic and Athletic Injuries.* 2nd ed. Philadelphia, PA: F.A. Davis; 2002.

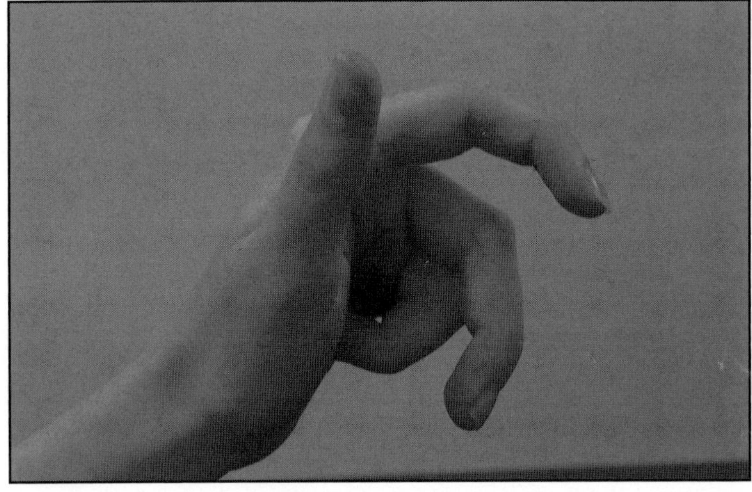

FIGURE 16-4

Claw Hand Deformity

Mechanism

Claw Hand Deformity results from loss of the intrinsic muscle activity, coupled with overaction of extensor muscles of the proximal phalanx.

Clinical Findings

The MCP joints are hyperextended, while the DIP and PIP joints are both flexed (Figure 16-5).

Diagnostic Procedures

This condition is best diagnosed upon visual inspection.

Special Considerations

In cases where the intrinsic musculature is completely lost, normal cupping of the hand cannot be performed and the longitudinal and transverse arches of the hand disappear due to muscle atrophy. This deformity is called an Intrinsic Minus Hand and is most often the result of combined median and ulnar nerve pathology.

References

Magee DJ. *Orthopedic Physical Assessment.* 4th ed. Philadelphia, PA: W.B. Saunders; 2002.

Starkey C, Ryan JL. *Evaluation of Orthopedic and Athletic Injuries.* 2nd ed. Philadelphia, PA: F.A. Davis; 2002.

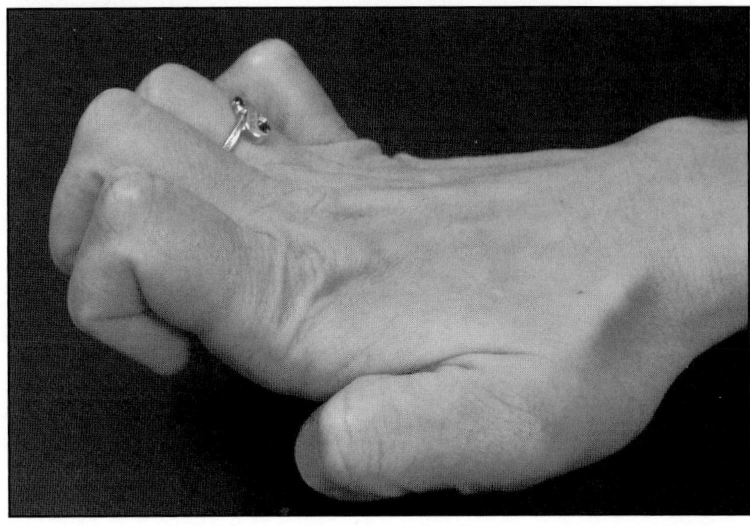

FIGURE 16-5

Chapter 17

Special Tests for the Upper Extremity

Adson's Test

Test Position

The patient is positioned in sitting or standing.

Action

The clinician palpates the distal radial pulse with the patient's arm at his or her side. The clinician maintains palpation of the radial pulse throughout the test procedure. The clinician passively positions the patient in shoulder external rotation and extension. The patient is instructed to take a deep breath while simultaneously extending and rotating his or her cervical spine toward the side of testing (Figure 17-1). This test should be performed bilaterally to compare findings.

Positive Finding

A positive finding is a diminished (rate or rhythm) or absent radial pulse, indicating Thoracic Outlet Syndrome. Reproduction of the patient's upper extremity symptoms during testing further confirms a diagnosis of Thoracic Outlet Syndrome.

Special Considerations

Although Thoracic Outlet Syndrome can involve neurologic and vascular structures, this test is primarily designed to assess compression of the subclavian artery between the scalenes and the pectoralis minor musculature. This test has a very high incidence, estimated at greater than 50%, of false-positives.

Historical Notes

This test is named for neurosurgeon Alfred Washington Adson.

Alternate Names

This test is also known as *Adson's Procedure* and *Adson's Maneuver*.

Specificity

No data available.

Sensitivity

No data available.

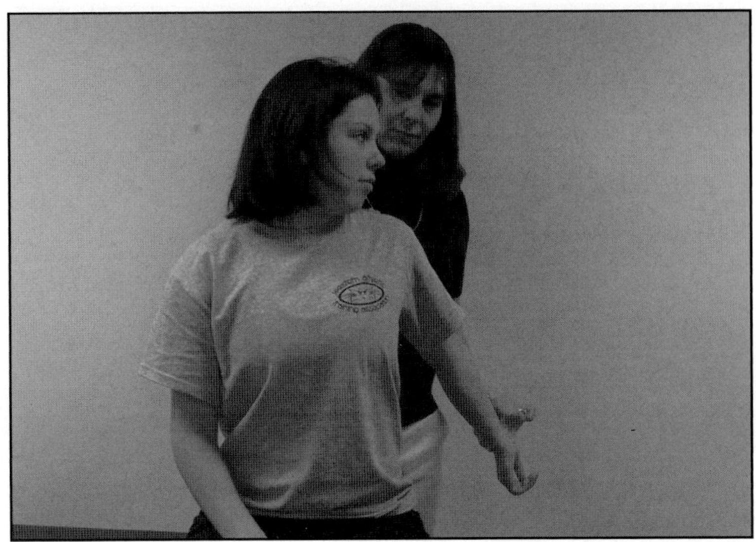

FIGURE 17-1

REFERENCES

Baker CL, Liu SH. Neurovascular injuries to the shoulder. *J Ortho Sports Phys Ther*. 1993;18(1):360-364.

Konin JG, Wiksten DL, Isear JA, Brader H. *Special Tests for Orthopedic Examination*. 3rd ed. Thorofare, NJ: SLACK Incorporated; 2006.

Magee DJ. *Orthopedic Physical Assessment*. 4th ed. Philadelphia, PA: W.B. Saunders; 2002.

Malanga GA, Landes P, Nadler SF. Provocative tests in cervical spine examination: historical basis and scientific analyses. *Pain Physician*. 2003;6(2):199-205.

Piewa MC, Delinger M. The false-positive rate of thoracic outlet syndrome shoulder maneuvers in healthy subjects. *Acad Emerg Med*. 1998;5(4):337-342.

Starkey C, Ryan JL. *Evaluation of Orthopedic and Athletic Injuries*. 2nd ed. Philadelphia, PA: F.A. Davis; 2002.

Allen's Test

Test Position

The patient is positioned in sitting or standing with the shoulder positioned in 90 degrees of abduction and 90 degrees of external rotation. The elbow is also flexed to 90 degrees.

Action

The clinician palpates the distal radial pulse and instructs the patient to rotate his or her cervical spine away from the test arm (Figure 17-2). This test should be performed bilaterally to compare findings.

Positive Finding

A positive finding is a diminished (rate or rhythm) or absent radial pulse, indicating Thoracic Outlet Syndrome. Reproduction of the patient's upper extremity symptoms during testing further confirms a diagnosis of Thoracic Outlet Syndrome.

Special Considerations

This test is designed to assess for compression of neurovascular structures by a tight pectoralis minor muscle. This test has a very high incidence, estimated at greater than 50%, of false-positives.

Historical Notes

This test is named for Edgar Van Nuys Allen, a professor of medicine at the Mayo Clinic, who published extensively on the topic of peripheral vascular disease.

Alternate Names

This test is also known as *Allen's Maneuver*.

Specificity

No data available.

Sensitivity

No data available.

References

Konin JG, Wiksten DL, Isear JA, Brader H. *Special Tests for Orthopedic Examination*. 3rd ed. Thorofare, NJ: SLACK Incorporated; 2006.

Magee DJ. *Orthopedic Physical Assessment*. 4th ed. Philadelphia, PA: W.B. Saunders; 2002.

Starkey C, Ryan JL. *Evaluation of Orthopedic and Athletic Injuries*. 2nd ed. Philadelphia, PA: F.A. Davis; 2002.

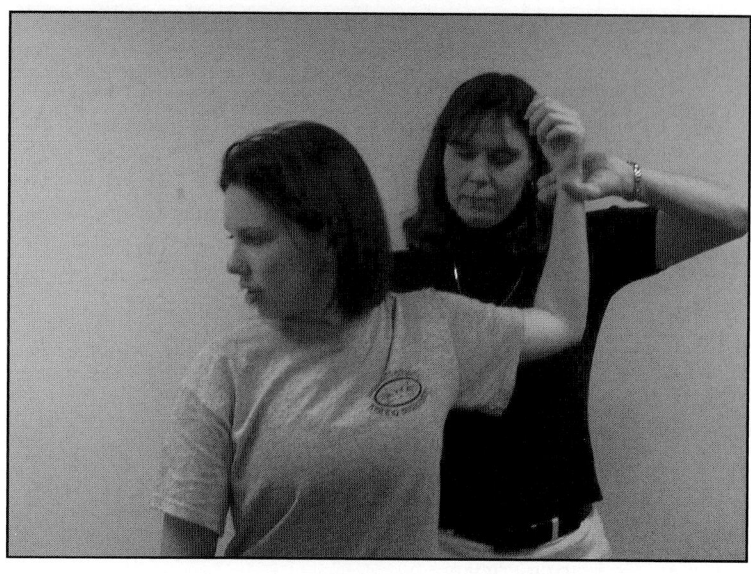

FIGURE 17-2

Military Brace Position

Test Position

The patient is positioned in standing in anatomical position.

Action

The clinician palpates the distal radial pulse with the patient's arm at his or her side and maintains palpation of the radial pulse throughout the test procedure. The clinician passively positions the involved shoulder in extension and abduction (30 degrees), while simultaneously instructing the patient to extend his or her cervical spine to end-range (Figure 17-3). This test should be performed bilaterally to compare findings.

Positive Finding

A positive finding is a diminished (rate or rhythm) or absent radial pulse, indicating Thoracic Outlet Syndrome.

Special Considerations

Although Thoracic Outlet Syndrome can involve neurologic and vascular structures, this test is primarily designed to assess compression of the subclavian artery as it passes under the clavicle and ribs.

Historical Notes

This test is a modification of the standing at attention position that is utilized in the military.

Alternate Names

This test is also known as the *Costoclavicular Syndrome Test, Scapular Posterior Depression Test,* and the *Costoclavicular Maneuver*.

Specificity

No data available.

Sensitivity

No data available.

References

Baker CL, Liu SH. Neurovascular injuries to the shoulder. *J Ortho Sports Phys Ther*. 1993;18(1):360-364.

Lain, TM. The military brace syndrome. A report of sixteen cases of Erb's palsy occurring in military cadets. *J Bone Joint Surg Am*. 1969;51(3):557–560.

Magee DJ. *Orthopedic Physical Assessment*. 4th ed. Philadelphia, PA: W.B. Saunders; 2002.

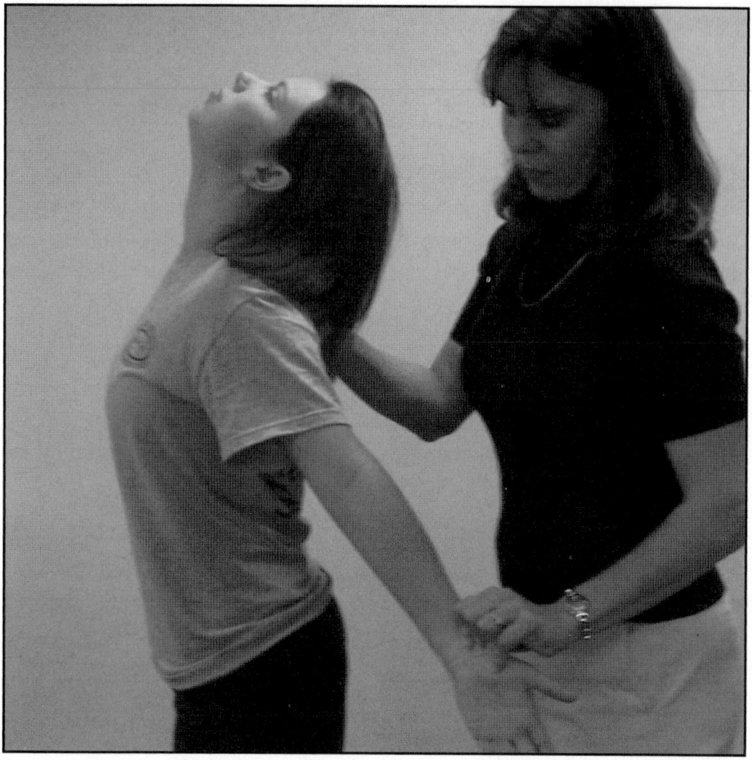

FIGURE 17-3

Piewa MC, Delinger M. The false-positive rate of thoracic outlet syndrome shoulder maneuvers in healthy subjects. *Acad Emerg Med*. 1998;5(4):337-342.

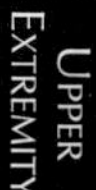

Hyperabduction Syndrome Test

Test Position

The patient is positioned in sitting or supine.

Action

The clinician palpates the distal radial pulse with the patient's arm at his side and maintains palpation of the radial pulse throughout the test procedure. The clinician passively abducts the shoulder 180 degrees with the shoulder externally rotated (Figures 17-4 through 17-6).

Positive Finding

A positive finding is a diminished (rate or rhythm) or absent radial pulse, indicating Thoracic Outlet Syndrome. Reproduction of the patient's upper extremity symptoms during testing further confirms a diagnosis of Thoracic Outlet Syndrome.

Special Considerations

The patient may be instructed to take a deep breath while simultaneously extending and rotating the cervical spine toward the involved side.

Historical Notes

This test was developed by Wright, but has since been modified to become the *Allen Maneuver*.

Alternate Names

This test is also known as the *Wright Test* and the *Wright Maneuver*.

Specificity

No data available.

Sensitivity

No data available.

References

Baker CL, Liu SH. Neurovascular injuries to the shoulder. *J Ortho Sports Phys Ther*. 1993;18(1):360-364.

Gagey OJ, Gagey N. The hyperabduction test. *J Bone Joint Surg*. 2001;83(1): 69-74.

Magee DJ. *Orthopedic Physical Assessment*. 4th ed. Philadelphia, PA: W.B. Saunders; 2002.

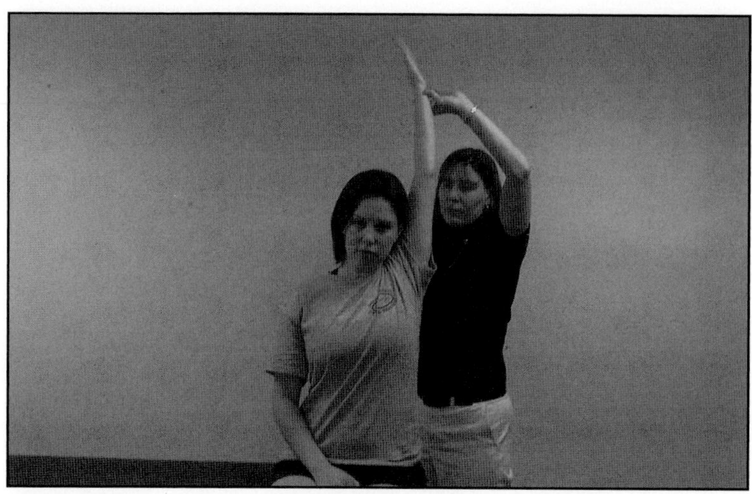

FIGURE 17-4

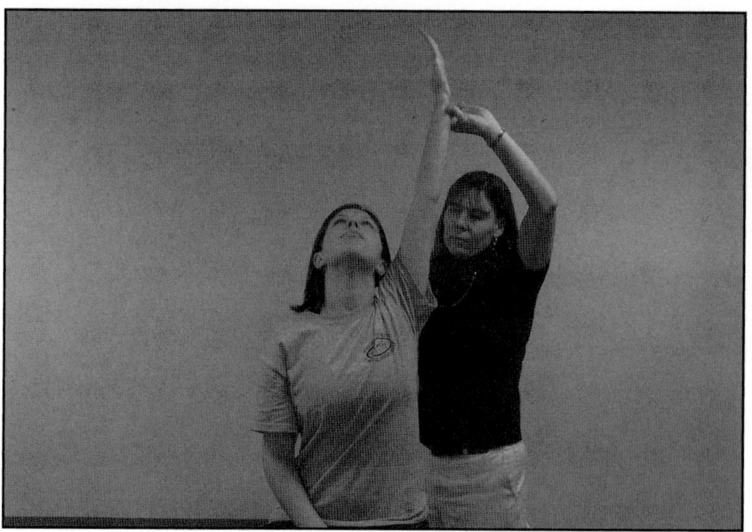

FIGURE 17-5

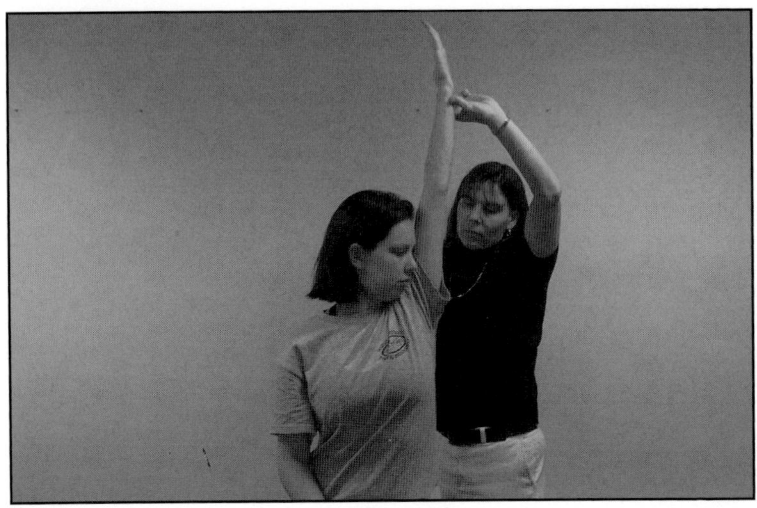

FIGURE 17-6

Halstead's Maneuver

Test Position

The patient is positioned in sitting or standing.

Action

The clinician palpates the distal radial pulse with the patient's arm at his or her side and maintains palpation of the radial pulse throughout the test procedure. The clinician applies downward traction on the involved upper extremity while instructing the patient to simultaneously extend and rotate his or her cervical spine to the opposite side of testing (Figure 17-7). This test should be performed bilaterally to compare findings.

Positive Finding

A positive finding is a diminished (rate or rhythm) or absent radial pulse, indicating Thoracic Outlet Syndrome.

Alternate Names

This test is also known as *Halstead's Test*.

Specificity

No data available.

Sensitivity

No data available.

References

Magee DJ. *Orthopedic Physical Assessment.* 4th ed. Philadelphia, PA: W.B. Saunders; 2002.

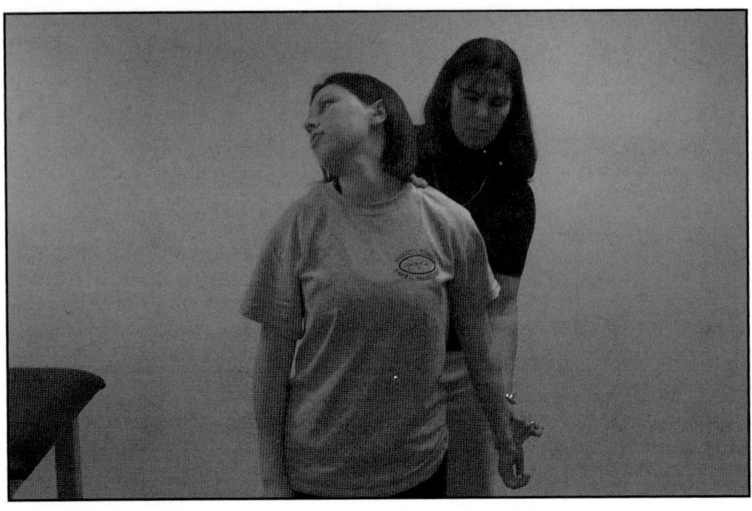

FIGURE 17-7

Roo's Test

Test Position

The patient is positioned in sitting or standing with both elbows and the shoulders positioned in 90 degrees of abduction and external rotation.

Action

The patient is instructed to rapidly open and close both hands repeatedly for 3 minutes (Figures 17-8 and 17-9).

Positive Finding

Positive findings are diminished motor function, pain and weakness in the hand, and/or loss of sensation into the upper extremity. Positive test results are indicative of Thoracic Outlet Syndrome.

Special Considerations

This test is designed to assess for compression of both neurovascular structures. Roo's Test is considered the most accurate test for assessing Thoracic Outlet Syndrome. Inability to complete the exam for 3 minutes may be considered a positive test.

Historical Notes

The test is named for physician David B. Roos, who first described the test during his study of Thoracic Outlet Syndrome causes.

Alternate Names

This test is also known as the *Roo's Stress Test, Elevated Arm Stress Test (EAST)*, the *Positive Abduction and External Rotation Position Test*, and the *Hands-Up Test*.

Specificity

No data available.

Sensitivity

No data available.

References

Konin JG, Wiksten DL, Isear JA, Brader H. *Special Tests for Orthopedic Examination.* 3rd ed. Thorofare, NJ: SLACK Incorporated; 2006.

Magee DJ. *Orthopedic Physical Assessment.* 4th ed. Philadelphia, PA: W.B. Saunders; 2002.

Starkey C, Ryan JL. *Evaluation of Orthopedic and Athletic Injuries.* 2nd ed. Philadelphia, PA: F.A. Davis; 2002.

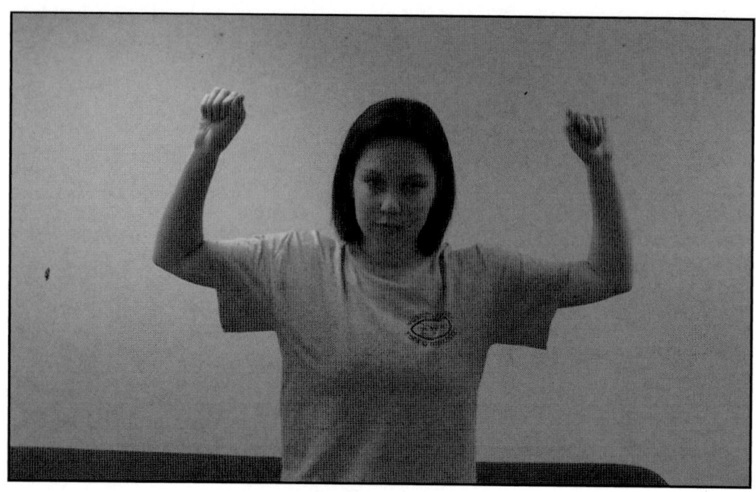

Figure 17-8

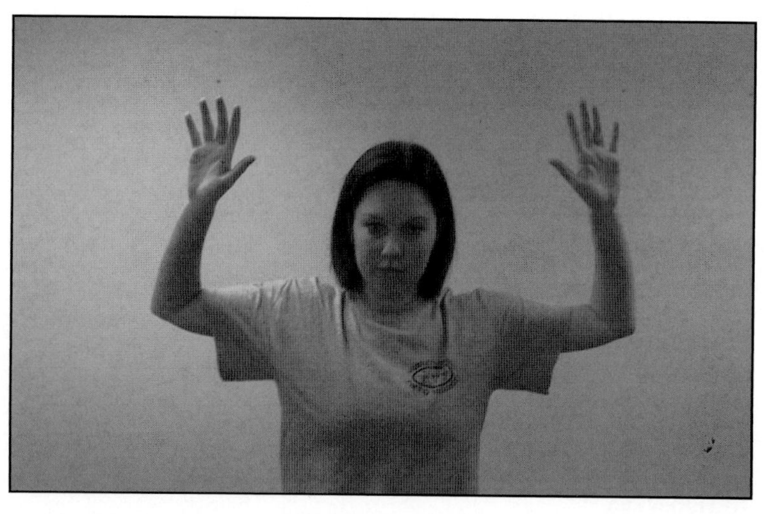

Figure 17-9

Tinel's Sign at the Elbow

Test Position

The patient is positioned in sitting with the elbow in slight flexion.

Action

The clinician stabilizes the wrist and taps the ulnar nerve in the cubital tunnel using the index finger (Figure 17-10).

Positive Finding

A positive finding is tingling along the ulnar nerve distribution (the medial side of the forearm and hand), indicative of ulnar nerve pathology.

Special Considerations

This test should be performed bilaterally for comparison of findings.

Historical Notes

This test is named for Jules Tinel, who, in 1915, described the process of nerve regeneration after injury and described a test that involved pressing on the nerve area. In reality, however, it was Paul Hoffmann who, also in 1915, originally described the tapping test to assess for median nerve injury in cases of Carpal Tunnel Syndrome.

Alternate Names

This test is also known as *Tinel's Test*.

Specificity

.76 – .98

Sensitivity

.68 – .70

Positive Likelihood Ratio

2.8 – 35

Negative Likelihood Ratio

.31 – .42

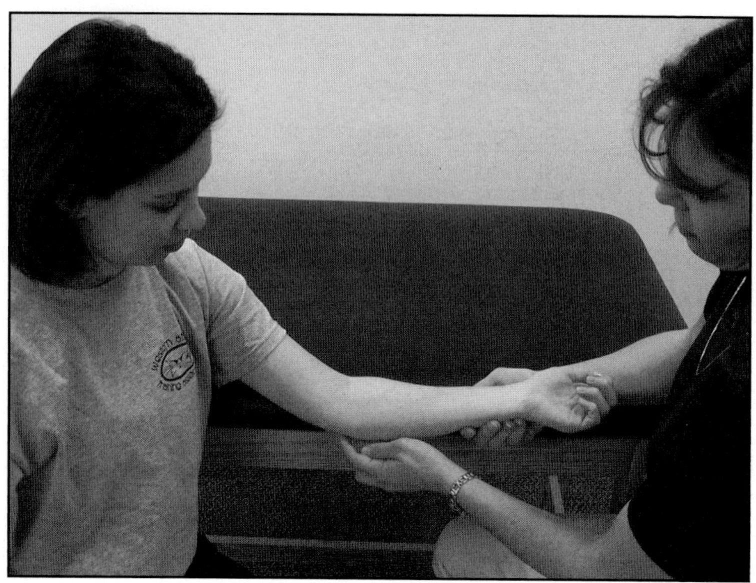

FIGURE 17-10

REFERENCES

Greenwald D, Blum LC, Adams D, Mercantonio C, Moffit M, Cooper B. Effective surgical treatment of cubital tunnel syndrome based on provocative clinical testing with electrodiagnostics. *Plast Reconstr Surg*. 2006;117(5):87-91.

Kingery WS, Park KS, Wu PB, Date ES. Electromyographic motor Tinel's sign in ulnar mononeuropathies at the elbow. *Am J Phys Med Rehab*. 1995;74:419-426.

Konin JG, Wiksten DL, Isear JA, Brader H. *Special Tests for Orthopedic Examination*. 3rd ed. Thorofare, NJ: SLACK Incorporated; 2006.

Magee DJ. *Orthopedic Physical Assessment*. 4th ed. Philadelphia, PA: W.B. Saunders; 2002.

Norkus SA, Meyers NC. Ulnar neuropathy of the elbow. *Sports Medicine*. 1994;17(3):189-199.

Novak CB, Lee GW, Mackinnon SE, Lay L. Provocative testing for cubital tunnel syndrome. *J Hand Surg [Am]*. 1994;19(5):817-820.

Elbow Flexion Test

Test Position

The patient is positioned in sitting or standing.

Action

The patient is instructed to actively flex his or her bilateral elbows to end-range with the wrists in full flexion and the forearms in supination. The patient holds this position for 3 to 5 minutes (Figure 17-11).

Positive Finding

A positive finding is radiating pain into the median nerve distribution (middle fingers and middle of hand), indicating compression of the median nerve in the cubital fossa. A second positive finding is radiating pain into the ulnar nerve distribution (medial border of forearm and hand), indicating ulnar nerve compression in the cubital tunnel.

Special Considerations

The patient may also be positioned with elbow flexion to end-range with wrist extension, forearm pronation, and shoulder depression and abduction (Figure 17-12).

Specificity

.99

Sensitivity

.75

Positive Likelihood Ratio

75

Negative Likelihood Ratio

.25

References

Konin JG, Wiksten DL, Isear JA, Brader H. *Special Tests for Orthopedic Examination*. 3rd ed. Thorofare, NJ: SLACK Incorporated; 2006.

Magee DJ. *Orthopedic Physical Assessment*. 4th ed. Philadelphia, PA: W.B. Saunders; 2002.

Norkus SA, Meyers NC. Ulnar neuropathy of the elbow. *Sports Medicine*. 1994;17(3):189-199.

Novak CB, Lee GW, Mackinnon SE, Lay L. Provocative testing for cubital tunnel syndrome. *J Hand Surg [Am]*. 1994;19(5):817-820.

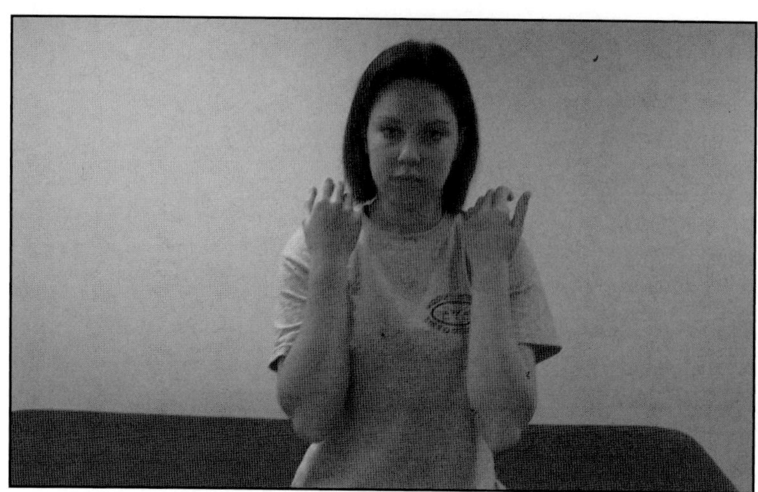

Figure 17-11

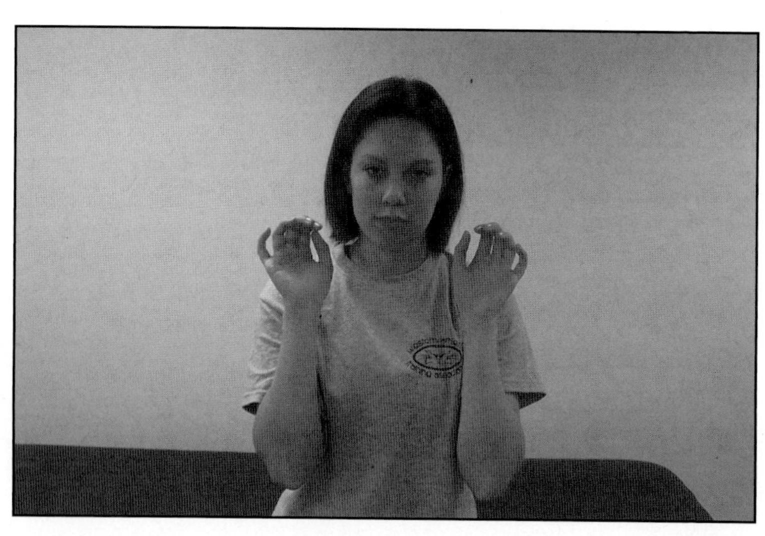

Figure 17-12

Pronator Teres Syndrome Test

Test Position

The patient is positioned in sitting with the elbow flexed to 90 degrees.

Action

The clinician resists forearm pronation while allowing active extension of the elbow (Figures 17-13 through 17-15).

Positive Finding

A positive finding is paresthesia in the median nerve distribution (middle fingers and middle of hand), indicating compression of the median nerve at the pronator teres.

Specificity

No data available.

Sensitivity

No data available.

References

Magee DJ. *Orthopedic Physical Assessment.* 4th ed. Philadelphia, PA: W.B. Saunders; 2002.

Mysiew WJ, Colachis SC. The pronator syndrome: an evaluation of dynamic maneuvers for improving electrodiagnostic sensitivity. *Am J Phys Med Rehab.* 1991;70(5):274-277.

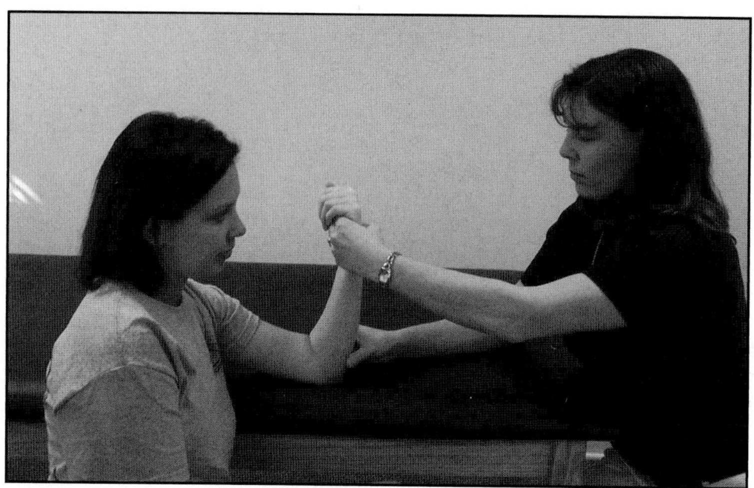

Figure 17-13

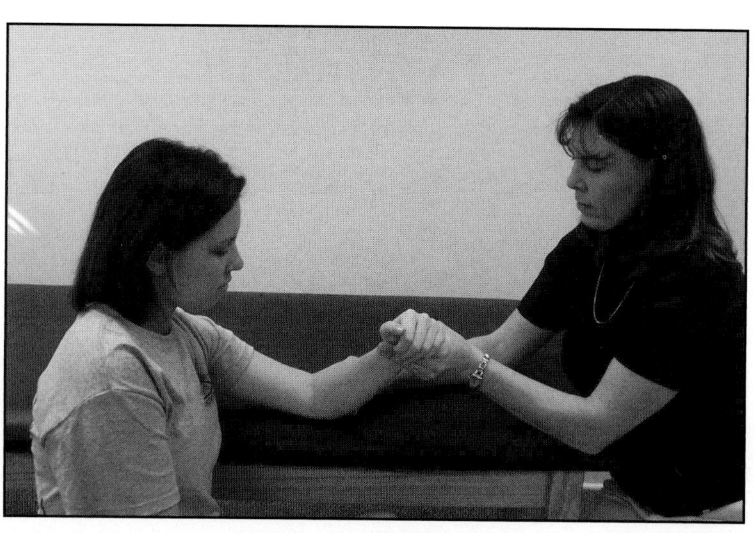

Figure 17-14

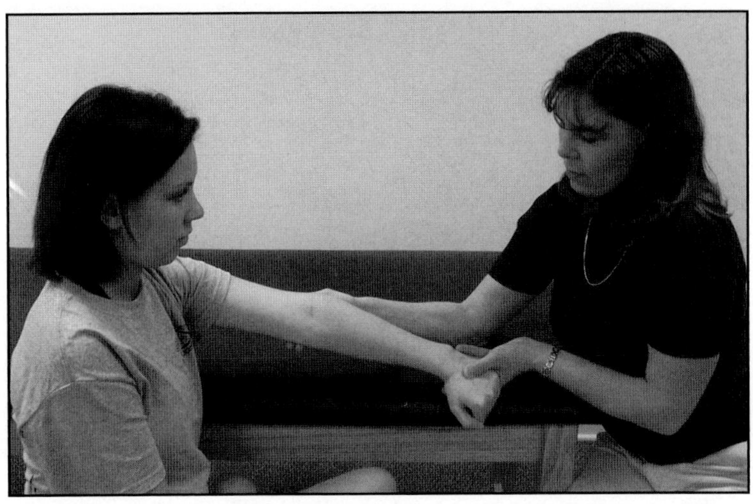

FIGURE 17-15

Wartenberg's Sign

Test Position

The patient is positioned in sitting with the palm of his or her hand resting on the table.

Action

The clinician passively abducts the patient's fingers (Figure 17-16). The patient is then instructed to actively adduct the fingers (Figure 17-17).

Positive Finding

A positive finding is an inability to adduct the fifth digit, indicating an ulnar nerve pathology (Figure 17-18).

Historical Notes

This test is named for neurologist Robert Wartenberg, who first described his findings in 1944.

Specificity

No data available.

Sensitivity

No data available.

References

Magee DJ. *Orthopedic Physical Assessment.* 4th ed. Philadelphia, PA: W.B. Saunders; 2002.

Voche P, Merle M. Wartenberg's sign: a new method of surgical correction. *J Hand Surg*. 1995;20(1):49-52.

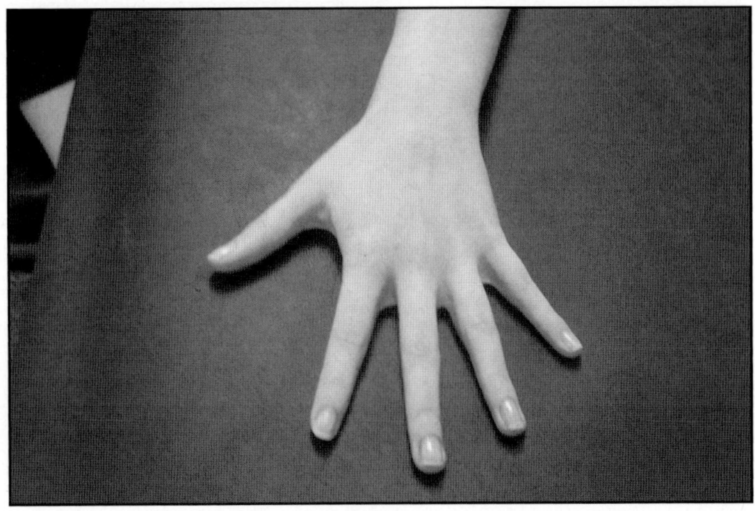

FIGURE 17-16

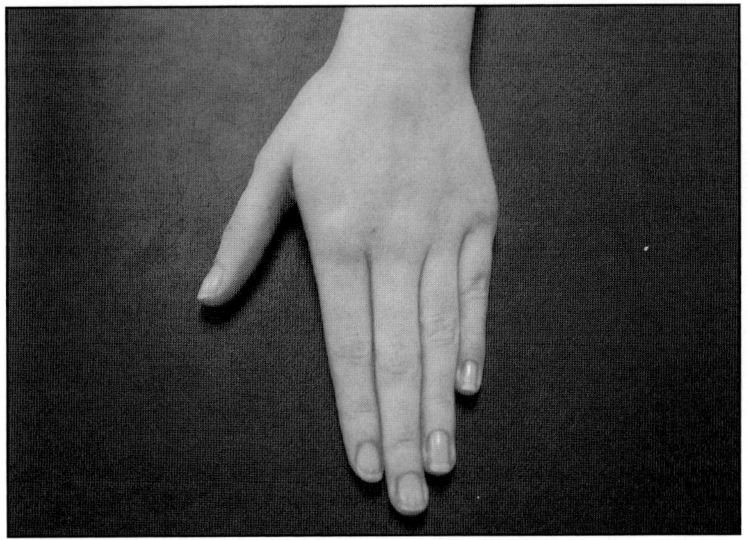

FIGURE 17-17

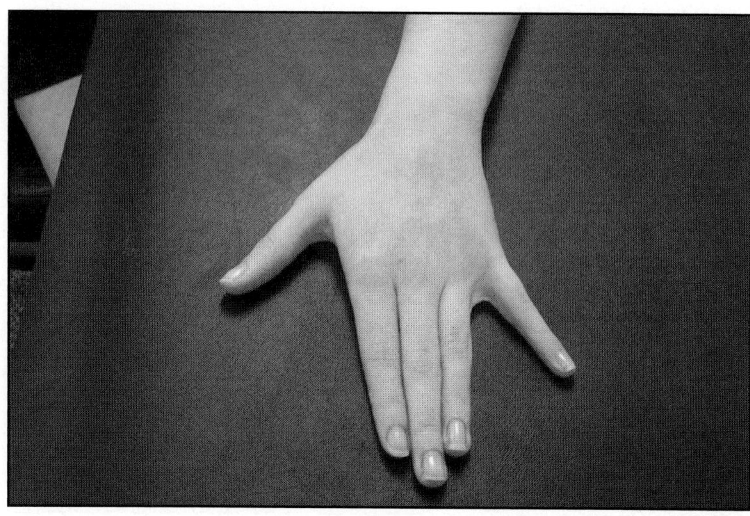

FIGURE 17-18

Phalen's Test

Test Position

The patient is positioned in sitting or standing.

Action

The clinician instructs the patient to place the dorsum of both hands together while placing the wrists in flexion. The patient is then instructed to apply compression of the hands through the forearms to maximally flex the wrists to end-range. This position is held for 1 minute (Figure 17-19).

Positive Finding

A positive finding is numbness and tingling in the median nerve distribution (middle of the hand and digits 2-4), indicative of Carpal Tunnel Syndrome, secondary to median nerve compression.

Special Considerations

The patient's forearms should be parallel to the shoulders while performing this exam. Positive test results may be further exacerbated by having the patient form an "O" using the index finger and thumb while completing Phalen's Test. Wrist pain without neurologic deficits is not a positive finding for Carpal Tunnel Syndrome.

Historical Notes

This test was developed by orthopedist George S. Phalen.

Alternate Names

This test is also known as *Phalen's Maneuver, Phalen's Sign,* and *Phalen's Position*.

Specificity

.40 – 1.0

Sensitivity

.34 – .88

Positive Likelihood Ratio

1.15 – 8.7

Negative Likelihood Ratio

.12 – .89

Reliability

Kappa values at the 95% confidence interval range from .79 – .88.

References

Cleland J. *Orthopaedic Clinical Examination: An Evidence-Based Approach for Physical Therapists*. Carlstadt, NJ: Icon Learning Systems; 2005.

Gellman H. Carpal tunnel syndrome: an evaluation of the provocative diagnostic tests. *J Bone Joint Surg*. 1986;68:734-737.

Ghavanini MR, Haghighat M. Carpal tunnel syndrome: reappraisal of five clinical tests. *Electromyogr Clin Neurophysiol*. 1998;38(7):437-441.

Konin JG, Wiksten DL, Isear JA, Brader H. *Special Tests for Orthopedic Examination*. 3rd ed. Thorofare, NJ: SLACK Incorporated; 2006.

Magee DJ. *Orthopedic Physical Assessment*. 4th ed. Philadelphia, PA: W.B. Saunders; 2002.

Marx RG, Hudak PL, Bombardier C, Graham B, Goldsmith C, Wright JG. The reliability of physical examination for carpal tunnel syndrome. *J Hand Surg*. 1998;23(4):499-502.

Starkey C, Ryan JL. *Evaluation of Orthopedic and Athletic Injuries*. 2nd ed. Philadelphia, PA: F.A. Davis; 2002.

Szabo RM, Slater RR, Farver TB, Stanton DB, Sharman WK. The value of diagnostic testing in carpal tunnel syndrome. *J Hand Surg*. 1999;24(4):704-714.

Walters C, Rice V. An evaluation of provocative testing in the diagnosis of carpal tunnel syndrome. *Military Medicine*. 2002;167(8):647-652.

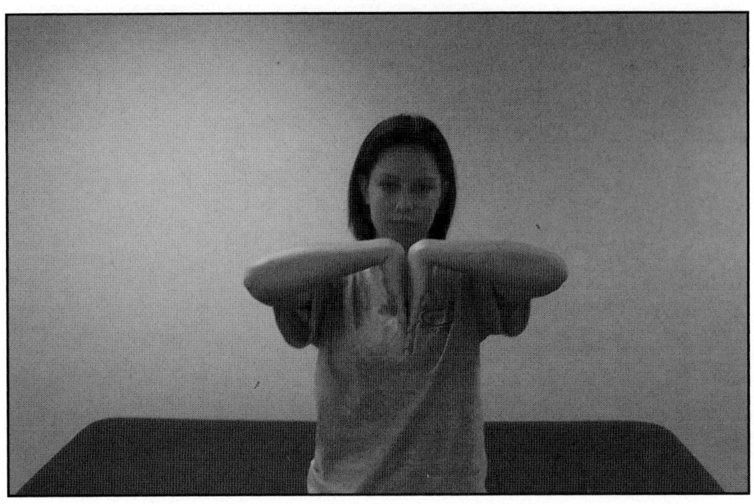

FIGURE 17-19

Reverse Phalen's Test

Test Position

The patient is positioned in sitting or standing.

Action

The clinician instructs the patient to place the palmar aspect of both hands together while placing the wrists in extension. The patient is then instructed to apply compression of the hands through the forearms to maximally extend the wrists to end-range. This position is held for 1 minute (Figure 17-20).

Positive Finding

A positive finding is numbness and tingling in the median nerve distribution (middle of the hand and digits 2-4), indicative of Carpal Tunnel Syndrome secondary to median nerve compression.

Special Considerations

The patient's forearms should be parallel to the shoulders while performing this exam. Wrist pain without neurologic deficits is not a positive finding for Carpal Tunnel Syndrome.

Historical Notes

This test was developed by orthopedist George S. Phalen.

Alternate Names

This test is also known as the *Wrist Extension Test, Reverse Phalen's Maneuver, Reverse Phalen's Sign,* and *Reverse Phalen's Position*.

Specificity

.82

Sensitivity

.55

Positive Likelihood Ratio

3.06

Negative Likelihood Ratio

.55

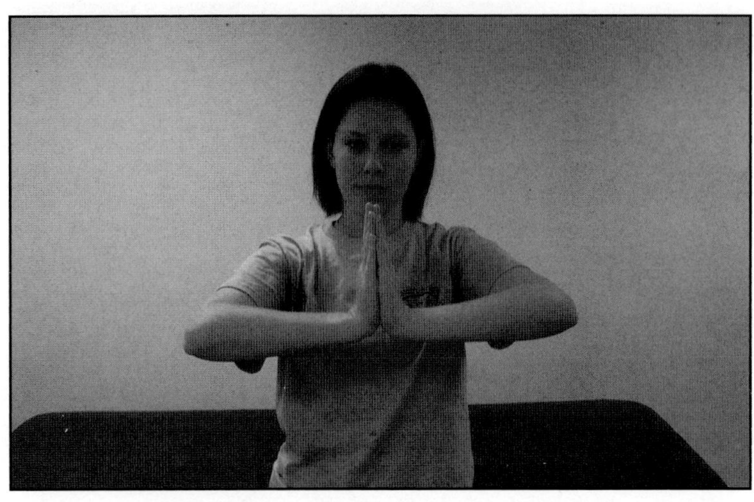

FIGURE 17-20

REFERENCES

Ghavanini MR, Haghighat M. Carpal tunnel syndrome: reappraisal of five clinical tests. *Electromyogr Clin Neurophysiol*. 1998;38(7):437-441.

Konin JG, Wiksten DL, Isear JA, Brader H. *Special Tests for Orthopedic Examination*. 3rd ed. Thorofare, NJ: SLACK Incorporated; 2006.

Magee DJ. *Orthopedic Physical Assessment*. 4th ed. Philadelphia, PA: W.B. Saunders; 2002.

Mondelli M, Passero S, Giannini F. Provocative tests in different stages of carpal tunnel syndrome. *Clin Neurol Neurosurg*. 2001;103:178-183.

Starkey C, Ryan, JL. *Evaluation of Orthopedic and Athletic Injuries*. 2nd ed. Philadelphia, PA: F.A. Davis; 2002.

Werner RA, Bir C, Armstrong TJ. Reverse Phalen's maneuver as an aid in diagnosing carpal tunnel syndrome. *Arch Phys Med Rehab*. 1994;75(7):783-786.

Tinel's Sign at the Wrist

Test Position

The patient is positioned in sitting with the forearm resting on a table.

Action

The clinician taps over the palmar surface of the subject's wrist at the carpal tunnel (Figure 17-21).

Positive Finding

A positive finding is tingling or parasthesia along the median nerve distribution (digits 2-4), indicative of median nerve pathology at the carpal tunnel.

Special Considerations

This test should be performed bilaterally to allow for comparison.

Historical Notes

This test is named for Jules Tinel, who, in 1915, described the process of nerve regeneration after injury and described a test that involved pressing on the nerve area. In reality, however, it was Paul Hoffmann who, also in 1915, originally described the tapping test to assess for median nerve injury in cases of Carpal Tunnel Syndrome.

Alternate Names

This test is also known as *Tinel's Test*.

Specificity

.56 – 1.0

Sensitivity

.23 – .74

Positive Likelihood Ratio

.93 – 8.22

Negative Likelihood Ratio

.29 – 1.05

Reliability

Kappa values at the 95% confidence interval range from .35 to .47.

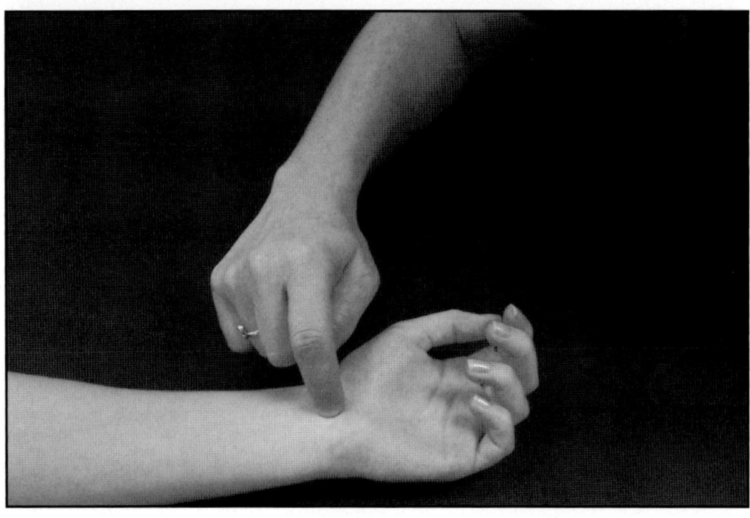

FIGURE 17-21

REFERENCES

Cleland J. *Orthopaedic Clinical Examination: An Evidence-Based Approach for Physical Therapists*. Carlstadt, NJ: Icon Learning Systems; 2005.

Konin JG, Wiksten DL, Isear JA, Brader H. *Special Tests for Orthopedic Examination*. 3rd ed. Thorofare, NJ: SLACK Incorporated; 2006.

Magee DJ. *Orthopedic Physical Assessment*. 4th ed. Philadelphia., PA: W.B. Saunders; 2002.

Marx RG, Hudak PL, Bombardier C, Graham B, Goldsmith C, Wright JG. The reliability of physical examination for carpal tunnel syndrome. *J Hand Surg*. 1998;23(4):499-502.

Mondelli M, Passero S, Giannini F. Provocative tests in different stages of carpal tunnel syndrome. *Clin Neurol Neurosurg*. 2001;103:178-183.

Priganc VW, Henry SM. The relationship among five common carpal tunnel syndrome tests and the severity of carpal tunnel syndrome. *J Hand Ther*. 2003;16(3):225-236.

Starkey C, Ryan JL. *Evaluation of Orthopedic and Athletic Injuries*. 2nd ed. Philadelphia, PA: F.A. Davis; 2002.

Szabo RM, Slater RR, Farver TB, Stanton DB, Sharman WK. The value of diagnostic testing in carpal tunnel syndrome. *J Hand Surg*. 1999;24(4):704-714.

Wainner RS, Fritz JM, Irrgang JJ, Delitto A, Allison S, Boninger ML. Development of a clinical prediction rule for the diagnosis of carpal tunnel syndrome. *Arch Phys Med Rehab*. 2005;86:609-618.

Carpal Compression Test

Test Position

The patient is positioned in sitting with the forearm resting on a table.

Action

The clinician uses his or her thumb to apply compression over the palmar surface of the subject's wrist at the carpal tunnel (Figure 17-22).

Positive Finding

A positive finding is tingling or parasthesia along the median nerve distribution (digits 2-4), indicative of median nerve pathology at the carpal tunnel.

Special Considerations

This test should be performed bilaterally to allow for comparison.

Specificity

.30 – .95

Sensitivity

.28 – .89

Positive Likelihood Ratio

.91 – 17.4

Negative Likelihood Ratio

.13 – 1.2

References

Cleland J. *Orthopaedic Clinical Examination: an Evidence-Based Approach for Physical Therapists*. Carlstadt, NJ: Icon Learning Systems; 2005.

Ghavanini MR, Haghighat M. Carpal tunnel syndrome: reappraisal of five clinical tests. *Electromyogr Clin Neurophysiol*. 1998;38(7):437-441.

Gonzalez del Pino J, Delgado-Martinez AD, Gonzalez-Gonzalez I, Lovic A. Value of the carpal compression test in the diagnosis of carpal tunnel syndrome. *J Hand Surg*. 1997;22(1):38-41.

Kaul MP, Pagel KJ, Wheatley MJ, Dryden JD. Carpal compression test and pressure provactive test in veterans with median-distribution parasthesias. *Muscle and Nerve*. 2001;24(1):107-111.

Magee DJ. *Orthopedic Physical Assessment*. 4th ed. Philadelphia, PA: W.B. Saunders; 2002.

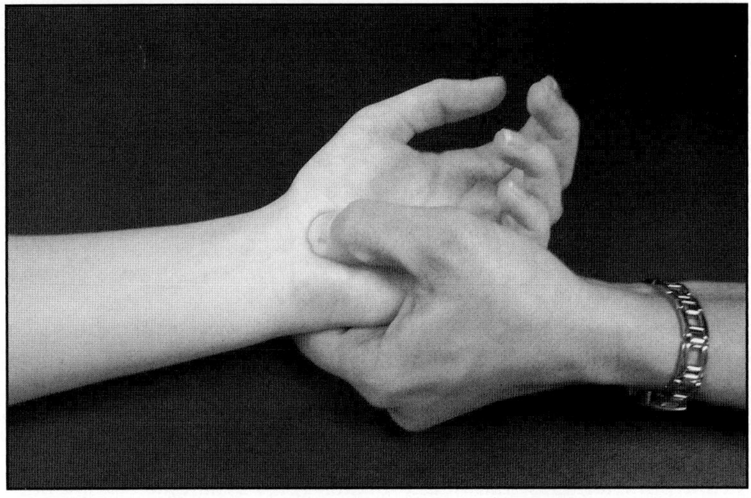

FIGURE 17-22

Massy-Westropp N, Grimmer K, Bain G. A systematic review of the clinical diagnostic tests for carpal tunnel syndrome. *J Hand Surg*. 2000;25(1):120-127.

Nathan PA, Keniston RC, Meadows KD, Lockwood LS. The value of carpal compression test as an alternative provocative clinical maneuver. *J Hand Surg*. 1997;22(6):823-825.

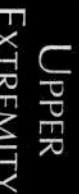

Pinch Grip Test

Test Position

The patient is positioned in sitting or standing.

Action

The clinician instructs the patient to pinch the tip of his or her thumb to the tip of his or her index finger, forming a circle (Figure 17-23).

Positive Finding

A positive finding is the patient demonstrating an inability to touch the thumb and index finger together using a tip-to-tip pinch. Rather, the patient with a positive finding will demonstrate a pad-to-pad grip of the index finger and thumb (Figure 17-24). A positive test is indicative of compression of the anterior interosseous branch of the median nerve at the pronator teres, known as Pronator Teres Syndrome.

Reliability

Kappa values at the 95% confidence interval range from .86 to .97 for intratester reliability and from .84 to .99 for intertester reliability.

References

Cleland J. *Orthopaedic Clinical Examination: An Evidence-Based Approach for Physical Therapists.* Carlstadt, NJ: Icon Learning Systems; 2005.

Magee DJ. *Orthopedic Physical Assessment.* 4th ed. Philadelphia, PA: W.B. Saunders; 2002.

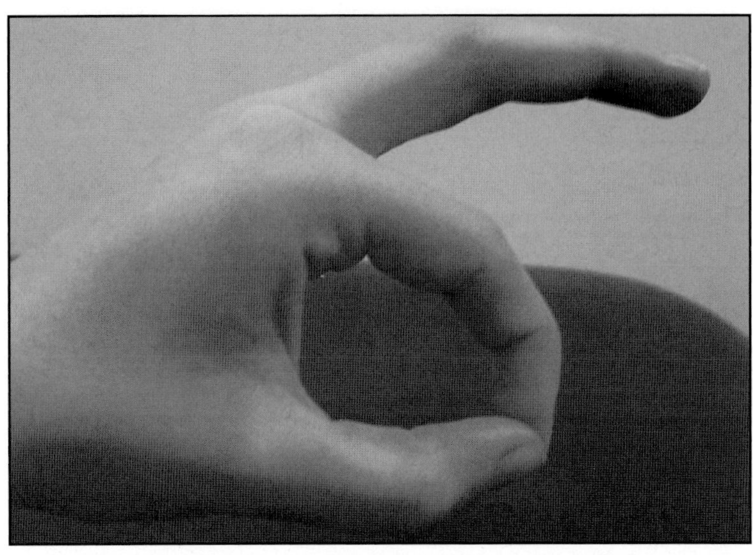

FIGURE 17-23

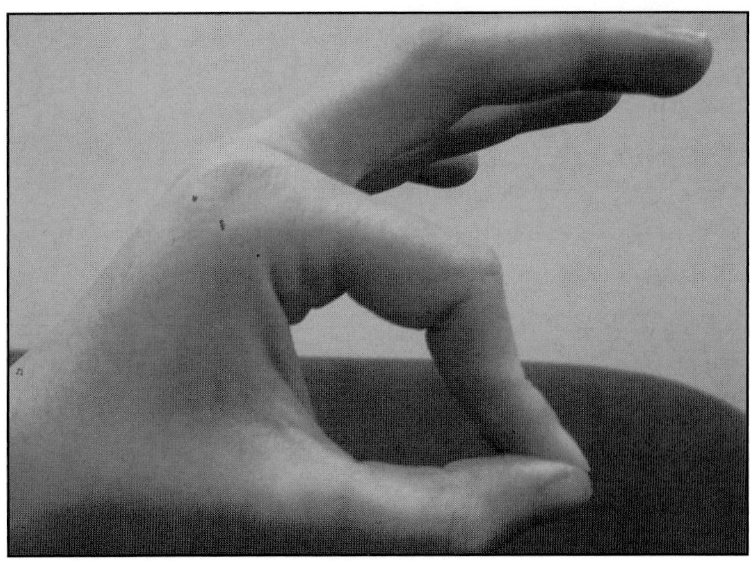

FIGURE 17-24

Froment's Sign

Test Position

The patient is positioned in sitting or standing.

Action

The clinician instructs the patient to hold a playing card, piece of paper, or piece of cardboard between the thumb and index finger, using a key grip pattern. The clinician instructs the patient to hold the object while the clinician attempts to remove the object from the patient's grip (Figure 17-25).

Positive Finding

A positive test is the patient demonstrating flexion of the interphalangeal joint of the thumb in order to hold the object (Figure 17-26). This finding is indicative of paralysis of adductor pollicis muscle secondary to ulnar nerve injury.

Special Considerations

Jeanne's Sign, hyperextension of the first MCP when performing this test, is also indicative of ulnar nerve injury.

Historical Notes

This test was first described in 1904 by Breeman, however the test is named for French internist Jules Froment.

Specificity

No data available.

Sensitivity

No data available.

References

Magee DJ. *Orthopedic Physical Assessment*. 4th ed. Philadelphia, PA: W.B. Saunders; 2002.

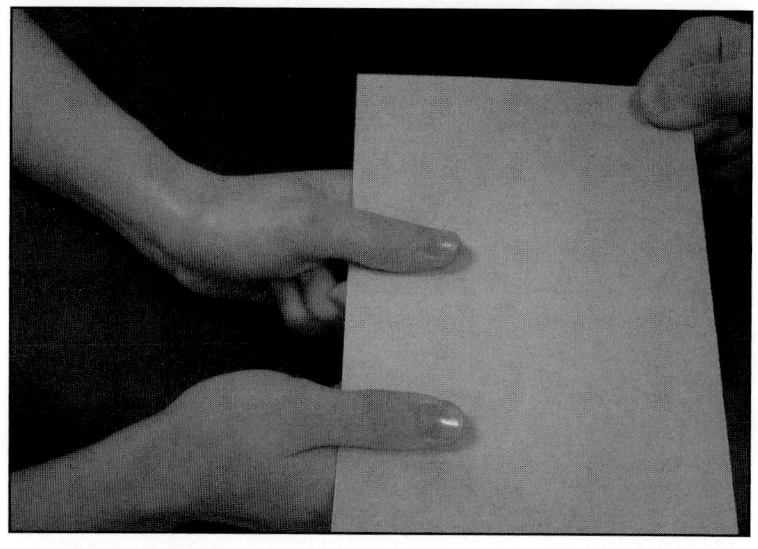

FIGURE 17-25

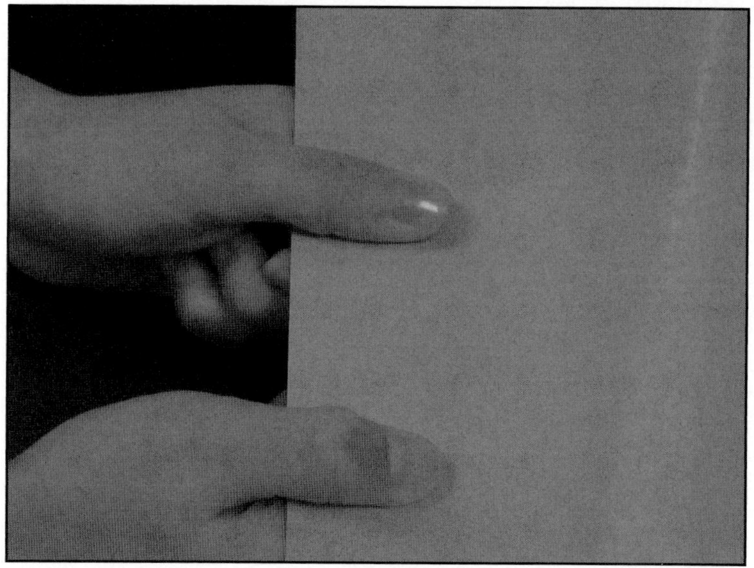

FIGURE 17-26

Egawa's Sign

Test Position

The patient is positioned in sitting.

Action

The clinician instructs the patient to flex his or her middle digit and then alternately radially and ulnarly deviate the wrist (Figures 17-27 through 17-29).

Positive Finding

A positive test is the patient's inability to maintain flexion of the middle finger while performing radial and ulnar deviation of the wrist. This finding is indicative of ulnar nerve pathology.

Special Considerations

Some patients without ulnar nerve pathology may have difficulty completing this test.

Specificity

No data available.

Sensitivity

No data available.

References

Magee DJ. *Orthopedic Physical Assessment.* 4th ed. Philadelphia, PA: W.B. Saunders; 2002.

Schreuders TAR, Roebroeck ME, Jaquet JB, Hovius SER, Stam HJ. Long-term outcome of muscle strength in ulnar and median nerve injury: comparing manual muscle strength testing, grip and pinch strength dynamometers and a new intrinsic muscle strength dynamometer. *J Rehab Med.* 2004;36(6):273-278.

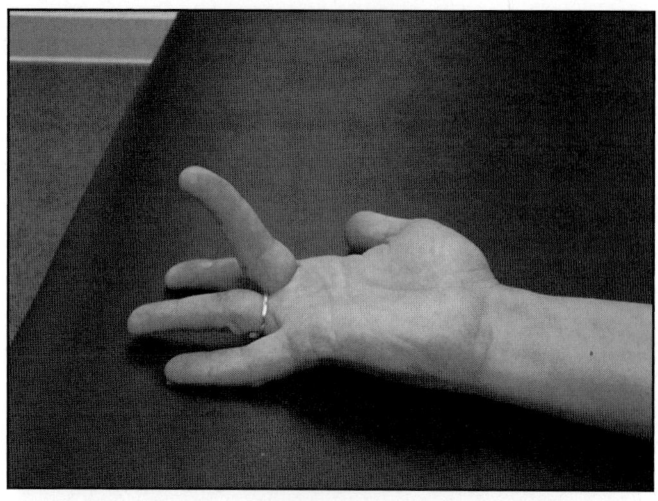

FIGURE 17-27

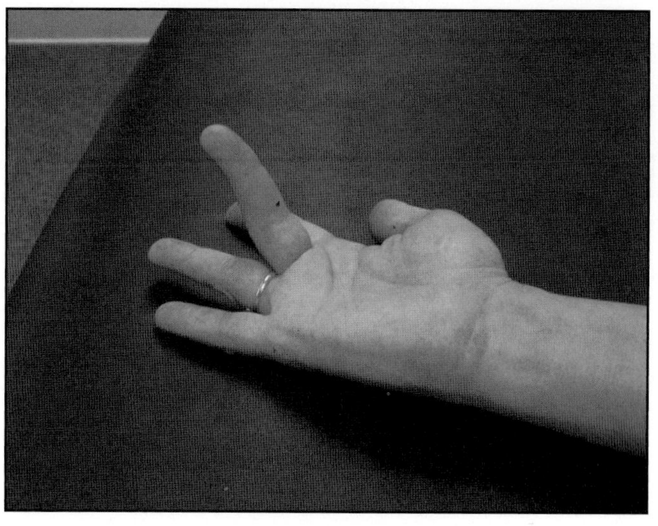

FIGURE 17-28

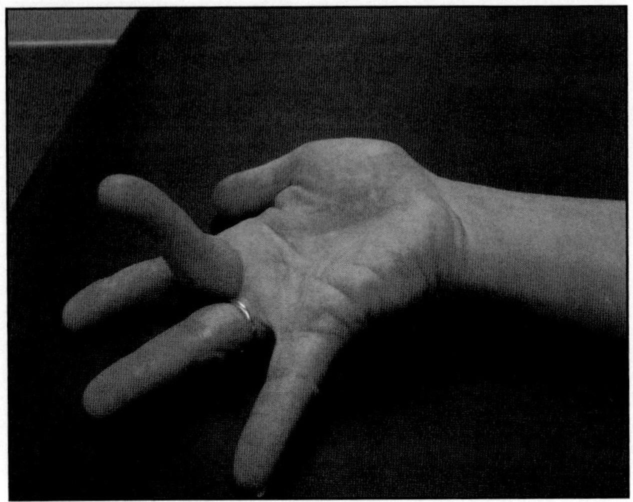

FIGURE 17-29

Wrinkle Test

Test Position

The patient is positioned in sitting next to a table.

Action

The patient is instructed to place his or her fingers in a glass of warm water for approximately 10 minutes. After 10 minutes, the clinician instructs the patient to remove his or her fingers from the water and the clinician assesses the patient's skin for wrinkling around the pulp (Figure 17-30).

Positive Finding

A positive test is an absence of wrinkling of the skin, indicative of tissue denervation.

Special Considerations

The clinician can perform this test on the fourth digit and utilize the findings to differentiate involvement of the median or ulnar nerves. The validity of this test is diminished several months after onset.

Alternate Names

This test is also known as the *Shrivel Test*.

Specificity

No data available.

Sensitivity

No data available.

References

Falanga V. The wrinkle test: Clinical use for detecting early epidermal resurfacing. *Journal of Dermatological Surgery and Oncology*. 1993;19(2):172-173.

Konin JG, Wiksten DL, Isear JA, Brader H. *Special Tests for Orthopedic Examination*. 3rd ed. Thorofare, NJ: SLACK Incorporated; 2006.

Magee DJ. *Orthopedic Physical Assessment*. 4th ed. Philadelphia, PA: W.B. Saunders; 2002.

Vasudevan TM, Van Rij AM, Mukada H, Taylor PK. Skin wrinkling for the assessment of sympathetic function in the limbs. *Aust N Z J Surg*. 2000;70(1):57-59.

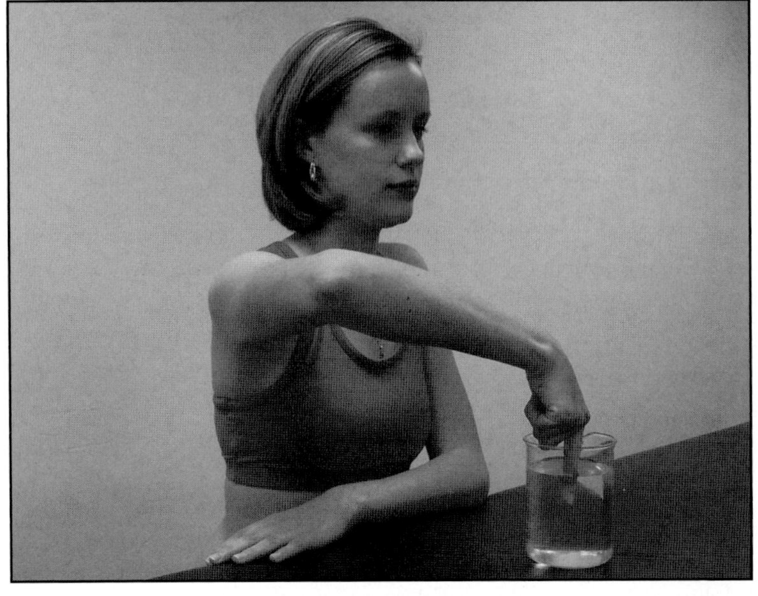

FIGURE 17-30

Ninhydrin Test

Test Position

The patient is positioned in sitting with his or her hand resting comfortably on the table.

Action

The clinician cleans the patient's fingertips thoroughly with an alcohol wipe. The patient is instructed to wait 5 to 30 minutes without touching any objects with fingertips. This time lapse allows the sweating process to occur. Next, the patient is instructed to press his or her fingers, using moderate pressure, against good quality bond paper that has not been touched. The fingertips are held in place for 15 seconds and traced with a pencil. The paper is then sprayed with Ninhydrin (triketohydrindene) spray reagent and allowed to dry for 24 hours. After drying, sweat areas will stain purple in color.

Positive Finding

If no color change occurs at the fingerprints, the test is considered positive for nerve lesion.

Special Considerations

This tests requires that the clinician have access to bond paper and Ninhydrin spray.

Historical Notes

This test is named for the chemical reagent that is sprayed on the bond paper.

Alternate Names

This test is also known as the *Ninhydrin Sweat Test*.

Specificity

No data available.

Sensitivity

No data available.

References

Magee DJ. *Orthopedic Physical Assessment.* 4th ed. Philadelphia, PA: W.B. Saunders; 2002.

Weber's Two-Point Discrimination Test

Test Position

The patient is positioned in sitting with his or her hand resting on the table.

Action

The clinician instructs the patient to close his or her eyes. The clinician assesses the patient's ability to distinguish one point from two points. The clinician repeats the test, moving the two points closer together or further apart depending upon the patient's response (Figures 17-31 and 17-32). The shortest distance between the two points that can be identified by the patient is recorded. Comparisons are made bilaterally to assess for sensory deficits.

Positive Finding

Variation in the shortest distance between the two points is indicative of sensory deficits.

Special Considerations

The clinician will need a two-point discriminator, two-point esthesiometer, caliper or clean, unused paperclip in order to complete this exam (see Figure 6-11).

Historical Notes

This test was developed in 1846 and is named for physiologist Ernst Weber.

Specificity

No data available.

Sensitivity

No data available.

References

Finnell JT, Knopp R, Johnson P, Holland PC, Schubert W. A calibrated paper clip is a reliable measure of two-point discrimination. *Academy of Emergency Medicine*; 2004;11(6):710-714.

Louis DS, Greene TL, Jacobson KE, Rasmussen C, Kolowich P, Goldstein SA. Evaluation of normal values for stationary and moving two-point discrimination in the hand. *J Hand Surg*. 1984;9(4):552-555.

Magee DJ. *Orthopedic Physical Assessment.* 4th ed. Philadelphia, PA: W.B. Saunders; 2002.

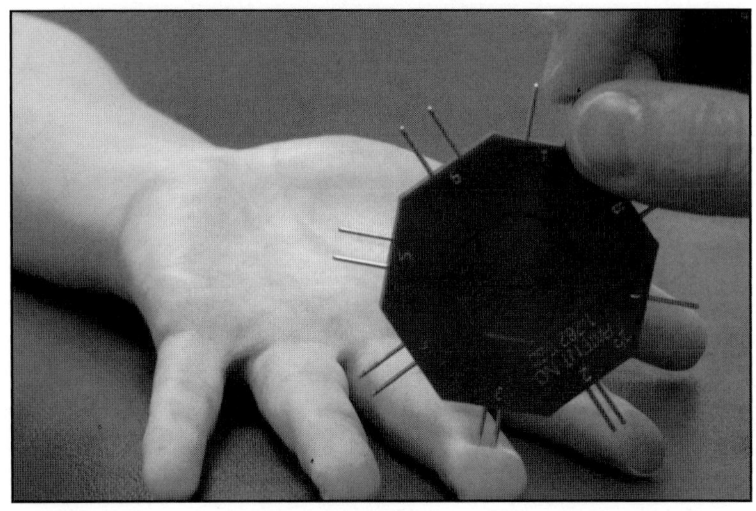

Figure 17-31

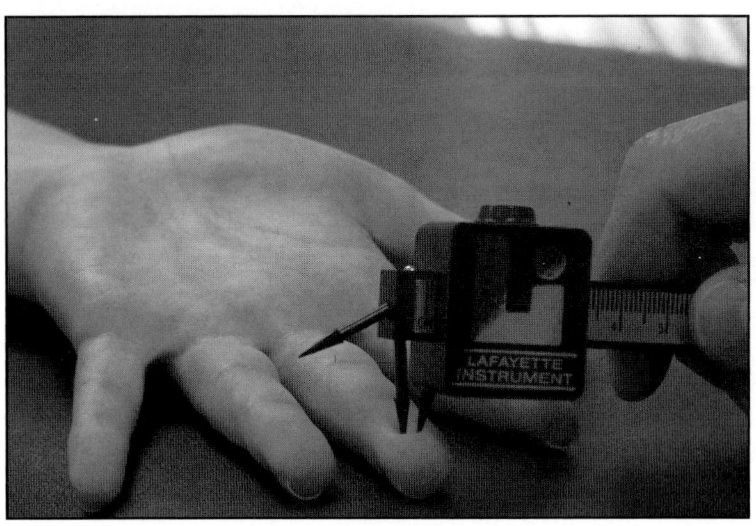

Figure 17-32

Section SIX

Lower Extremity

Chapter 18

Peripheral Nerve Pathology of the Lower Extremity

Morton's Neuroma

Mechanism

A Morton's Neuroma is caused by swelling, entrapment, or thickening of the nerve between the metatarsal heads. The most commonly involved structures are the medial and lateral branches of the plantar nerves between the third and fourth metatarsal heads. This region of the foot is a primary area for pressure and friction during weight-bearing activity. This repeated trauma results in the formation of fibrous tissue around the nerve.

Clinical Findings

The most common symptoms associated with Morton's Neuroma are pain with weight-bearing (particularly when weight-bearing on the forefoot) and narrow fitting footwear. The patient may also report neurologic symptoms, such as burning, tingling, numbness, and radiating pain, in the forefoot and into the toes. Morton's Neuroma is more commonly found in patients who demonstrate an excessively pronated gait pattern.

Diagnostic Procedures

The most appropriate special tests to apply in diagnosing Morton's Neuroma are the Pencil Test and the Interdigital Neuroma Test (see Chapter 19).

Special Considerations

This condition is also commonly referred to as a *plantar neuroma* or an *interdigital neuroma*.

References

Brukner P, Khan K. *Clinical Sports Medicine.* 3rd ed. Auckland, NZ: McGraw-Hill Book Co; 2006.

Gallaspy J, May JD. *Signs and Symptoms of Athletic Injuries*. Boston, MA: McGraw-Hill; 1996.

Magee DJ. *Orthopedic Physical Assessment.* 4th ed. Philadelphia, PA: W.B. Saunders; 2002.

Starkey C, Ryan JL. *Evaluation of Orthopedic and Athletic Injuries.* 2nd ed. Philadelphia, PA: F.A. Davis; 2002.

Common Fibular Nerve Injury

Mechanism

The common fibular nerve is most commonly injured due to compression at the proximal fibula. Common mechanisms include direct trauma to the nerve at the proximal fibula, fibular head fracture or excessive pressure from a brace, wrap, tape, or a cast. Additionally, the nerve can be injured in association with injury to the posterior lateral ligaments of the knee.

Clinical Findings

The most tell-tale sign of Common Fibular Nerve Injury is a weakening or paralysis of the lower leg muscles responsible for ankle dorsiflexion and eversion. This condition is commonly referred to as drop foot, due to the patient's inability to hold the ankle in a neutral position. Additional signs and symptoms may include pain and tenderness over the proximal fibula, as well as neurologic symptoms over the anterior, lateral lower leg, and the dorsum of the foot.

Diagnostic Procedures

The best diagnostic test to confirm common fibular nerve palsy is manual muscle testing in ankle dorsiflexion and eversion. The clinician may also assess for a loss of sensation in the common fibular nerve distribution. The condition can be confirmed through EMG and NCV studies.

Special Considerations

The common fibular nerve was formerly known as the common peroneal nerve. Common Fibular Nerve Injury may occur as a result of prolonged ice and compression treatment to the lateral aspect of the knee or the proximal aspect of the lateral lower leg. Caution should be taken to protect the common fibular nerve at the fibular head.

References

Brukner P, Khan K. *Clinical Sports Medicine.* 3rd ed. Auckland, NZ: McGraw-Hill Book Co; 2006.

Gallaspy J, May JD. *Signs and Symptoms of Athletic Injuries.* Boston, MA: McGraw-Hill; 1996.

Magee DJ. *Orthopedic Physical Assessment.* 4th ed. Philadelphia, PA: W.B. Saunders; 2002.

Peterson L, Renstrom L. *Sports Injuries: Their Prevention and Treatment.* Champaign, IL: Human Kinetics; 2001.

Starkey C, Ryan JL. *Evaluation of Orthopedic and Athletic Injuries.* 2nd ed. Philadelphia, PA: F.A. Davis; 2002.

Tarsal Tunnel Syndrome

Mechanism

Tarsal tunnel syndrome is the term used to describe entrapment of the posterior tibial nerve in the tunnel formed between the flexor retinaculum and the medial malleolus. The posterior tibial nerve transverses the tarsal tunnel along with the tendons of the flexor digitorum, flexor hallicus, and tibialis posterior. The most common cause is overuse of the tendons caused by excessive pronation. The condition may also be the result of trauma.

Clinical Findings

Commonly observed signs and symptoms include medial ankle pain, paresthesia, medial longitudinal arch pain, and medial heel pain. Tenderness upon palpation of the tarsal tunnel may also be noted. The condition is worsened with activity such as running, walking, and standing.

Diagnostic Procedures

Tinel's Sign at the Tarsal Tunnel will be positive in the presence of Tarsal Tunnel Syndrome. The condition can be confirmed through EMG and NCV studies.

Special Considerations

Tarsal Tunnel Syndrome is most commonly observed in patients who demonstrate excessive pronation during gait. Tarsal tunnel may present with heel pain similar to that of plantar fasciitis, particularly when the plantar nerve branches of the posterior tibial nerve are involved.

References

Brukner P, Khan K. *Clinical Sports Medicine.* 3rd ed. Auckland, NZ: McGraw-Hill Book Co; 2006.

Gallaspy J, May JD. *Signs and Symptoms of Athletic Injuries.* Boston, MA: McGraw-Hill; 1996.

Magee DJ. *Orthopedic Physical Assessment.* 4th ed. Philadelphia, PA: W.B. Saunders; 2002.

Peterson L, Renstrom L. *Sports Injuries: Their Prevention and Treatment.* Champaign, IL: Human Kinetics; 2001.

Starkey C, Ryan JL. *Evaluation of Orthopedic and Athletic Injuries.* 2nd ed. Philadelphia, PA: F.A. Davis; 2002.

Anterior Compartment Syndrome

Mechanism

Anterior Compartment Syndrome can be caused by direct trauma to the anterior compartment of the lower leg or by repetitive microtrauma to the structures housed within the anterior compartment.

Clinical Findings

Common signs of Anterior Compartment Syndrome include swelling in the lower leg, tenderness over the anterior compartment, and a loss of sensation over the dorsal webspace of the first and second toes. In the presence of Anterior Compartment Syndrome, the patient will demonstrate weakness in ankle dorsiflexion and great toe extension. In severe cases, foot drop may be present. The patient will also report pain with active and resistive ankle dorsiflexion and passive, end-range ankle plantarflexion. Pain will be exacerbated by activities such as running.

Diagnostic Procedures

Testing for anterior compartment syndrome should include an assessment of sensation to the dorsum of the foot. Additionally, the dorsal pedal pulse should be assessed. Finally, active and resistive range of motion in ankle dorsiflexion and passive range of motion in plantarflexion should be performed.

References

Brukner P, Khan K. *Clinical Sports Medicine.* 3rd ed. Auckland, NZ: McGraw-Hill Book Co; 2006.

Gallaspy J, May JD. *Signs and Symptoms of Athletic Injuries*. Boston, MA: McGraw-Hill; 1996.

Magee DJ. *Orthopedic Physical Assessment.* 4th ed. Philadelphia, PA: W.B. Saunders; 2002.

Peterson L, Renstrom L. *Sports Injuries: Their Prevention and Treatment.* Champaign, IL: Human Kinetics; 2001.

Starkey C, Ryan JL. *Evaluation of Orthopedic and Athletic Injuries.* 2nd ed. Philadelphia, PA: F.A. Davis; 2002.

Piriformis Syndrome

Mechanism

The sciatic nerve passes, partially or in whole, through the piriformis muscle in approximately 11% of the population, significantly increasing the risk of piriformis syndrome. In these individuals, spasm, hypertrophy or inflammation of the piriformis muscle will result in compression of the sciatic nerve.

Clinical Findings

The classic presentation of sciatic nerve compression is pain radiating from the buttock, down the posterior thigh, and into the lateral lower leg and lateral foot. Burning, numbness, and tingling may accompany this lower extremity pain. In the presence of true sciatica, that caused by Piriformis Syndrome, the symptoms should be exacerbated by contracting or elongating the involved piriformis muscle.

Diagnostic Procedures

The Piriformis Test will be positive in the presence of Piriformis Syndrome. The clinician can further differentiate Piriformis Syndrome from lumbar spine pathology by utilizing repeated range of motion testing in trunk flexion and extension and also by applying lumbar spine special tests such as the Straight Leg Raise Test, the Well Straight Leg Raise Test, and Valsalva's Maneuver. Additionally, sciatic nerve compression in the popliteal space should be differentiated from Piriformis Syndrome through the use of special tests such as the Tension Sign and the Bowstring Test.

Special Considerations

Piriformis syndrome is six times more common in women than men. Sciatica-type symptoms are also commonly found in the presence of lumbar spine disc herniation or lumbar spine nerve root compression.

References

Gallaspy J, May JD. *Signs and Symptoms of Athletic Injuries*. Boston, MA: McGraw-Hill; 1996.

Magee DJ. *Orthopedic Physical Assessment*. 4th ed. Philadelphia, PA: W.B. Saunders; 2002.

Starkey C, Ryan JL. *Evaluation of Orthopedic and Athletic Injuries*. 2nd ed. Philadelphia, PA: F.A. Davis; 2002.

Meralgia Paresthetica

Mechanism

Meralgia Paresthetica is the result of pressure or entrapment of the lateral femoral cutaneous nerve as the nerve passes under the inguinal ligament. Causes include trauma, as might occur from a safety belt during a motor vehicle accident, by tight clothing compressing the nerve, or as a complication of hernia surgery.

Clinical Findings

The lateral femoral cutaneous nerve is sensory only, so the patient will report sensory loss and burning sensation over the lateral aspect of the thigh.

Diagnostic Procedures

The clinician should complete a thorough assessment of sensation over the L1 and L2 dermatomes, looking for loss of sensation over the lateral aspect of the thigh.

References

Brukner P, Khan K. *Clinical Sports Medicine.* 3rd ed. Auckland, NZ: McGraw-Hill Book Co; 2006.

Magee DJ. *Orthopedic Physical Assessment.* 4th ed. Philadelphia, PA: W.B. Saunders; 2002.

Peterson L, Renstrom L. *Sports Injuries: Their Prevention and Treatment.* Champaign, IL: Human Kinetics; 2001.

Ilioinguinal Nerve Entrapment

Mechanism

The ilioinguinal nerve is another commonly entrapped nerve at the hip and groin. Injury may occur due to spasm of the transverse abdominus muscle or as a complication following hernia surgery.

Clinical Findings

Symptoms include sensory alterations or loss to the anterior thigh, the groin and the scrotum (in men) and the labia (in women). The pain is exacerbated by ipsilateral hip extension and contralateral trunk rotation. The patient may also complain of groin, hip and back pain.

Diagnostic Procedures

The clinician should complete a thorough assessment of sensation over the L1, L2 and L3 dermatomes, looking for loss of sensation over the anterior thigh, the groin and the genital region.

Special Considerations

Entrapment of the ilioinguinal nerve is also commonly referred to as Hockey Player's Syndrome.

References

Brukner P, Bradshaw C, McCroy P. Obturator neuropathy. *Phys Sportsmed.* 1999;27(5):62-65.

Brukner P, Khan K. *Clinical Sports Medicine.* 3rd ed. Auckland, NZ: McGraw-Hill Book Co; 2006.

Lacroix VJ. A complete approach to groin pain. *Phys Sportsmed.* 2000;28(1):1-17.

Magee DJ. *Orthopedic Physical Assessment.* 4th ed. Philadelphia, PA: W.B. Saunders; 2002.

Peterson L, Renstrom L. *Sports Injuries: Their Prevention and Treatment.* Champaign, IL: Human Kinetics; 2001.

Chapter

19

Special Tests for the Lower Extremity

Tinel's Sign for Tarsal Tunnel

Test Position

The patient is positioned in supine, long sitting, or sitting.

Action

The clinician uses one finger to tap over the most superficial location of the posterior tibial nerve, just posterior to the medial malleolus in the tarsal tunnel (Figure 19-1).

Positive Finding

A positive finding is pain or tingling along the posterior tibial nerve pathway, indicating irritation of the posterior tibial nerve, known as Tarsal Tunnel Syndrome.

Special Considerations

Tarsal Tunnel Syndrome can result from compression or reaction of the posterior tibial nerve. Pain may be noted over the medial longitudinal arch and the medial plantar aspect of the heel in the presence of Tarsal Tunnel Syndrome.

Historical Notes

This test is named for Jules Tinel, who, in 1915, described the process of nerve regeneration after injury and described a test that involved pressing on the nerve area. In reality, however, it was Paul Hoffmann who, also in 1915, originally described the tapping test to assess for median nerve injury in cases of Carpal Tunnel Syndrome.

Alternate Names

This test is also known as *Tinel's Test*.

Specificity

No data available.

Sensitivity

No data available.

References

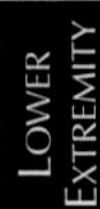

Bailie DS, Kelikian AS. Tarsal tunnel syndrome: diagnosis, surgical technique and functional outcome. *Foot Ankle Int*. 1998;19(2):65-72.

Konin JG, Wiksten DL, Isear JA, Brader H. *Special Tests for Orthopedic Examination*. 3rd ed. Thorofare, NJ: SLACK Incorporated; 2006.

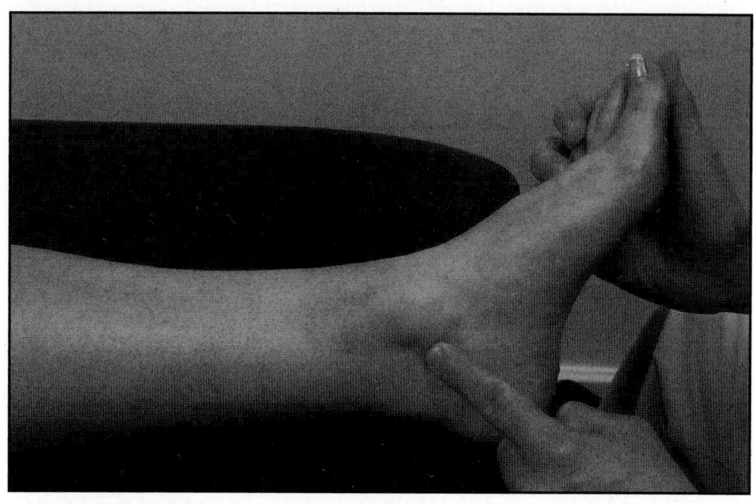

FIGURE 19-1

Magee DJ. *Orthopedic Physical Assessment.* 4th ed. Philadelphia, PA: W.B. Saunders; 2002.

Starkey C, Ryan JL. *Evaluation of Orthopedic and Athletic Injuries.* 2nd ed. Philadelphia, PA: F.A. Davis; 2002.

Pencil Test

Test Position

The patient is positioned in supine, long sitting, or sitting.

Action

The clinician uses a pen or the eraser end of a pencil to apply a compressive force to the intermetatarsal space between the third and fourth metatarsals (Figure 19-2).

Positive Finding

A positive finding is pain or reproduction of neurologic symptoms, indicating a Morton's Neuroma.

Special Considerations

Morton's Neuromas are most commonly found between metatarsals three and four, but can also occur between the second and third metatarsals. Therefore, this test should also be performed at the second and third intermetatarsal space.

Alternate Names

This test is also known as the *Test for Intertarsal Neuroma*.

Specificity

No data available.

Sensitivity

No data available.

References

Shultz SJ, Hoglum PA, Perrin DH. *Assessment of Athletic Injuries*. Champaign, IL: Human Kinetics; 2000.

Starkey C, Johnson G. *Athletic Training and Sports Medicine*. 4th ed. Boston, MA: Jones and Bartlett; 2005.

Starkey C, Ryan JL. *Evaluation of Orthopedic and Athletic Injuries*. 2nd ed. Philadelphia, PA: F.A Davis; 2002.

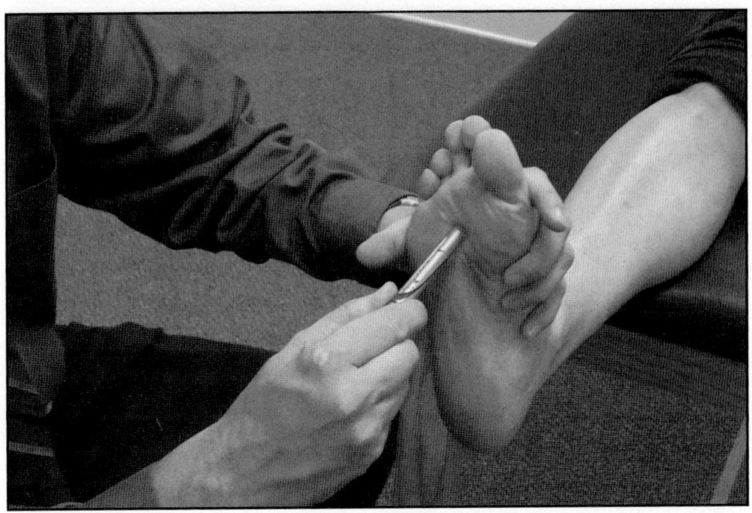

FIGURE 19-2

Interdigital Neuroma Test

Test Position

The patient is positioned in supine, long sitting, or sitting.

Action

The examiner grasps the metatarsal heads and squeezes the bones together, holding for 1 to 2 minutes (Figure 19-3).

Positive Finding

A positive finding is pain, numbness, and tingling into the foot or toes that is exacerbated with squeezing and relieved upon release. A positive test indicates an interdigital neuroma or Morton's Neuroma.

Special Considerations

This test may also be positive for pain in the presence of a metatarsal stress fracture.

Alternate Names

This test is also known as the *Squeeze Test*.

Specificity

No data available.

Sensitivity

No data available.

References

Giannini S, Bacchini P, Ceccarelli F, Vannini F. Interdigital neuroma: clinical examination and histopathological results in 63 cases treated with excision. *Foot Ankle Int*. 2004;25(2):79-84.

Konin JG, Wiksten DL, Isear JA, Brader H. *Special Tests for Orthopedic Examination*. 3rd ed. Thorofare, NJ: SLACK Incorporated; 2006.

Magee DJ. *Orthopedic Physical Assessment*. 4th ed. Philadelphia, PA: W.B. Saunders; 2002.

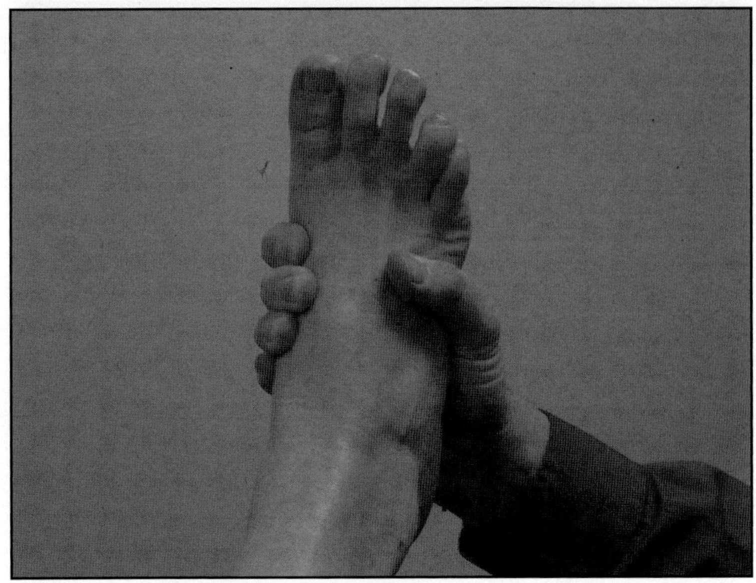

FIGURE 19-3

Duchenne Test

Test Position

The patient is positioned in supine with the knees in extension.

Action

The clinician applies force to plantar surface of the foot at the first metatarsal, forcing the ankle into dorsiflexion (Figure 19-4). The patient is then instructed to plantarflex the ankle against the clinician's resistance (Figure 19-5).

Positive Finding

A positive finding is plantarflexion force production on the lateral aspect of the foot with no plantarflexion force produced on the medial side of the foot.

This finding indicates either a lesion of the superficial fibular nerve or injury to the L4, L5, or S1 nerve roots.

Specificity

No data available.

Sensitivity

No data available.

References

Magee DJ. *Orthopedic Physical Assessment.* 4th ed. Philadelphia, PA: W.B. Saunders; 2002.

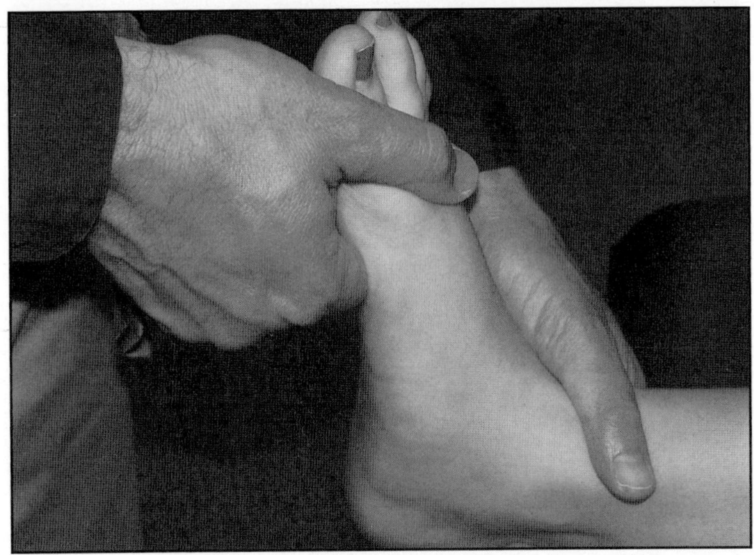

FIGURE 19-4

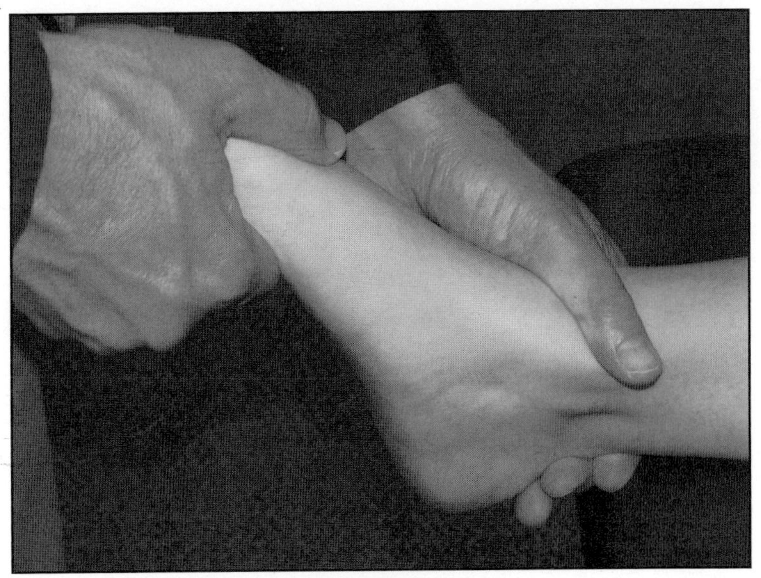

FIGURE 19-5

Piriformis Test

Test Position

The patient is positioned in sidelying on the uninvolved hip. This test may also be performed with the patient in supine.

Action

The patient is instructed to flex the involved hip 60 degrees with the knee flexed. The examiner stabilizes the involved hip with one hand, while applying downward pressure toward the table at the knee (Figure 19-6).

Positive Finding

A positive finding is pain in the buttocks, indicating a tight piriformis muscle, and/or peripheral pain in the sciatic nerve distribution, indicating Piriformis Syndrome (sciatic nerve compression secondary to piriformis tightness).

Special Considerations

The sciatic nerve passes, partially or in whole, through the piriformis muscle in approximately 11% of the population, significantly increasing the risk of Piriformis Syndrome. When completing this test, the clinician may also instruct the patient to attempt to externally rotate the involved hip against resistance to further exacerbate the patient's sciatica.

Alternate Names

This test is also known as the *FAIR Position*.

Specificity

.88

Sensitivity

.83

Positive Likelihood Ratio

5.2

Negative Likelihood Ratio

1.4

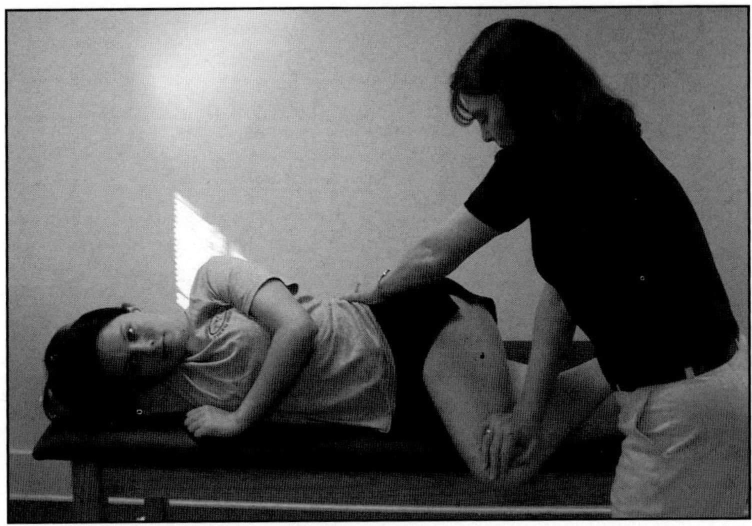

FIGURE 19-6

REFERENCES

Fishman L, Dombi G, Michaelson C, et al. Piriformis syndrome: diagnosis, treatment and outcome: a 10-year study. *Arch Phys Med Rehab.* 2002;83(5):295-301.

Konin JG, Wiksten DL, Isear JA, Brader H. *Special Tests for Orthopedic Examination.* 3rd ed. Thorofare, NJ: SLACK Incorporated; 2006.

Magee DJ. *Orthopedic Physical Assessment.* 4th ed. Philadelphia, PA: W.B. Saunders; 2002.

Yeoman's Test

Test Position

The patient is positioned in prone.

Action

The clinician flexes the involved knee to 90 degrees while simultaneously extending the involved hip (Figure 19-7). If possible, the clinician should stabilize the pelvis during the performance of this test.

Positive Finding

A positive finding is anterior thigh paresthesia, indicating femoral nerve pathology or tightness. Other positive findings include anterior thigh discomfort relating to hip flexor tightness, sacroiliac joint pain indicating pathology of the anterior sacroiliac ligaments, and lumbar spine pain resulting from lumbar spine pathology.

Special Considerations

This test can be modified to include hip extension with knee extension (Figure 19-8), primarily for use in assessing lumbar spine pain.

Alternate Names

This test is also known as the *Femoral Nerve Stretch Test*.

Specificity

No data available.

Sensitivity

No data available.

References

Konin JG, Wiksten DL, Isear JA, Brader H. *Special Tests for Orthopedic Examination*. 3rd ed. Thorofare, NJ: SLACK Incorporated; 2006.

Magee DJ. *Orthopedic Physical Assessment*. 4th ed. Philadelphia, PA: W.B. Saunders; 2002.

Starkey C, Ryan JL. *Evaluation of Orthopedic and Athletic Injuries*. 2nd ed. Philadelphia, PA: F.A. Davis; 2002.

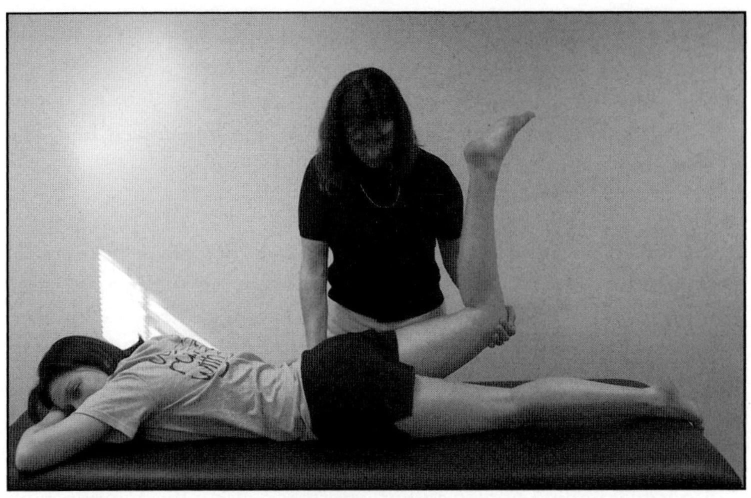

FIGURE 19-7

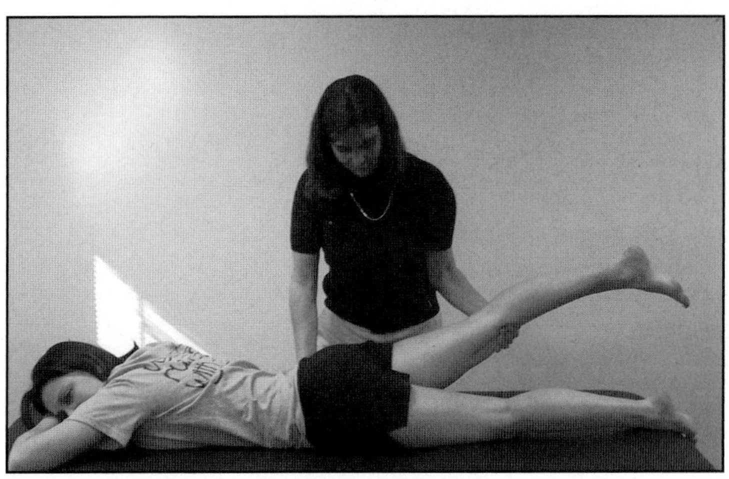

FIGURE 19-8

Femoral Nerve Traction Test

Test Position

The patient is positioned in sidelying on the uninvolved hip. The involved hip and knee are positioned in slight flexion.

Action

The clinician instructs the patient to actively flex his or her cervical spine slightly. The clinician stabilizes the pelvis on the involved side with one hand, while simultaneously extending the knee to end-range and extending the hip approximately 15 degrees with the other hand. The examiner then flexes the knee, assessing for patient reports of discomfort (Figures 19-9 and 19-10).

Positive Finding

A positive finding of pain and/or paresthesia along the anterior thigh is indicative of femoral nerve pathology or tightness.

Special Considerations

The patient's lumbar spine should remain in neutral flexion/extension during the performance of this test. This test may also be positive for involvement of lumbar nerve roots L2–L4.

Alternate Names

This test is also known as the *Femoral Nerve Tension Test.*

Specificity

No data available.

Sensitivity

No data available.

References

Dyck P. The femoral nerve traction test with lumbar disc protrusions. *Surg Neurol.* 1976;3:163-166.

Konin JG, Wiksten DL, Isear JA, Brader H. *Special Tests for Orthopedic Examination.* 3rd ed. Thorofare, NJ: SLACK Incorporated; 2006.

Magee DJ. *Orthopedic Physical Assessment.* 4th ed. Philadelphia, PA: W.B. Saunders; 2002.

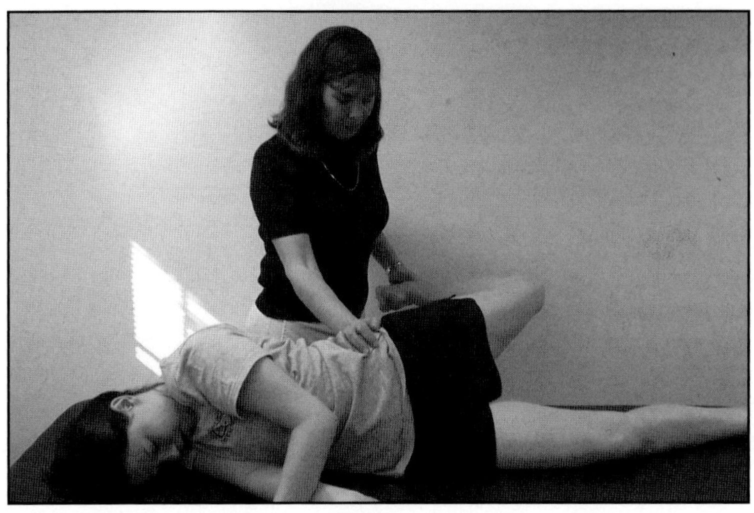

FIGURE 19-9

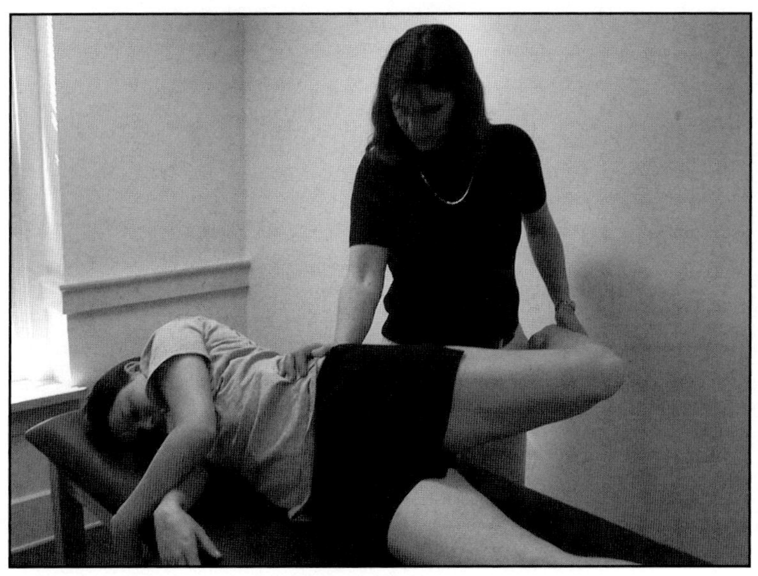

FIGURE 19-10

Index